AJPH
A PUBLICATION OF THE
AMERICAN PUBLIC HEALTH ASSOCIATION

AMERICAN JOURNAL of PUBLIC HEALTH
OCTOBER 2024
Issue 10

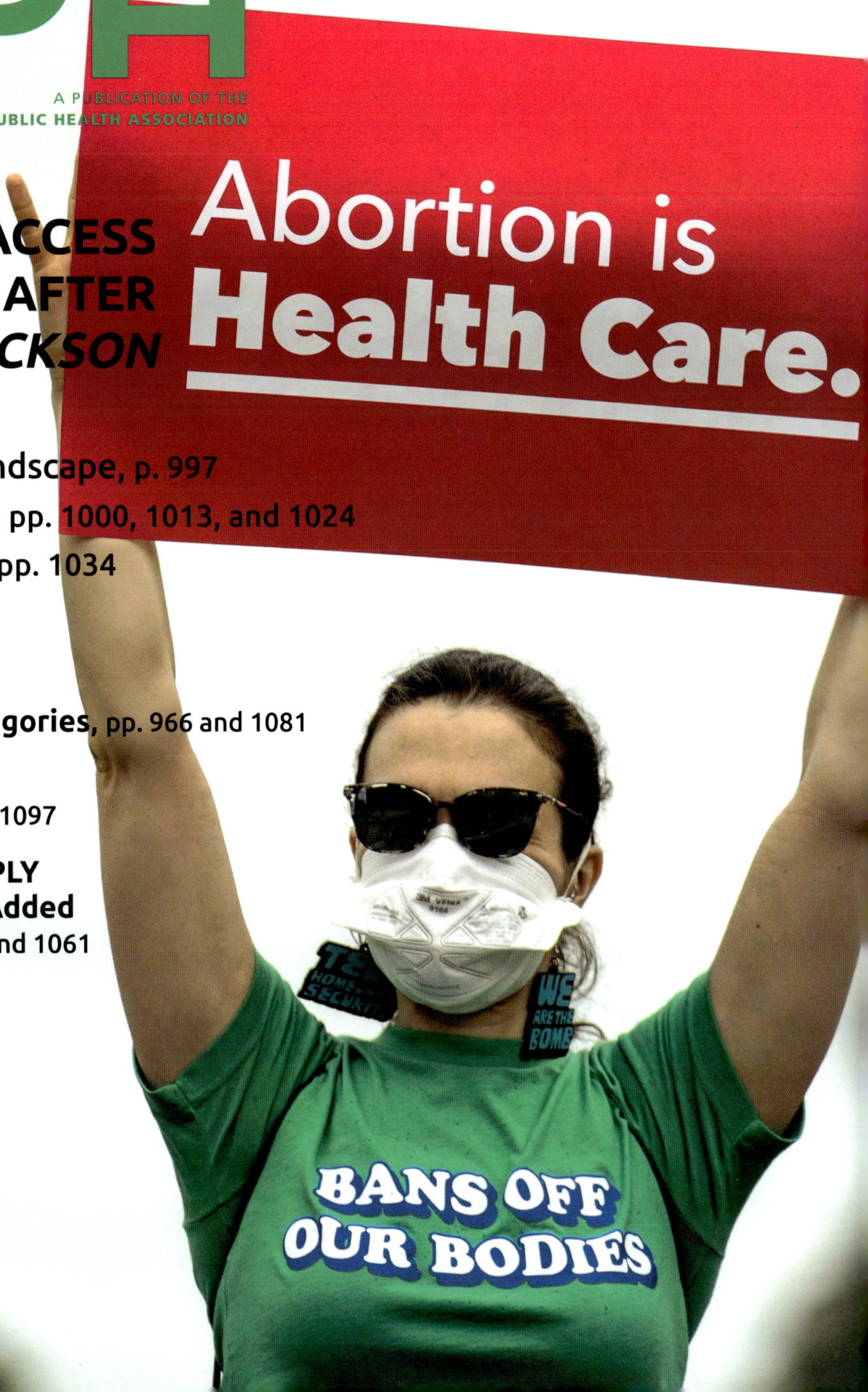

ABORTION ACCESS TWO YEARS AFTER *DOBBS V JACKSON* RULING

The New Legal Landscape, p. 997
The Case of Texas, pp. 1000, 1013, and 1024
The Case of Ohio, pp. 1034

Also in this issue:

OVERDOSE
Trends by Drug Categories, pp. 966 and 1081

FIREARMS
Pediatric Injuries, p. 1097

HUMAN FOOD SUPPLY
FDA Regulation of Added Substances, pp. 968 and 1061

APHA
AMERICAN PUBLIC HEALTH ASSOCIATION
For science. For action. For health.

AJPH®, published monthly, is the official Journal of the American Public Health Association®, 800 I St NW, Washington, DC 20001-3710; (202) 777- APHA; TDD (202) 777-2500. APHA is a nongovernmental professional society founded in 1872, representing all disciplines and specialties in public health.

The *American Journal of Public Health*® (*AJPH*) (print ISSN: 0090-0036; electronic ISSN: 1541- 0048), first published in 1911, is the official journal of the American Public Health Association® (APHA). The oldest and largest organization of public health professionals in the world, APHA represents approximately 30 000 members from more than 50 occupations of public health.

Submissions: Visit www.editorialmanager.com/ajph or ajph.edmgr.com for online manuscript preparation and submission guidelines. Contributions of original unpublished research, social science analyses, scholarly essays, critical commentaries, departments, and letters to the editor are welcome. Questions? Write ajph.submissions@apha.org or call APHA at (202) 777-2469.

Print plus online subscriptions: Institutional price (print copy with online access for a single institution and all authorized users, regardless of geographic location) varies by size of organization and ranges from $993–$1445 for US organizations, and $1073–$1526 for international organizations (air delivery); multiple campuses not permitted without special arrangement. Details of the tiered pricing system at https://subscriptionoffice.com/pages/apha-landing-page. To order, write apha.subscriptions@apha.org.

Online-only subscriptions: Institutional price for one institution and its authorized users (regardless of geographic location) is $878–$1307. To order, write apha.subscriptions@apha.org. For academic consortia or multisite corporate subscriptions, contact apha.subscriptions@apha.org.

Print-only subscriptions: Institutional price is US $701, $782 international.

Back print issues: A limited number of print issues are for sale. Single copies are US $49, $55 international (air delivery). Shipping included; prepay only. To order, write apha.subscriptions@apha.org.

Reprints: For prices and ordering information on 50 or more reprints, check the Reprints section at www.ajph.org. To order smaller quantities of reprints (rush delivery), use the "Purchase Article" link on the article site itself.

Electronic access: Online articles more than 10 years old are available free for personal use at www.ajph.org. Recent articles are available through pay-per-view: single PDF article for $24, single issue access for 24 hours for $33, or entire site access for 24 hours for $38.

Postal information: Periodicals postage paid at Washington, DC, and additional mailing offices. Postmaster: Send address changes to American Journal of Public Health, 800 I St NW, Washington, DC 20001-3710.

Address changes: Send to AJPH, Membership Department (members) or AJPH Subscriptions (subscribers), APHA, 800 I St NW, Washington, DC 20001-3710. Or write to membership.mail@apha. org (members) or apha.subscriptions@apha.org (subscribers).

Advertising: For pricing and other information, see www.ajph.org. Please write to ashell.alston@apha.org or call (202) 777-2470 for other advertising opportunities. Ask about special exhibit packages and sponsorships. Acceptance of advertising by the *Journal* does not imply endorsement of products.

Indexes: Publications that index or abstract articles from *AJPH* include the following: Ageline, Assia (Applied Social Science Index and Abstracts), Biological Abstracts, Chemical Abstracts, CINAHL, Criminal Justice Abstracts, EMBASE, EMCare, Environmental Abstracts, e-psyche, ERIC, ETOH (Alcohol and Alcohol Problems Science Database), Excerpta Medica, Food Science and Technology, General Science Index, Grateful Med, Hospital Literature Index, Human Resources Abstracts, International Pharmaceutical Abstracts (IPA), Medline, Physical Education Index, Pollution Abstracts, Psychological Abstracts, PsychINFO, Safety Science Abstracts, Sage Family Studies Abstracts, Sage Human Resources Abstracts, Science Citation Index, SCOPUS, SIIC Data Bases, Social Work Research and Abstracts, and Statistical Reference Index (SRI)/LexisNexis.

AJPH

A PUBLICATION OF THE
AMERICAN PUBLIC HEALTH ASSOCIATION

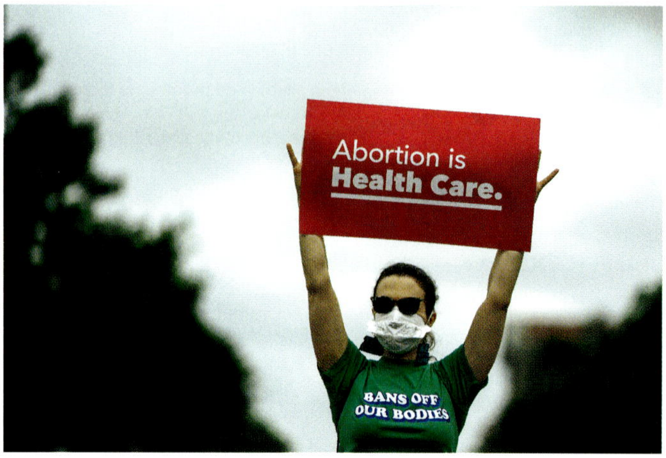

COVER: Abortion rights activists participate in a Bans Off Our Bodies rally and march to the US Supreme Court on Saturday, May 14, 2022, in Washington, DC. Abortion rights supporters are holding rallies across the country urging lawmakers to codify abortion rights into law after a leaked draft from the Supreme Court revealed a potential decision to overturn the precedent set by landmark *Roe v Wade*.

Cover concept and selection by Aleisha Kropf. Photo by Kent Nishimura/ Los Angeles Times via Getty. Printed with permission.

APHA
AMERICAN PUBLIC HEALTH ASSOCIATION
For science. For action. For health.

Promoting public health research, policy, practice, and education is the *AJPH* mission. As we widen our scope to embrace global issues, we also sharpen our focus to support the needs of public health practitioners. We invite contributions of original unpublished research, opinion and commentary, and letters to the editor.

The *Journal* is printed on acid-free recycled paper.

OPEN ACCESS ONLINE ONLY PODCAST DATA SUPPLEMENT AVAILABLE

EDITOR'S CHOICE

958 Nuclear Weapons Kill People Even When Not Used
J. M. Samet

OPINIONS, IDEAS, & PRACTICE

EDITORIALS

960 What Should the Public Health Policy Response Be to Harmful Exposure to Oil and Gas Development?
É. Caron-Beaudoin, A. Aker, and M. J. McGregor

963 The Challenge of Mortality Surveillance in Pandemics—Imperfect Perceptions of Reality
A. C. K. Lee

966 New Insights on Trends in Overdose Deaths by Intent and Drug Involvement From Improved Public Health Monitoring
A. S. B. Bohnert and S. Sen

968 Contesting Deregulation and Medicalization to Revitalize Public Health
D. G. Aaron

971 Restricting Immigrant Access to Pregnancy-Related Insurance Has Public Health Consequences
T. Janevic, E. Weber, and A. Fox

974 Polarization, Partisanship, and Political Alignment Threaten Public Health: A Public Health of Consequence, October 2024
F. Kapadia

PERSPECTIVES

977 Deep Reform and Targeted Investment: Essential Strategies for Preparing for the Next Health Emergency in Europe and Elsewhere
F. Vandenbroucke and P. Facon

980 Social Media and Adolescent Health
J.-P. Allem

983 The Dire Need for Surveillance of Vaccine Hesitancy in the United States
D. M. Higgins and S. T. O'Leary

986 Reenvisioning Title X to Meet Early Pregnancy Needs
K. Vinekar, A. Abernathy, and K. L. Rising

991 Recommitting to Ventilation Standards for Healthy Indoor Air Quality
J. G. Allen

ABORTION ACCESS 2 YEARS AFTER *DOBBS V JACKSON* RULING

994 Understanding the Post-*Dobbs* Landscape for Abortion Care in the United States
F. Kapadia, L. Ferguson, and W. E. Parmet

997 The Post-*Dobbs* Legal Landscape
M. Ziegler

1000 Collective Persistence, Care, and Advocacy Amid Repeated Attacks on Reproductive Freedom
W. S. Rice, S. A. Hartwig, H. V. McMahon, C. Irwin, N. Quinones, S. K. Redd, and K. A. Singh

1003 Latin American Nations Once Lagged on Abortion Rights: Now Some Present Role Models for the United States
C. Roth and M. M. Jones

1008 "To Anyone Reading in the Future You Are Not Alone": How Patients Seeking Abortion in a Surge State Use Their Stories to Support Each Other
M. McQuade, B. Banwarth-Kuhn, V. Trujillo, and A. Truehart

RESEARCH & ANALYSIS

ABORTION ACCESS 2 YEARS AFTER *DOBBS V JACKSON* RULING

1013 Abortion Return Rates and Wait Times Before and After Texas' Executive Order Banning Abortion During COVID-19
B. Whitfield, G. Sierra, K. Lerma, V. Goyal, L. Thaxton, B. Kumar, A. Gilbert, and K. White

1024 Unequal Spatial Consequences of Abortion Restrictions in Texas, 2021–2023
S. R. Sauter, M. E. Wallace, and J. H. Hernandez

1034 Longitudinal Impact of *Dobbs v Jackson Women's Health Organization* on Abortion Service Delivery in Ohio, 2022–2023
M. H. Smith, M. L. McGowan, C. Kerestes, D. Bessett, and A. H. Norris

1043 Post-*Dobbs* Abortion Restrictions and the Families They Leave Behind
N. Madden, E. Trawick, K. Watson, and L. M. Yee

LAW & ETHICS

1051 Navigating the Labyrinth of Pregnancy-Related Coverage for Undocumented Immigrants: An Assessment of Current State and Federal Policies
A. DiMeo, R. Logendran, B. D. Sommers, A. Beecroft, Y. P. Herencia, M. Bazan, C. Wade, J. Sprankle, M. M. Sullivan, and R. L. Molina

1061 Regulation of Added Substances in the Food Supply by the Food and Drug Administration Human Foods Program
J. L. Pomeranz, E. M. Broad Leib, and D. Mozaffarian

HEALTH MONITORING

1071 Mortality Surveillance for the COVID-19 Pandemic: Review of the Centers for Disease Control and Prevention's Multiple System Strategy
D. Khan, M. Park, P. Grillo, L. Rossen, B. C. Lyons, S. David, M. D. Ritchey, F. B. Ahmad, A. D. McNaghten, A. V. Gundlapalli, and A. B. Suthar

1081 Trends in Drug Overdose Deaths by Intent and Drug Categories, United States, 1999–2022
A. Nguyen, J. Wang, K. M. Holland, D. C. Ehlman, L. E. Welder, K. D. Miller, and D. M. Stone

OPEN-THEMED RESEARCH

1086 The War on Drugs, Racialized Capitalism, and Health Care Utilization Among White People Who Use Drugs in 22 Rural Appalachian Counties
H. L. F. Cooper, M. "Douglas" Livingston, N. D. Crawford, J. Feinberg, C. L. Ford, V. Go, U. Ibragimov, T. Jahangir, A. Mullany, W. C. Miller, S. Peddireddy, L. Salas-Hernandez, G. Smith, A. M. Young, W. Zule, and A. Sewell

1097 Preinjury and Event-Related Characteristics of Pediatric Firearm Injuries: The American College of Surgeons Firearm Study, United States, March 2021–February 2022
K. T. Flynn-O'Brien, C. Sathya, M. Kotagal, S. Banks, L. L. Agoubi, D. A. Kuhls, A. Nathens, A. B. Hink, and F. P. Rivara

1110 Structural Stigma and Disparities in Long-Term Health Conditions Among Australians in Same-Sex Relationships: 2021 Australian Census
K. Saxby, Y. Zhang, and Z. Aitken

BACKMATTER

LETTERS & RESPONSES

1123 Community Engagement: The Missing Link in Public Health Leadership
Y. Wu and C. Lin

1124 Helm-Murtagh and Erwin Respond
S. C. Helm-Murtagh and P. C. Erwin

1125 Strategies to Improve COVID-19 Vaccination in a Pregnant, Marginalized Population: Correspondence
H. Daungsupawong and V. Wiwanitkit

1126 Bakhai et al. Respond
S. Bakhai, J. Jordan, and J. A. Stoll

OTHER DEPARTMENTS

1128 Subscription Form

Nuclear Weapons Kill People Even When Not Used

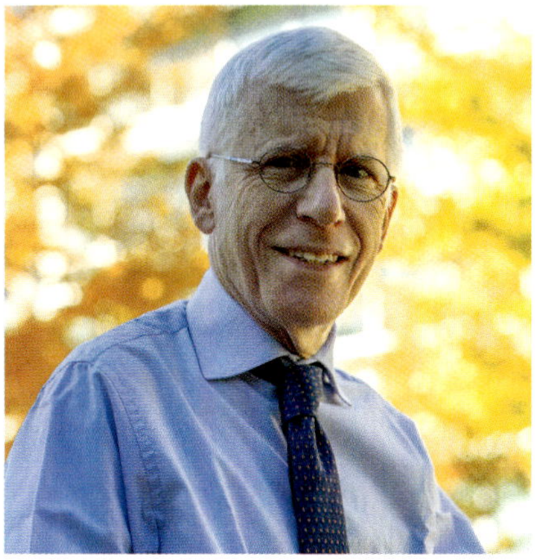

Jonathan M. Samet, MD, MS
Colorado School of Public Health

Most likely those reading this editorial will have seen *Oppenheimer*, the 2024 Academy Award–winning film about J. Robert Oppenheimer, who led the Manhattan Project as it developed the first atomic bombs and launched the atomic age. Beyond the tragic consequences of the Hiroshima and Nagasaki bombings, the nuclear age that began with the Manhattan Project has had profound implications for the health of nuclear workers and the public throughout the world.

Let's start with the atomic bomb survivors, many participating in epidemiological studies that began in the late 1940s. The survivors receive medical care and other support under the Japanese government's Atomic Bomb Survivors' Support Law. They, and their children, have contributed to the world by allowing their health to be tracked. We have learned from them how radiation increases cancer risk; that information has long been the foundation for radiation protection. Following the bombings, the survivors experienced an almost immediate epidemic of acute leukemia followed later by a radiation dose–related rise in risks of most adult cancers.

Decades after the blasts, the survivors experienced an unexpected increase in heart disease risk and a general shortening of their life spans. For the survivors' children, a critical and still incompletely addressed question is whether they will experience transgenerational effects. These studies are carried out by a unique Japan–US binational organization, the Radiation Effects Research Foundation. Looking forward, the foundation's researchers will build on the survivors' legacy by using 21st century science and more than 2 million biological samples (e.g., blood) to deepen understanding of how radiation injures the body.

The starting point for making nuclear weapons is uranium. After World War II, demand for uranium soared as the nuclear arms race drove the buildup of ever larger stockpiles of bombs. The launching of nuclear power added to the need for uranium. By the 1950s, thousands

Continued on page 959...

HISTORY CORNER

53 YEARS AGO

Abortion—1970

The recent changes in the abortion laws have opened a veritable Pandora's Box from which myriads of problems are spewing forth. These are urgent problems requiring rapid solutions—solutions that will tax the ingenuity of the consumer, the health professional, the legal and administrative community, and government, at national, state, and local levels. Can the public be adequately served? Can professional standards be maintained in the face of increasing demand? Are current patterns of health care delivery and current patterns of payment for services still applicable or are they now outmoded? Do we go the in-hospital route or the "come-and-go" outpatient route? Is professional manpower sufficiently available to cope with demand? Is there need for a new type of health professional? Will conventional maternity care and family planning services suffer a relapse? Will illegitimacy, unwanted pregnancy, and illegal induced abortion be reduced or eliminated? Will legal abortion be available and within the financial reach of all socioeconomic and ethnic groups? It was to these questions that the symposium, "Abortion-1970," directed itself.

From *AJPH*, March 1971, pp. 487–488

worked underground as miners and aboveground as millers, operating the mills that produced yellowcake.

As uranium mining took off in the Colorado Plateau, historical evidence indicted radon as a potential cause of lung cancer, and the US Public Health Service undertook an epidemiological study of miners in the region. By the early 1960s, that study showed excess lung cancer. Because all uranium was mined for the Atomic Energy Commission through 1971, the US government had jurisdiction for protecting the miners' health but did not do enough. A radon exposure standard for miners was eventually implemented but too late, and it was not low enough to prevent a still ongoing lung cancer epidemic among the former miners. The millers were exposed to radon and also to uranium and are at risk for cancer as well as lung and kidney problems. There is also a legacy of environmental contamination at uranium-mining and -milling sites, a particular concern for the Navajo Nation.

There are other points for radiation exposure in the cycle of producing and testing nuclear weapons. At the start of the atomic age, there were fatal accidents during the Manhattan Project at Los Alamos, New Mexico. Workers were exposed to radiation in other Manhattan Project facilities. Workers at Rocky Flats were exposed to plutonium and beryllium. Military personnel, stationed as observers at test blasts, are another broad class of exposed individuals, as are people (the downwinders) in communities where the fallout drifted. Nuclear fallout spread globally from testing by the United States and five other countries.

Thus, nuclear weapons have harmed the health of diverse groups in the United States: the "atomic veterans," the downwinders, the Atomic Energy Commission and later Department of Energy workers, and uranium miners and millers. Compensation schemes are in place for these groups, albeit too late for many. The Department of Energy workers are covered for beryllium-related problems and radiogenic cancers. The Atomic Veterans can participate in a Veterans Administration program and are also eligible for compensation from the Radiation Exposure Compensation Act (RECA).

RECA, first passed in 1990, was amended in 2000, and was extended for two years in 2022. It expired in 2024. It covered downwinders, those exposed to radiation at test sites, and uranium miners (and later millers). It includes an apology: "The Congress apologizes on behalf of the Nation to the individuals described in subsection (a) and their families for the hardships they have endured." That apology was included because the government had not acknowledged the risks to the downwinders or protected the uranium miners and millers.

Unfortunately, it is clear that the production of nuclear weapons will continue—in the United States and elsewhere. There are currently nine countries with nuclear weapons, totaling almost 13 000. The existence of nuclear weapons has been posed as a deterrent to major conflicts and wars because the consequences of their use is civilization ending. We have enough postapocalyptic fiction and film to help imagine the planet after an exchange of atomic weapons. For the present, there are people who have been harmed by the production and testing of nuclear weapons; many were bystanders. We should continue fair and just compensation. AJPH

DOI: https://doi.org/10.2105/AJPH.2024.307829

ORCID iD:
Jonathan M. Samet https://orcid.org/0000-0001-5676-9175

HISTORY CORNER

53 YEARS AGO

Logistic Problems of Legal Abortion

Traditionally, therapeutic abortions in the United States have been carried out by qualified obstetrician-gynecologists with admission of the patient to an accredited hospital for two to three days, and with adjudication of her case by appropriate consultation. The latter two requirements are part of the restrictiveness of even the new, liberalized California law, since it requires the use of an accredited hospital and adjudication of the case by a two- two- or three-member hospital committee. Where then are California hospitals suddenly to find about 120,000 extra bed-days this year, and the personnel necessary to man-hospital committees and to carry out the procedures? . . . [M]any hospitals have found their usual hospital and operating room activities disrupted. . .Hospital committees have been overwhelmed by the numbers of cases to review. . . . Already, however, we are seeing material public health benefits. A recent study at our county hospital in San Francisco documents a precipitous drop in the incidence of septic abortion patients. And, for the first time in that hospital's history, during the year 1969 there were no abortion-related maternal deaths-which had heretofore been the most common single type of maternal death in California.

From AJPH, *March 1971, pp. 496–498*

What Should the Public Health Policy Response Be to Harmful Exposure to Oil and Gas Development?

Élyse Caron-Beaudoin, PhD, Amira Aker, PhD, and Margaret J. McGregor, MD

ABOUT THE AUTHORS

Élyse Caron-Beaudoin is with the Department of Health and Society, University of Toronto Scarborough, Toronto, ON, and the Dalla Lana School of Public Health, University of Toronto, Toronto, ON. Amira Aker is with the Centre Hospitalier Universitaire de Québec, Université Laval, QC. Margaret J. McGregor is with the Centre for Clinical Epidemiology and Evaluation, Vancouver Coastal Health Research Institute, Vancouver, BC, and the Department of Family Practice, Faculty of Medicine, University of British Columbia, Vancouver, BC.

AJPH October 2024, Vol. 114, No. 10

It is estimated that 17.6 million people in the United States live within one mile of oil and gas development. In Canada, the province of British Columbia alone currently houses 35 000 oil and gas wells, of which approximately one third are unconventional wells. Unconventional wells use hydraulic fracturing, which involves vertical and horizontal drilling for several kilometers under fresh and saline water aquifers. Unconventional oil and gas extraction has been rapidly expanding in both countries over the past decade: hydraulically fractured wells now produce between 65% and 80% of US natural gas and crude oil. In northeastern British Columbia, residents can live with up to 368 unconventional wells within 10 kilometers of their home, which makes us ask how "unconventional" the practice truly is.

Hydraulic fracturing is a well stimulation technique that injects pressurized fluid to fracture rock formations to extract fossil fuels such as natural gas. The wastewaters generated during this process contain a variety of toxic compounds, including chemicals used in the hydraulic fracturing fluid (biocides, friction reducers, scale inhibitors, surfactants, acids, corrosion inhibitors, gelling agents, etc.), heavy metals, volatile compounds, and radioactive elements naturally occurring in the rock formation,[1] potentially contaminating the environment through spills and wastewater evaporation. Oil and gas development can result in air pollutant emissions, including, for example, volatile organic compounds.[2,3] Other important emission sources include machinery and gas flaring.

Many chemicals used in the hydraulic fracturing fluid are known toxicants. Toxicological studies using human cells or rodents have shown deleterious effects, such as endocrine disruption, cytotoxicity, carcinogenicity, behavioral changes, and metabolic health disruptions. This evidence of "biological plausibility" is aligned with the growing epidemiological literature pointing to the various adverse health effects associated with living near oil and gas development.

Earlier this year, we published a review of 52 studies examining the health outcomes of people living close to unconventional wells, and the results are less than reassuring.[4] Perinatal outcomes were most often studied, and of these studies, the majority reported adverse neonatal outcomes among pregnant people living nearby these sites, including preterm birth, low birthweight, impaired fetal growth, and congenital malformations. Other studies found that living near these sites was associated with higher risk of asthma exacerbations, adverse cardiovascular outcomes, childhood cancers, and overall mortality, among other health issues.[4]

In the United States and Canada, there is also consistent evidence that unconventional oil and gas operations disproportionately affect systematically and structurally disadvantaged communities. A 2019 analysis of sociodemographic characteristics of people living close to drilling and hydraulic fracturing operations in the states of Colorado, Oklahoma, Pennsylvania, and Texas found strong evidence that minorities, especially African Americans, disproportionately live near unconventional wells.[5] Additionally, biomonitoring studies in northeastern British Columbia that our group has published demonstrate that exposure to trace elements and volatile organic compounds is higher among cohorts of pregnant individuals than among the general population; this exposure is also higher among Indigenous than non-Indigenous participants.[6–8]

In the September 2024 issue of *AJPH*, Willis et al. discuss their study in which they recruited participants who answered questionnaires on their mental health (i.e., perceived stress, major depression symptoms, use of medications for anxiety, depression, and sleep disorders) and evaluated the associations between proximity and density of active oil and gas development sites within 20 kilometers of the participant's address during preconception (a critical window of vulnerability) and perceived stress, symptoms of depression, and the use of psychotropic medication in women living in the United States and Canada.[9] The study adds to the literature by using a large study across the United States and Canada that deployed social media to recruit a large sample of women during the preconception period. The authors used national oil and gas databases to assign each individual a series of exposure metrics based on the proximity and density of active or new oil and gas wells around their residence and at various preconception time windows. Willis et al. observed that oil and gas development intensity was associated with moderate to high perceived stress, moderate to severe depressive symptoms, and psychotropic medication use. Notably, associations with perceived stress and depressive symptoms were strongest among those living closest to oil and gas development sites, further highlighting the impact of oil and gas development on the health of local communities.

Hypothesized pathways for the observed associations include the documented increase in noise, vibrations, light pollution, traffic, crime, and stressed infrastructures, which may cause increased psychosocial stress and loss of community cohesion, as previously documented in regions undergoing oil and gas booms.[10,11] Community members may experience increased stress and anxiety related to concerns regarding the pollutants released from the oil and gas operations. A direct chemical effect is also plausible: air pollution, for example, has been linked with adverse mental health outcomes.[12] Furthermore, increased chronic stress before and during pregnancy is known to contribute to negative birth outcomes, such as low birth weight.

The study by Willis et al., along with the accumulating evidence from multiple other studies, generate an urgency to act. Just as Finkel and Law commented in the pages of this journal 11 years ago,[13] we must consider exercising the precautionary principle when it comes to this industry. US President Biden has announced a pause on the permitting of all new liquefied natural gas exports, which will help decrease the number of people exposed to these industrial activities, and this is a policy we encourage our Canadian government to emulate. However, there remain thousands of communities currently living near these developments that we must protect. We suggest that governments consider the following.

First, setbacks for homes, schools, and daycares need to be informed by the best available evidence. Setbacks are the minimum distances allowed between homes and an oil extraction site. In their publication, Willis et al. reported an association between adverse mental outcomes and residential distance to the industry of 2 to 18 kilometers.[9] They further highlighted the wide range of setbacks across jurisdictions from as low as 100 meters (as is the case in British Columbia) to up to 970 meters in California. Our current understanding indicates that setbacks need to be further defined by the number of active wells in a given spatial boundary in addition to the distance between a site and an infrastructure.

Second, the same evidence that informs setbacks needs to be uniformly adopted across states and provinces so that one area doesn't become a "sacrifice zone" for industry expansion owing to lower standards. Third, reporting of all chemicals in hydraulic fracturing fluid should be mandatory, without exceptions for trade secrets. Reporting the use of these chemicals should also not be limited to the hydraulic fracturing phase and needs to include all phases of the industrial process.

Finally, there should be mandated industry funding for credible and independent third-party environmental monitoring to prospectively measure the quality of air, water, soil, and human health outcomes of communities living near this industry. This process should include meaningful participation of the exposed communities in the monitoring process consistent with environmental justice principles. Likewise, the industry should fund remediation of significant pollution when identified.

Given the growing evidence of human harm associated with this industry including that which Willis et al. show, it is time for public health policymakers in all jurisdictions to work together to increase oversight, protect human health, and minimize environmental harm. AJPH

CORRESPONDENCE

Correspondence should be sent to Élyse Caron-Beaudoin, 1265 Military Trail, Toronto, ON M1C 1A4, Canada (e-mail: elyse.caronbeaudoin@utoronto.ca). Reprints can be ordered at https://www.ajph.org by clicking the "Reprints" link.

PUBLICATION INFORMATION

Full Citation: Caron-Beaudoin É, Aker A, McGregor MJ. What should the public health policy response be to harmful exposure to oil and gas development? *Am J Public Health*. 2024;114(10):960–962.

Acceptance Date: July 2, 2024.

DOI: https://doi.org/10.2105/AJPH.2024.307797

ORCID iDs:
Amira Aker https://orcid.org/0000-0002-0063-7955

Margaret J. McGregor https://orcid.org/0000-0002-0553-7240

CONTRIBUTORS

É. Caron-Beaudoin led the drafting of the editorial. A. Aker and M. J. McGregor contributed to the writing and editing. All authors performed the literature search and conceptualized and reviewed the editorial.

CONFLICTS OF INTEREST

The authors report no potential or actual conflicts of interest from funding or affiliation-related activities pertinent to this editorial.

REFERENCES

1. Chittick EA, Srebotnjak T. An analysis of chemicals and other constituents found in produced water from hydraulically fractured wells in California and the challenges for wastewater management. *J Environ Manage*. 2017;204(pt 1): 502–509. https://doi.org/10.1016/j.jenvman.2017.09.002
2. Macey GP, Breech R, Chernaik M, et al. Air concentrations of volatile compounds near oil and gas production: a community-based exploratory study. *Environ Health*. 2014;13:82. https://doi.org/10.1186/1476-069X-13-82
3. Gilman JB, Lerner BM, Kuster WC, de Gouw JA. Source Signature of volatile organic compounds from oil and natural gas operations in northeastern Colorado. *Environ Sci Technol*. 2013;47(3): 1297–1305. https://doi.org/10.1021/es304119a
4. Aker AM, Friesen M, Ronald LA, et al. The human health effects of unconventional oil and gas development (UOGD): a scoping review of epidemiologic studies. *Can J Public Health*. 2024;115(3): 446–467. [Erratum in: Aker AM, Friesen M, Ronald LA, et al. Correction: The human health effects of unconventional oil and gas development (UOGD): a scoping review of epidemiologic studies. *Can J Public Health*. Online ahead of print June 21, 2024. https://doi.org/10.17269/s41997-024-00913-6]. https://doi.org/10.17269/s41997-024-00860-2
5. Zwickl K. The demographics of fracking: a spatial analysis for four US states. *Ecol Econ*. 2019;161:202–215. https://doi.org/10.1016/j.ecolecon.2019.02.001
6. Caron-Beaudoin É, Bouchard M, Wendling G, et al. Urinary and hair concentrations of trace metals in pregnant women from northeastern British Columbia, Canada: a pilot study. *J Expo Sci Environ Epidemiol*. 2019;29(5):613–623. https://doi.org/10.1038/s41370-019-0144-3
7. Caron-Beaudoin É, Whyte KP, Bouchard MF, et al. Volatile organic compounds (VOCs) in indoor air and tap water samples in residences of pregnant women living in an area of unconventional natural gas operations: findings from the EXPERIVA study. *Sci Total Environ*. 2022;805:150242. https://doi.org/10.1016/j.scitotenv.2021.150242
8. Claustre L, Bouchard M, Gasparyan L, et al. Assessing gestational exposure to trace elements in an area of unconventional oil and gas activity: comparison with reference populations and evaluation of variability. *J Expo Sci Environ Epidemiol*. 2023;33(1):94–101. https://doi.org/10.1038/s41370-022-00508-8
9. Willis MD, Campbell EJ, Selbe S, et al. Residential proximity to oil and gas development and mental health in a North American preconception cohort study: 2013–2023. *Am J Public Health*. 2024;114(9):923–934. https://doi.org/10.2105/AJPH.2024.307730
10. Casey JA, Wilcox HC, Hirsch AG, Pollak J, Schwartz BS. Associations of unconventional natural gas development with depression symptoms and disordered sleep in Pennsylvania. *Sci Rep*. 2018;8(1):11375. https://doi.org/10.1038/s41598-018-29747-2
11. Aker AM, Whitworth KW, Bosson-Rieutort D, et al. Proximity and density of unconventional natural gas wells and mental illness and substance use among pregnant individuals: an exploratory study in Canada. *Int J Hyg Environ Health*. 2022;242:113962. https://doi.org/10.1016/j.ijheh.2022.113962
12. Bhui K, Newbury JB, Latham RM, et al. Air quality and mental health: evidence, challenges and future directions. *BJPsych Open*. 2023;9(4):e120. https://doi.org/10.1192/bjo.2023.507
13. Finkel ML, Law A. The rush to drill for natural gas: a public health cautionary tale. *Am J Public Health*. 2011;101(5):784–785. https://doi.org/10.2105/AJPH.2010.300089

The Challenge of Mortality Surveillance in Pandemics—Imperfect Perceptions of Reality

Andrew C. K. Lee, MD, MPH, MBChB

ABOUT THE AUTHOR

Andrew C. K. Lee is with the Division of Population Health, University of Sheffield, Sheffield, UK, and the UK Health Security Agency, Leeds, UK.

See also Khan et al., p. 1071.

Outbreaks of emerging infectious diseases, especially those with pandemic potential, generate considerable demand for information that will aid in understanding the spread and severity of the infectious disease. This vital intelligence informs the dynamic risk assessment of the public health threat posed by the pathogen, which in turn influences public health advice and disease control measures.[1]

Disease-specific mortality is one of the key indicators of disease severity and is accordingly a priority parameter gathered. The value of disease mortality data was apparent during the COVID-19 pandemic, during which many countries used their mortality surveillance systems to study and track the pandemic as it unfolded.[2,3] The resulting intelligence gathered enabled public health decisionmakers to understand the natural history of the disease, identify who and what settings were at risk, anticipate the timing needed to implement public health and social measures, and gauge those measures' efficacy and the pandemic's impact.

However, in most countries such endeavors involved herculean efforts to corral, link up, and analyze the various clinical, public health surveillance, and vital statistics data systems. The scale and pace required to reengineer these systems involved massive undertakings that were usually invisible to the public. In their article in this issue of *AJPH* (p. 1071), Khan et al. discuss the US Centers for Disease Control and Prevention's (CDC's) multiple system strategy for mortality surveillance during the COVID-19 pandemic. Their work is a timely and important record of the efforts taken and challenges faced and provides invaluable insights that can inform preparations for future pandemics during which the need to compile robust mortality surveillance data undoubtedly will arise.

Some critics may question the accuracy, completeness, and timeliness of the CDC's strategy for mortality surveillance. However, it is important to recognize that all forms of surveillance have limitations. Surveillance data are frequently delayed, inaccurate, and subject to surveillance bias.[4] Such data are a proxy of reality and, depending on the strength of surveillance systems used, may be incomplete. For example, studies from Europe in 2020 observed that, for every COVID-19 case reported, between 9 and 12 cases were missed by the surveillance systems.[4]

The true incidences of disease and disease mortality at any given time were difficult to determine with exact certainty because of variable coverage of COVID-19 testing and varying accuracy of clinical diagnoses. Public health–seeking behavior also affected the detection of cases. Even in death, which should be an objective and incontrovertible indicator, confirmation of COVID-19 as cause of death was not always possible, was frequently delayed, and was even missed.[5] Consequently, reported COVID-19 numbers were only ever imperfect estimations. For those who were basing public health decisions on this information, it was akin to steering a car while looking through a cracked and distorted rearview mirror.

So how does the CDC's approach compare with those used in other countries? International comparisons are difficult, as contexts and systems differ considerably between countries. Such comparisons are flawed because of the variation in case definitions used for COVID-19 between countries but also because of changes to case definitions and the emergence of new SARS-CoV-2 (severe acute respiratory syndrome coronavirus 2) variants over time.

Moreover, surveillance issues were especially challenging in countries with more fragmented or less well-developed surveillance systems.[6] Health data and civil registration and vital statistics systems often exist independently, with limited interconnectivity or semantic consistency between them.[7] Crucially, the robustness of surveillance systems and their data outputs were only ever as good as the clinical and laboratory reporting and surveillance data collection systems that formed the foundation of those surveillance systems. Where frontline clinicians have poor access to lab facilities, or lack the means or motivation to report, significant underdetection and underreporting of cases will occur.

Completeness of surveillance was also affected by public health–seeking and –reporting behaviors, which were in turn influenced by variable public awareness, social media, cultural norms and stigma, media misinformation and disinformation, reporting fatigue, and effects of at-home testing, as reported by Khan et al.

Also notable is the diversity of stakeholders interested in surveillance outputs. Traditionally, interest in these outputs has been narrowly thought of in terms of upward reporting to decision-makers and politicians. However, during the COVID-19 pandemic, it also emerged that the public was interested in surveillance outputs, which may have influenced behavior.[8] In the contemporary social media age, it must be recognized that members of the public are not passive receptacles of information but active consumers who choose who and what to believe and modify their behaviors accordingly. Going forward, we need to better understand how data consumerism operates and can be influenced for the good of public health.

Another emergent phenomenon during the recent pandemic was the plurality of lay interpretations, including by so-called armchair epidemiologists, that were widely shared through social media. These nonexpert analyses or interpretations of surveillance data were often inaccurate or taken out of context, highlighting a deficiency in public epidemiological literacy. Although public misinformation has always been a public health challenge, social media amplified its reach and speed of spread.[9]

It is also worth recognizing that politicians could and did politicize surveillance information to suit their political agendas, sometimes leading to misinformation or disinformation that undermined public trust.[10] The diversity of opinions and interpretations of data does not help public confidence in official information, and discrepancies and changes in official reported mortality numbers may lead some to question the veracity of official figures.

Although there is the inherent danger of misinterpretation of mortality surveillance data, these data, however imperfect, have important utility, as highlighted earlier. The challenge is how to optimize the data's utility. The CDC's strategies of greater use of open source data, automated processes such as Web scraping, and synergies with third-party data aggregators are pragmatic approaches that worked. However, efforts elsewhere to integrate disease surveillance systems around the world have seen mixed results.[7]

Moreover, the pursuit for ever greater accuracy, coverage, and depth of detail of surveillance data comes with increasing cost. Similarly, attaining close to real-time data often necessitates a trade-off that relies on incomplete, provisional data.[4] Consequently, the key questions that need to be answered are how much information is enough and what level of detail and accuracy can we afford? The latter will no doubt be guided by the risk posed by the pathogen but may be skewed by political appetite and public interest rather than by actual public health value. A pragmatic approach requires the consideration of the opportunity cost of investing precious public health resources in strengthening surveillance efforts versus the actual return on investment to guide public health decisions.

As we prepare for the next pandemic, further efforts are needed to strengthen and better link up surveillance systems. Beyond data system integration, we also need to consider functional integration, but this does not mean just database linkages.[7] Triangulation of trends from various sources, as was done by the CDC and national public health agencies elsewhere, did help provide a more timely and complete picture.

In addition, there is considerable value in bringing in subject matter experts, surveillance epidemiologists, data scientists, public health professionals, and others to collectively add depth and context to provide data interpretations that best fit reality. This requires multidisciplinary and multisectoral collaboration at all levels from subnational to international.[11] Most importantly, we must not forget the role of surveillance—surveillance exists to guide public health action. If it does not do that, it is pointless. AJPH

CORRESPONDENCE

Correspondence should be sent to Andrew C. K. Lee, University of Sheffield, Regent Court, Regent St, Sheffield S1 4DA, UK (e-mail: andrew.lee@sheffield.ac.uk). Reprints can be ordered at https://www.ajph.org by clicking the "Reprints" link.

PUBLICATION INFORMATION

Full Citation: Lee ACK. The challenge of mortality surveillance in pandemics—imperfect perceptions of reality. *Am J Public Health*. 2024;114(10): 963–965.

Acceptance Date: July 15, 2024.

DOI: https://doi.org/10.2105/AJPH.2024.307808

ORCID iD:

Andrew C. K. Lee https://orcid.org/0000-0002-9795-3793

CONFLICTS OF INTEREST

The author has previously undertaken work with the International Association of National Public Health Institutions on global disease surveillance and response, which was funded by the Bill and Melinda Gates Foundation. The author has no other conflicts of interest from funding or affiliation-related activities to declare.

REFERENCES

1. Setel P, AbouZahr C, Atuheire EB, et al. Mortality surveillance during the COVID-19 pandemic. *Bull World Health Organ.* 2020;98(6):374. https://doi.org/10.2471/BLT.20.263194
2. Allan M, Lièvre M, Laurenson-Schafer H, et al. The World Health Organization COVID-19 surveillance database. *Int J Equity Health.* 2022;21(S3, suppl 3):167. [Erratum in: Allan M, Lièvre M, Laurenson-Schafer H, et al. Correction to: The World Health Organization COVID-19 surveillance database. *Int J Equity Health.* 2023;22:95. https://doi.org/10.1186/s12939-023-01870-1]. https://doi.org/10.1186/s12939-022-01767-5
3. Adebisi YA, Rabe A, Lucero-Prisno DE III. COVID-19 surveillance systems in African countries. *Health Promot Perspect.* 2021;11(4):382–392. https://doi.org/10.34172/hpp.2021.49
4. Tancredi S, Cullati S, Chiolero A. Surveillance bias in the assessment of the size of COVID-19 epidemic waves: a case study. *Public Health.* 2024;234:98–104. https://doi.org/10.1016/j.puhe.2024.06.006.
5. Rosenbaum JE, Stillo M, Graves N, Rivera R. Timeliness of provisional United States mortality data releases during the COVID-19 pandemic: delays associated with electronic death registration system and weekly mortality. *J Public Health Policy.* 2021;42(4):536–549. https://doi.org/10.1057/s41271-021-00309-7
6. Carter ED, Stewart DE, Rees EE, et al. Surveillance system integration: reporting the results of a global multicountry survey. *Public Health.* 2024;231:31–38. https://doi.org/10.1016/j.puhe.2024.03.004
7. Lee AC, Iversen BG, Lynes S, et al. The state of integrated disease surveillance globally: synthesis report of a mixed methods study. *Public Health.* 2024;228:85–91. https://doi.org/10.1016/j.puhe.2024.01.003
8. Focacci CN, Lam PH, Bai Y. Choosing the right COVID-19 indicator: crude mortality, case fatality, and infection fatality rates influence policy preferences, behaviour, and understanding. *Humanit. Soc. Sci. Commun.* 2022;9(1):1–8. https://doi.org/10.1057/s41599-021-01032-0
9. Gabarron E, Oyeyemi SO, Wynn R. COVID-19-related misinformation on social media: a systematic review. *Bull World Health Organ.* 2021;99(6):455–463, 463A. https://doi.org/10.2471/BLT.20.276782
10. Muhammed TS, Mathew SK. The disaster of misinformation: a review of research in social media. *Int J Data Sci Anal.* 2022;13(4):271–285. https://doi.org/10.1007/s41060-022-00311-6
11. Archer BN, Abdelmalik P, Cognat S, et al. Defining collaborative surveillance to improve decision making for public health emergencies and beyond. *Lancet.* 2023;401(10391):1831–1834. https://doi.org/10.1016/S0140-6736(23)01009-7

New Insights on Trends in Overdose Deaths by Intent and Drug Involvement From Improved Public Health Monitoring

Amy S. B. Bohnert, PhD, and Srijan Sen, MD, PhD

ABOUT THE AUTHORS

Amy S. B. Bohnert is with Michigan Medicine and the Opioid Research Institute and Srijan Sen is with Michigan Medicine and the Eisenberg Family Depression Center, University of Michigan, Ann Arbor.

AJPH October 2024, Vol. 114, No. 10

See also Nguyen et al., p. 1081.

Overdose deaths have emerged as an important North American health crisis of the early 21st century. Despite recent declines,[1] the rate of overdoses in the United States is exponentially higher than the rate was in 2000. Clearly, solving this crisis is a public health priority.

A unique challenge of the overdose crisis is the rapid evolution of the problem over a relatively short period of time. Most notably, the substances driving overdoses have shifted in "waves" defined by opioid types—first with a period of increasing prescription opioid-related deaths, followed by a brief period of heroin as the dominant driver of increases, followed by years of soaring rates of illicitly manufactured fentanyl overdoses.[2] These shifts in the nature of the overdose epidemic have important implications for prevention. For example, the potential impact of novel prescription opioid formulations that deter abuse diminished substantially once heroin and illicit fentanyl became the drivers of overdoses. These rapid changes may help explain why responses to the crisis, formulated over time and often with dated information, have been largely ineffective in addressing the problem.

In this issue of *AJPH*, a report by Nguyen et al. (p. 1081) details drug overdose deaths by both intent and involved drugs for the period 1999 to 2022. Traditional reporting of overdose mortality statistics has grouped deaths by the intent of the overdose or the substances involved in the overdose, but rarely by both factors together. The results of the analysis indicate several important emerging trends, such as increases in benzodiazepine- and stimulant-involved overdoses, including an especially concerning increase in psychostimulants for intentional overdoses. This analysis also highlights the value of highly detailed mortality data for public health monitoring, which has been the focus of significant investments by the Centers for Disease Control and Prevention.[3] These improvements may be reflected most clearly in the substantial decrease in overdoses with "miscellaneous" reported as the drug type after 2010, as seen in the article's Figure 1.

Understanding epidemiological trends in overdose stratified by intent in a timely manner is critical for prevention, as there are distinct (although also some shared) prevention tools for overdoses that are intentional versus unintentional.[4] However, determining the intent of an overdose can be challenging for medical examiners and coroners, who create the raw data that eventually become coded mortality data. Specifically, in the absence of a suicide note, the burden of evidence for ruling an overdose a suicide tends to be higher than for other mechanisms of external injury.[5] Consequently, it is likely that some overdoses classified as unintentional were in fact intentional.

Further, caution should be taken in interpreting the relationships identified here between intent and drug involvement. It remains unclear how much the drugs identified during toxicology testing by medical examiners and coroners may influence their decisions about ruling a death intentional or unintentional. For example, if there is no opioid involved, medical examiners and coroners may be more likely to assume that the overdose was the result of self-harm, given the higher lethality of opioids over other drugs (and the same for fentanyl vs prescription opioids). Although this may be a reasonable approach to individual cases, it results in misclassification.

Given the difficulty in accurately distinguishing unintentional overdoses and suicides, it is worth looking at overdose deaths collectively. The increasing presence of synthetic opioids, stimulants, and benzodiazepines over the past few years indicates that these substances deserve particular attention. Given the population-level reductions in the coprescribing of opioids and benzodiazepines,[6] the findings indicate that changes to prescribing have been an insufficient response. In addition to continuing the many efforts to address opioid overdoses, new approaches that prevent overdoses from other drugs are increasingly important.

It remains unclear what proportion of overdose deaths are attributable to prescribed use versus nonprescribed use of the drug for those drug types that have medical use. Further, it is also unknown how often the decedent knew they were using all of the drugs identified via toxicology, or when a drug's presence was the result of drug contamination. These distinctions are important to prevention, but data are limited or out of date. These limitations further highlight the need for continued improvement in the granularity and timeliness of data of the kind used in this study. AJPH

CORRESPONDENCE

Correspondence should be sent to Amy S. B. Bohnert, PhD, 2800 Plymouth Rd, Bldg 16, Ann Arbor, MI 48109 (e-mail: amybohne@med.umich.edu). Reprints can be ordered at https://www.ajph.org by clicking the "Reprints" link.

PUBLICATION INFORMATION

Full Citation: Bohnert ASB, Sen S. New insights on trends in overdose deaths by intent and drug involvement from improved public health monitoring. *Am J Public Health.* 2024;114(10):966–967.

Acceptance Date: July 15, 2024.

DOI: https://doi.org/10.2105/AJPH.2024.307811

ORCID iD:
Amy S. B. Bohnert https://orcid.org/0000-0002-4426-1136

CONTRIBUTORS

Both authors contributed equally to this editorial.

CONFLICTS OF INTEREST

The authors have no conflicts of interest to disclose.

REFERENCES

1. Centers for Disease Control and Prevention, National Center for Health Statistics. US overdose deaths decrease in 2023, first time since 2018. CDC Online Newsroom. 2024. Available at: https://www.cdc.gov/nchs/pressroom/nchs_press_releases/2024/20240515.htm#:~:text=Provisional%20data%20from%20CDC's%20National,111%2C029%20deaths%20estimated%20in%202022. Accessed July 27, 2024.
2. Jalal H, Buchanich JM, Roberts MS, Balmert LC, Zhang K, Burke DS. Changing dynamics of the drug overdose epidemic in the United States, 1979–2016. *Science.* 2018;361(6408):eaau1184. https://doi.org/10.1126/science.aau1184
3. Centers for Disease Control and Prevention, National Center for Injury Prevention and Control. Opioid overdose prevention: using data to drive action. Enhanced state opioid overdose surveillance (ESOOS). Available at: https://www.cdc.gov/overdose-prevention/media/pdfs/CDC-NCIPC-ESOOSReport-508.pdf. Accessed July 27, 2024.
4. Bohnert ASB, Ilgen MA. Understanding links among opioid use, overdose, and suicide. *N Engl J Med.* 2019;380(1):71–79. https://doi.org/10.1056/NEJMra1802148
5. Rockett IRH, Caine ED, Stack S, et al. Method overtness, forensic autopsy, and the evidentiary suicide note: a multilevel National Violent Death Reporting System analysis. *PLoS One.* 2018;13(5):e0197805. https://doi.org/10.1371/journal.pone.0197805
6. Zhang K, Strahan AR, Guy GP, Larochelle MR. Trends in concurrent opioid and benzodiazepine prescriptions in the United States, 2016 to 2019. *Ann Intern Med.* 2022;175(7):1051–1053. https://doi.org/10.7326/M21-4656

Contesting Deregulation and Medicalization to Revitalize Public Health

Daniel G. Aaron, MD, JD

ABOUT THE AUTHOR

Daniel G. Aaron is associate professor of law, S. J. Quinney College of Law, University of Utah, Salt Lake City.

See also Pomeranz et al., p. 1061.

The US Food and Drug Administration (FDA) is charged with overseeing food additives in the United States. In this issue of *AJPH*, Pomeranz et al. (p. 1061) describe the regulatory failure that this regime embodies. Their research highlights one corner of a growing trend toward the disempowerment of agencies that protect health and the environment and raises questions about how we can reverse course.

On June 28, 2024, the Supreme Court overturned its superprecedent *Chevron USA Inc v National Resources Defense Council Inc*, dealing a structural blow to the deference usually afforded administrative agencies. The overturning of *Chevron* is part of a larger project to subvert federal agencies.[1] Interestingly, however, courts played a minor role in the fall of FDA food additives regulation.

FOOD AND DRUG ADMINISTRATION'S FOOD ADDITIVES REGIME

There are at least four structural forces, other than judicial scrutiny, that have assailed the effectiveness of the FDA across its regulatory areas.[2] These include congressional statutory defects, presidential micromanagement, resource constraints, and ideological capture.[2]

Pomeranz et al. rightly point to resources and a congressional statutory loophole as the seeds of regulatory failure for food additives. Today, FDA exerts minimal oversight of food additives, instead allowing a statutory loophole to subsume almost the entire regime. The loophole, called "generally recognized as safe" (GRAS), is an exemption to the definition of food additive.[2] Because the vast majority of food additives enter the market through the GRAS pathway, almost all substances added to food are, oddly, not "food additives," at least legally speaking.[2] And FDA allows companies to self-certify their substances as GRAS—and insert them into our food supply—without oversight.[3] A federal court upheld FDA's approach in *Center for Food Safety v Becerra* (SDNY 2021). FDA has admitted that additional resources would be needed to review food additives in house.

Unfortunately, FDA's anemic oversight of GRAS substances creates a problem of unknown unknowns. With companies not required to inform FDA about the substances they are adding to the food supply,[3] it is difficult to synthesize comprehensive evidence about their public health impact.

Despite this uncertainty, several substances deemed GRAS appear to be associated with major morbidity and mortality burdens. An obesity epidemic driven significantly by excess sugar consumption could be mitigated if FDA declared certain uses or levels of sugar "not GRAS." Salt, for its part, costs about 58 000 American lives each year, and the American Medical Association and other groups have urged FDA to declare certain levels of salt "not GRAS."[2] FDA has not budged. Other lesser-known GRAS substances, like butylated hydroxyanisole and propylparaben, have been found to pose risks of endocrine disruption or cancer.

REPAIRING THE FOOD ADDITIVE REGULATORY FRAMEWORK

Pomeranz et al. explain that FDA already has substantial authority to regulate GRAS substances to promote the public health. Given its limited resources, it might target additives known to cause the highest morbidity and mortality in the United States, particularly sugar and salt. The agency could use preexisting authorities to rein in excess quantities of food additives, adopt transparency measures, and curb conflicts of interest in corporate GRAS panels.

More structurally, Congress could infuse the regime with resources or replace the GRAS process with something more robust—perhaps a "new framework."

Ultimately, structural reform by Congress is the only true salve for our food additive regime given the resource constraints that would impair any sincere FDA effort to survey substances added to food in the United States. Yet this poses a quandary at a historical moment when congressional politics are heavily influenced by regulated industry.[2] This long-recognized problem has led FDA to

AJPH October 2024, Vol. 114, No. 10

take action on its own in some instances—for example, with regard to laboratory-developed tests, which largely went unregulated until FDA took decisive action in May 2024. FDA seems disinterested in bold action in the food additive regulatory space, perhaps because it might have to pilfer funding from other food regulatory efforts. (On the other hand, the hope with laboratory-developed tests is that, by regulating them as devices, FDA will receive proportionate increases in user fees.) So, while Pomeranz et al. pose excellent suggestions for improving the framework, it may be challenging to secure a statutory rework that would empower FDA with ample resources and authority.

UNDERCURRENTS OF PRIVATIZATION AND CORPORATE POWER

The failed oversight system for food additives highlights an important lesson: that corporations can exploit structural weaknesses in regulatory frameworks[4,5] to undermine a seemingly large grant of regulatory authority. Antiregulatory actors have generally fought increased funding for FDA food regulation,[6] leading to FDA's regime gradually eroding into the emaciated system it is today.[2]

Intriguingly, we see a contrast with medical approaches, which are flush with funding to mitigate downstream disease. For example, while in 2022 the United States spent $4500 billion in national health expenditures, $944 billion for Medicare, $1300 billion for private insurance, and $634 billion on prescription drugs, the FDA food budget was shrimpy at $1.1 billion—despite diet being the leading risk factor for death in the United States.[7] Likewise, the "astounding amount" of financial investment in Food Is Medicine efforts has been critiqued for leaving unaddressed core problems leading to diet-related disease, including food industry conduct, the low price of ultraprocessed food, and aggressive marketing.[8] So, it is not that the government lacks the funds to properly invest in public health but that it spends its funds on expensive, individualized, downstream treatment rather than preventing disease for the entire community.

The "privatization" of our health—emphasizing corporate solutions like drugs and devices and the medical model, instead of government oversight[9]—reflects a neoliberal approach to social problems. Neoliberalism is a framework that favors market solutions over government-enabled communal guarantees.[10] This approach, which we have largely adopted in the United States, clashes with the original purpose of the Food Additives Amendment—and a host of other laws largely stemming from the 1960s and 1970s empowering government to protect public health, ranging from the Occupational Safety and Health Act of 1970, to the Clean Air Act of 1970, to the Kefauver–Harris Amendment of 1962 (which amplified FDA drug regulation), to the Medical Device Amendments of 1976. These laws generally sought to prevent, not treat, public health harms.

How do we restore the spirit of good government, reawaken social solidarity, and reaffirm the importance of public health? This is a vital question public health experts must increasingly consider. Akbar suggests that solving core social problems "must be a bottom-up project" that cannot be entrusted to political parties; she stresses the importance of social movements.[11(p97)] Lantz et al. argue public health researchers and journalists should educate the public about the perils of medicalization.[9] Public health itself tends to focus on biomedical approaches; internal change within the public health community may be integral.[12]

The article by Pomeranz et al. sparks a larger conversation about the current state of administrative regulation and how to ensure it operates on behalf of the public's health. By forming alliances with grassroots movements and refocusing on systemic approaches to the leading causes of disease—food and tobacco—public health could participate in revitalizing regulatory frameworks like the GRAS system that fail to appropriately check corporate power. AJPH

CORRESPONDENCE

Correspondence should be sent to Daniel G. Aaron, 383 South University St, Salt Lake City, UT 84112 (e-mail: daniel.aaron@law.utah.edu). Reprints can be ordered at https://www.ajph.org by clicking the "Reprints" link.

PUBLICATION INFORMATION

Full Citation: Aaron DG. Contesting deregulation and medicalization to revitalize public health. *Am J Public Health*. 2024;114(10):968–970.

Acceptance Date: July 18, 2024.

DOI: https://doi.org/10.2105/AJPH.2024.307817

ORCID iD:
Daniel G. Aaron https://orcid.org/0000-0003-4490-7504

CONFLICTS OF INTEREST

The author declares no conflicts of interest.

REFERENCES

1. Aaron DG, Emery AE. US Supreme Court limits on the power of US health agencies. *JAMA*. 2024; 331(17):1441. https://doi.org/10.1001/jama.2024.3723
2. Aaron DG. The fall of FDA review. *Yale J Health Policy Law Ethics*. 2023;22(1):95–191.
3. Faustman C, Aaron D, Negowetti N, Leib EB. Ten years post-GAO assessment, FDA remains uninformed of potentially harmful GRAS substances in foods. *Crit Rev Food Sci Nutr*. 2021;61(8):1260–1268. https://doi.org/10.1080/10408398.2020.1756217
4. Aaron DG, Wallace CR, Sinha MS. Including E-cigarettes in the FDA rule limiting nicotine. *JAMA*. 2023;330(12):1129. https://doi.org/10.1001/jama.2023.14254

5. Aaron DG, Cohen IG, Adashi EY. Medicare Advantage under fire: public criticism and implications. *J Gen Intern Med.* 2024; epub ahead of print June 26, 2024. https://doi.org/10.1007/s11606-024-08876-7
6. Zimmerman S. House Republicans set up partisan food fight with proposed USDA, FDA budget cuts. *Agriculture Dive.* June 12, 2024. Available at: https://www.agriculturedive.com/news/usda-fda-busget-congress-fy25-biden/718739. Accessed July 5, 2024.
7. Mokdad AH, Ballestros K, Echko M, et al. The US Burden of Disease Collaborators. The state of US health, 1990–2016: burden of diseases, injuries, and risk factors among US States. *JAMA.* 2018; 319(14):1444–1472. https://doi.org/10.1001/jama.2018.0158
8. Moran AJ, Roberto CAA. "Food Is Medicine" approach to disease prevention: limitations and alternatives. *JAMA.* 2023;330(23):2243–2244. https://doi.org/10.1001/jama.2023.24472
9. Lantz PM, Goldberg DS, Gollust SE. The perils of medicalization for population health and health equity. *Milbank Q.* 2023;101(suppl 1):61–82. https://doi.org/10.1111/1468-0009.12619
10. Britton-Purdy J, Grewal DS, Kapczynski A, Rahman KS. Building a law-and-political-economy framework: beyond the twentieth-century synthesis. *Yale Law J.* 2020;129(6):1784–1835.
11. Akbar AA. Demands for a democratic political economy. *Harv Law Rev.* 2020;134:90–118.
12. Lacy-Nichols J, Marten R, Crosbie E, Moodie R. The public health playbook: ideas for challenging the corporate playbook. *Lancet Glob Health.* 2022; 10(7):e1067–e1072. https://doi.org/10.1016/S2214-109X(22)00185-1

Restricting Immigrant Access to Pregnancy-Related Insurance Has Public Health Consequences

Teresa Janevic, PhD, MPH, Ellerie Weber, PhD, MBA, and Ashley Fox, PhD, MA

ABOUT THE AUTHORS

Teresa Janevic is with the Columbia University Mailman School of Public Health. New York, NY. Ellerie Weber is with the Icahn School of Medicine at Mount Sinai, New York, NY. Ashley Fox is with the Rockefeller College of Public Affairs and Policy, Albany, NY.

See also DiMeo et al., p. 1051.

In the article "Navigating the Labyrinth of Pregnancy-Related Coverage for Undocumented Immigrants: An Assessment of Current State and Federal Policies," DiMeo et al. (p. 1051) outline state and federal policies regarding public health insurance coverage for nonqualified immigrants, highlighting substantial gaps in eligibility, leaving many pregnant immigrants without insurance coverage. For those eligible, the authors further describe barriers to obtaining coverage, including knowledge, awareness, and administrative burden. In this commentary, we build on these findings to describe consequences to the nation's public health and review possible policy solutions.

POPULATION IMPACT

The demographic profile of the United States implies that, by numbers alone, restricting immigrant access to pregnancy-related insurance is likely to have a large population impact. As the authors point out, it is estimated that 22% of immigrants to the United States are unauthorized.[1] Centers for Disease Control and Prevention Wide-Ranging Online Data for Epidemiologic Research (CDC WONDER) reports 832 728 births to immigrants in the United States in 2022. Therefore, if the proportion of birthing immigrants that are unauthorized is similar to the total population estimate, approximately 183 200 births were to unauthorized people. Although births to unauthorized immigrants occur in all 50 states, states with a large population of unauthorized immigrants are especially affected. For example, in Texas, it is estimated that 30% of immigrants are unauthorized, so of 104 269 births to immigrants in 2022,[2] 31 280 were to unauthorized immigrants. However, even in states with smaller immigrant populations, because newer immigrants tend to live in ethnic enclaves,[3] large proportions of certain neighborhoods are likely severely affected by restrictive policies, as are the health facilities serving them. Therefore, states with both large and small unauthorized immigrant populations experience important public health consequences.

INADEQUATE CARE BEFORE, DURING, AND AFTER PREGNANCY

Beyond the numbers, one of the most apparent public health consequences of gaps in health insurance eligibility for immigrants is inadequate prenatal and postpartum care. Research has demonstrated that immigrant birthing people have lower rates of preconception care,[4] timely prenatal care,[4,5] and postpartum care. Likewise, expanding prenatal health insurance to nonqualified immigrants resulted in increased prenatal care.[6] Inadequate care has a negative influence on both maternal and infant outcomes, and is also important for optimizing long-term health. Contrary to the prevailing notion of the "healthy immigrant effect," which implies that immigrants are not at risk for poor maternal and infant outcomes, immigrants are at an increased risk compared with native-born women of maternal morbidities such as gestational diabetes, and at-risk subgroups are also at increased risk of poor infant outcomes. Therefore, restricting access to pregnancy-related insurance deters achieving Healthy People 2030 goals for women and infants.

BURDEN ON PATIENTS AND HEALTH SYSTEMS

A critical aspect of the "labyrinth" of pregnancy-related coverage for immigrants, the lack of online access to eligibility and information on state agency websites, worsens administrative burden with public health consequences on both pregnant patients and health systems.[7] One consequence identified by DiMeo et al. is that even eligible immigrant persons may not enroll because of lack of awareness of eligibility

AJPH October 2024, Vol. 114, No. 10

on either the patient or provider side. Administrative burden may also have more direct health consequences. For the patient, battling the labyrinth can create stress and anxiety during a perinatal period that is physically and psychologically demanding. Stress can increase the risk of adverse pregnancy outcomes, such as low birth weight, preterm birth, and hypertensive disorders.[8] On the health system side, lack of transparency regarding eligibility criteria makes it arduous for health care providers, administrators, and social workers to connect their clients to services and increases workload and burnout.[9]

The social and political context likely moderates the consequences of immigrant restrictions on public health. In cities and states with a more favorable climate, information about pathways to coverage for immigrant women may be more freely advertised, whereas in restrictive climates, agencies and community-based organizations may be hesitant because of concern of calling attention to the services. DiMeo et al. rightly point out the "chilling effect" of immigrant exclusions from Medicaid. There is mounting evidence of the magnitude of the chilling effect, including its spillover effects onto otherwise eligible populations such as children who may reside in mixed-status households.[10] Because immigrants often receive information about health through community-based social networks, the reluctance to advertise coverage on the system side, and reluctance to engage on the patient side, can disrupt the vital flow of information in immigrant communities needed to access care and optimize pregnancy outcomes.

Finally, restricting immigrant access to pregnancy-related insurance has consequences on the health care system that go beyond immigrant communities. Studies consistently find that the cost of uncompensated care is higher in states with higher rates of uninsurance and that uninsurance increases uncompensated hospital care expenditures.[11] Safety-net hospitals are facing severe financial strain, and large hospital systems are consolidating, leaving even greater gaps in the already limited avenues for accessing care for immigrant populations. The decentralized and fragmented patchwork approach to covering pregnant immigrants is grossly inefficient, leading to duplicated efforts and spending by local communities and regional and state administrators, who may be independently trying to ensure that pregnant immigrants get the care needed. More thoughtful, coordinated approaches in Medicaid policy vis-à-vis pregnant immigrants, even within states, could simultaneously lower costs and improve outcomes and, thus, would be cost effective.

POLICY LEVERS TO INCREASE ACCESS

Policy solutions exist to increase health insurance coverage and access for pregnant and postpartum immigrants. Federally mandated universal access to public health insurance for all pregnant people is ideal, but other stop-gap measures exist. Legislative efforts to lift the federal 5-year waiting period to qualify for benefits would result in increased access for qualified pregnant people, although this would not increase access for unauthorized people. States have the option to create Medicaid look-alike programs for which unauthorized pregnant immigrants are eligible, as California and New York have done, and often provide more comprehensive care. States could also create legislation to allow peripartum individuals access to inexpensive, Affordable Care Act–compliant individual health plans. Options exist as well to increase postpartum coverage for immigrants. Currently, 47 of 50 states and the District of Columbia have extended Medicaid coverage postpartum, but in only 11 states does this extended coverage include unauthorized immigrants. For example, states that cover pregnant unauthorized immigrants using the Children's Health Insurance Program might continue coverage postpartum using Health Service Initiative funds, as some states (e.g., Illinois) currently do. Finally, states could increase access to care among those immigrants already eligible by streamlining application and eligibility determination processes and procedures (e.g., shorter applications and presumed eligibility) and conducting greater outreach to immigrant communities.

Restricting immigrant access to pregnancy-related insurance, either intentionally through policy or unintentionally because of lack of information and a confusing, patchwork system, is harmful to the nation's public health. Increasing access to pregnancy-related insurance can aid progress toward Healthy People 2030 goals while strengthening the US health care system and public health workforce. AJPH

CORRESPONDENCE

Correspondence should be sent to Teresa Janevic, PhD, MPH, Columbia University Mailman School of Public Health, 722 W 168th St, Rm 728, New York, NY 10032 (e-mail: tmj2101@cumc.columbia.edu). Reprints can be ordered at https://www.ajph.org by clicking the "Reprints" link.

PUBLICATION INFORMATION

Full Citation: Janevic T, Weber E, Fox A. Restricting immigrant access to pregnancy-related insurance has public health consequences. *Am J Public Health*. 2024;114(10):971–973.

Acceptance Date: July 23, 2024.

DOI: https://doi.org/10.2105/AJPH.2024.307828

ORCID iDs:

Ellerie Weber https://orcid.org/0000-0003-3179-7035

Ashley Fox https://orcid.org/0000-0003-4106-7853

CONTRIBUTORS

T. Janevic wrote the first draft and made final edits. E. Weber and A. Fox wrote a portion of the text and reviewed the final draft.

ACKNOWLEDGMENTS

Work contributing to this commentary was funded in part by the Robert Wood Johnson Foundation (grant 79625).

We thank Annabelle Ng, MPH, and Frances A. Howell, MA, for their contributions to our Postpartum Outcomes After Extension of Medicaid Study team.

CONFLICTS OF INTEREST

The authors report no conflicts of interest.

REFERENCES

1. Passel JS, Krogstad JM. What we know about unauthorized immigrants living in the US. Pew Research Center. November 16, 2023. Available at: https://www.pewresearch.org/short-reads/2023/11/16/what-we-know-about-unauthorized-immigrants-living-in-the-us. Accessed July 12, 2024.
2. National Center for Health Statistics, Centers for Disease Control and Prevention. About natality, 2007–2022. CDC WONDER. Available at: https://wonder.cdc.gov/natality-current.html. Accessed August 7, 2024.
3. Ellis M, Wright R, Parks V. The immigrant household and spatial assimilation: partnership, nativity, and neighborhood location. *Urban Geogr*. 2006;27(1):1–19. https://doi.org/10.2747/0272-3638.27.1.1
4. Maru S, Glenn L, Belfon K, et al. Utilization of maternal health care among immigrant mothers in New York City, 2016–2018. *J Urban Health*. 2021;98(6):711–726. https://doi.org/10.1007/s11524-021-00584-5
5. Janevic T, Weber E, Howell FM, Steelman M, Krishnamoorthi M, Fox A. Analysis of state Medicaid expansion and access to timely prenatal care among women who were immigrant vs US born. *JAMA Netw Open*. 2022;5(10):e2239264. https://doi.org/10.1001/jamanetworkopen.2022.39264
6. Swartz JJ, Hainmueller J, Lawrence D, Rodriguez MI. Oregon's expansion of prenatal care improved utilization among immigrant women. *Matern Child Health J*. 2018;23(2):173–182. https://doi.org/10.1007/s10995-018-2611-1
7. Herd P, Moynihan D. How administrative burdens can harm health. October 2, 2020. *Health Affairs Brief*. Available at: https://www.healthaffairs.org/do/10.1377/hpb20200904.405159/full. Accessed July 19, 2024.
8. Traylor CS, Johnson JD, Kimmel MC, Manuck TA. Effects of psychological stress on adverse pregnancy outcomes and nonpharmacologic approaches for reduction: an expert review. *Am J Obstet Gynecol MFM*. 2020;2(4):100229. https://doi.org/10.1016/j.ajogmf.2020.100229
9. Welles CC, Tong A, Brereton E, et al. Sources of clinician burnout in providing care for underserved patients in a safety-net healthcare system. *J Gen Intern Med*. 2023;38(6):1468–1475. https://doi.org/10.1007/s11606-022-07896-5
10. Barofsky J, Vargas A, Rodriguez D, Barrows A. Spreading fear: the announcement of the public charge rule reduced enrollment in child safety-net programs. *Health Aff (Millwood)*. 2020;39(10):1752–1761. https://doi.org/10.1377/hlthaff.2020.00763
11. Flavin L, Zallman L, McCormick D, Boyd JW. Medical expenditures on and by immigrant populations in the United States: a systematic review. *Int J Health Serv*. 2018;48(4):601–621. https://doi.org/10.1177/0020731418791963

Polarization, Partisanship, and Political Alignment Threaten Public Health: A Public Health of Consequence, October 2024

Farzana Kapadia, PhD, MPH

ABOUT THE AUTHOR

Farzana Kapadia is the deputy editor of AJPH *and professor of epidemiology at the School of Global Public Health, New York University, New York.*

See also Higgins and O'Leary, p. 983, Pomeranz et al., p. 1061, and Saxby et al., p. 1110.

AJPH October 2024, Vol. 114, No. 10

Modern US politics are defined by hyperpartisanship and polarization, and the November 2024 elections present concerns about a potential political alignment of highly conservative lawmakers at federal and state levels. The ensuing political divisiveness has fueled mistrust in government institutions. For example, during the height of the COVID-19 pandemic, partisanship, polarization, and political alignment drove inconsistent enactment and implementation of COVID-19 mitigation strategies, including social distancing, masking, and vaccination.[1] A conservative political alignment following the November 2024 elections could prompt legislative and policy changes with significantly harmful effects on population health and well-being in the United States.

As evidenced by the Supreme Court's conservative majority ruling in *Dobbs v Jackson Women's Health Organization* (*Dobbs*)[2] and other recent decisions, partisanship plays a major role in judicial decisions that have serious population health consequences. In this issue of *AJPH*, several articles address the consequences of the *Dobbs* decision. In addition to abortion rights, vaccination policy, LGBTQIA+ (lesbian, gay, bisexual, transgender/-sexual, queer or questioning, intersex, asexual, and all subsects) rights, marriage equality, environmental health, and food safety could come under attack with a conservative political alignment in 2024.

VACCINATION POLICY

Over the past two decades, Democratic and Republican lawmakers have become deeply divided on vaccination policy. Estep et al. describe partisan polarization between 1995 and 2020 on sponsorship of bills regarding immunization during public health emergencies, childhood vaccine exemptions, and specific vaccines, such as human papillomavirus.[3] Sustained polarization and partisanship in vaccination efforts will undermine scientifically justified and evidence-based public health policy and ultimately increase vaccine preventable morbidity and mortality.

Additionally, conservative legislators and antivaccination agitators have fueled vaccine hesitancy and supported antivaccine legislation under the pretext of protecting individual liberty from government meddling. In this issue of *AJPH*, Higgins and O'Leary (p. 983) call for robust monitoring of vaccine hesitancy in the United States that measures "complacency, convenience, and confidence"—three underlying determinants of hesitancy. Given the political wrangling that has fueled vaccine hesitancy, additional measures of political party affiliation and partisanship, as recommended by Pacheco et al., can offer perspectives on government mistrust, individualism, public health mistrust, and antiscience attitudes that drive the ideology fueling vaccine hesitancy.[4]

LGBTQIA+ RIGHTS AND MARRIAGE EQUALITY

During his tenure, former President Donald Trump appointed three of the Supreme Court's current roster of six conservative justices and more than 200 federal judges who the Human Rights Campaign has cited as being hostile to LGBTQIA+ rights.[5] Such a partisan judiciary poses real threats to the hard-fought rights, dignity, and humanity of LGBTQIA+ people. Evidence of this is clearly seen in Justice Clarence Thomas's concurring opinion on the Supreme Court's six to three partisan ruling in *Dobbs*. Justice Thomas advocated a reconsideration of "all of this Court's substantive due process precedents, including *Griswold*, *Lawrence*, and *Obergefell*" and claimed that the court had a "duty" to "overrul[e] these demonstrably erroneous decisions."[2] Taken together, these three major rulings ensured the legality of access to contraception for married couples,[6] decriminalized consensual sex between same-sex people,[7] and required all states to license and recognize same-sex marriage.[8]

Despite popular opinion in favor of marriage equality, a spate of recent state-level legislation has attacked the rights of transgender people by pushing bathroom bills, transgender athlete bans, and the highly repugnant child–parent separation law proposed by Governor Greg Abbott of Texas that would allow child welfare agencies to investigate parents and doctors providing gender-affirming care to transgender youths. In addition, in the 2021 decision in *Fulton v City of Philadelphia*,[9] the Supreme Court ruled in favor of a religious foster care agency to deny married same-sex couples the right to serve as foster parents. Not only do these legislative efforts and court rulings threaten the rights of transgender people and same-sex couples, but they signal that the rights of LGBTQIA+ individuals, including marriage equality, are subject to future challenge.

The potential for rolling back these rights and codifying sexual orientation– and gender identity–based discrimination will undoubtedly pose serious harms to the health of LGBTQIA+ communities. And as shown in numerous previous publications, structural stigma and discrimination against LGBTQIA+ persons—in the United States and elsewhere in the world—seriously harms the health of sexual and gender minority populations. In this issue, Saxby et al. (p. 1110) provide yet more evidence that residing in a region with greater structural stigma, defined as one where a majority of the populace voted against legalizing same-sex marriage, was associated with poorer long-term health outcomes among Australians in same-sex relationships.

ENVIRONMENTAL HEALTH AND FOOD SAFETY

In *Loper Bright Enterprise v Raimondo* (*Loper*),[10] the Supreme Court's six to three ruling along partisan lines eliminated the *Chevron* deference—a 40-year-old precedent—which required judges to defer to a federal agency's interpretation of relevant laws when its regulations are challenged in court. In overruling *Chevron*, courts can now "exercise their independent judgment in deciding whether an agency has acted in its statutory authority, and courts may not defer to an agency interpretation of the law simply because a statute is ambiguous."[10]

Following this ruling, several conservative Republican legislators are already spearheading efforts to strip federal agencies, including the Centers for Medicare & Medicaid Services, the Occupational Safety and Health Administration, the Environmental Protection Agency, the Centers for Disease Control and Prevention, and the Food and Drug Administration (FDA), of their regulatory authority and put it back into the hands of Congress and the courts. Overruling the *Chevron* deference undermines the ability of these agencies to ensure that the latest scientific evidence supports health policy and related regulations that these agencies set. Instead, judges and legislators that lack the scientific expertise will now have power over these regulatory statutes. Therefore, efforts to undermine bedrocks of our environmental protections (e.g., the clean air and clean water acts) will come under attack.

Pomeranz et al. (p. 1061) describe a unique example of how the *Loper* decision may affect the complex process involved in evaluating and regulating substances added to food products. Currently, because of gaps in FDA oversight over substances in the food supply, states have started to act to fill the regulatory void. However, with the overturning of the *Chevron* doctrine, it will now be up to Congress and the courts to decide whether the FDA has the regulatory authority to review any food additives. Given the high prevalence of ultraprocessed food consumption, it is likely that food industry lobbyists will mount challenges to such decisions.

CONCLUSIONS

We are actively witnessing how polarization, partisanship, and political alignment across the executive, legislative, and judicial branches of government are reshaping public health policy, health behaviors, and attitudes. Moreover, increasing partisanship and political alignment are emboldening states to follow their own health policy agendas.

The lack of bipartisanship at both federal and local levels will continue to jeopardize enactment and enforcement of health policies that can help, and not harm, our communities. Partisan divides and polarization along party lines will further undermine our already fragile and fragmented health care system. The possibility of a conservative political alignment after the fall 2024 election cannot be ignored as the state of our population's health and well-being are on the line. AJPH

CORRESPONDENCE

Correspondence should be sent to Farzana Kapadia, PhD, MPH, New York University, School of Global Public Health, 708 Broadway, Room 729, New York, NY 10003 (e-mail: farzana.kapadia@nyu.edu). Reprints can be ordered at https://www.ajph.org by clicking the "Reprints" link.

PUBLICATION INFORMATION

Full Citation: Kapadia F. Polarization, partisanship, and political alignment threaten public health: a public health of consequence, October 2024. *Am J Public Health*. 2024;114(10):974–976.

Acceptance Date: July 22, 2024.

DOI: https://doi.org/10.2105/AJPH.2024.307826

ORCID iD:

Farzana Kapadia https://orcid.org/0000-0003-3459-767X

CONFLICTS OF INTEREST

The author has no conflicts of interest to disclose.

REFERENCES

1. Barry CL, Anderson KE, Han H, Presskreischer R, McGinty EE. Change over time in public support for social distancing, mask wearing, and contact tracing to combat the COVID-19 pandemic among US adults, April to November 2020. *Am J Public Health*. 2021;111(5):937–948. https://doi.org/10.2105/AJPH.2020.306148
2. *Dobbs v Jackson Women's Health Organization*, 142 S. Ct. 2228 (2022). Available at: https://www.supremecourt.gov/opinions/21pdf/19-1392_6j37.pdf. Accessed July 27, 2024.
3. Estep K, Muse A, Sweeney S, Goldstein ND. Partisan polarization of childhood vaccination policies, 1995–2020. *Am J Public Health*. 2022;112(10):1471–1479. https://doi.org/10.2105/AJPH.2022.306964
4. Pacheco J, Gollust SE, Callaghan T, Motta M. A call for measuring partisanship in US public health research. *Am J Public Health*. 2024;114(8):772–776. https://doi.org/10.2105/AJPH.2024.307691
5. Human Rights Campaign. The real list of Trump's "unprecedented steps" for the LGBTQ community. Available at: https://www.hrc.org/news/the-list-of-trumps-unprecedented-steps-for-the-lgbtq-community. Accessed July 15, 2024.
6. *Griswold v Connecticut*, 381 US 479 (1965).
7. *Lawrence v Texas*, 539 US 558 (2003).
8. *Obergefell v Hodges*, 576 US 644 (2015).
9. *Fulton v City of Philadelphia*, 141 S. Ct. 1868 (2021).
10. *Loper Bright Enterprises v Raimondo*, 45 F.4th 61 (2d Cir. 2022).

Deep Reform and Targeted Investment: Essential Strategies for Preparing for the Next Health Emergency in Europe and Elsewhere

Frank Vandenbroucke, PhD, and Pedro Facon, MPS

ABOUT THE AUTHORS

Frank Vandenbroucke is Belgian deputy prime minister and minister of social affairs and public health, Brussels as well as chair of the Organization for Economic Cooperation and Development (OECD) 2024 Health Ministerial Meeting. Pedro Facon is deputy CEO of the Belgian National Institute for Health and Disability Insurance, Brussels and a member of the OECD Health Committee.

On January 24, 2024, health ministers of 50 countries, social partners, and international organizations convened in Paris, France, for the first Organization for Economic Cooperation and Development (OECD) Health Ministerial Meeting in more than five years. The aim was to take stock of health systems after three disruptive years of COVID-19 and to define new policy orientations. Our conclusions were anchored in a declaration on building better policies for more resilient health systems, as well as a renewed health system performance assessment framework.[1]

THE TOUGH LESSONS OF THE PANDEMIC

COVID-19 taught us a tough lesson on the need for crisis preparedness and response. Although health systems have demonstrated flexibility in swiftly finding solutions to the continuous flow of challenges during the pandemic, a high toll of excess mortality, morbidity and long-term health effects has been paid. An overstretched health system led to lasting fatigue for many health care professionals.

Clearly, institutions for health emergency preparedness and response must be strengthened, both at the national and regional level. The mandates of the European Centre for Disease Prevention and Control and the European Medicines Agency have been expanded, and a new Health Emergency Preparedness and Response Authority, modeled after the US Biomedical Advanced Research and Development Authority, was created at the European Union level. At the World Health Organization (WHO) level, negotiations on a pandemic treaty were launched, which are still ongoing. A point of concern is that less attention is paid to the "soft" dimensions of preparedness through which a risk culture is developed, with policymakers, health system actors, and citizens. Also, our focus may be too much on a respiratory infectious disease type of emergency, while other crises, related to climate; incidents of chemical, biological, radiological and nuclear nature; data; or war should equally be considered—or even a fully unexpected "black swan" event.

HEALTH SYSTEM RESILIENCE AND ITS FOUNDATIONS

Moreover, there is more to resilience than preparedness and response capacity. The extent to which health systems were effective in their response to COVID-19 was linked to their long-standing strengths and weaknesses. These flaws concern not only the health and care sector but also the larger social and economic environment people live in. Health crisis response can only be successful in reasonably well functioning social structure, public health systems, and society's communication systems.[2] Moreover, trust from citizens in policymakers, and trust from policymakers in scientific advisors, experts, and civil servants are all important variables in effective health crisis management.

It suffices to dive into the results of international and national health systems' performance assessments of the past decade to understand better why some things went well, while others went terribly wrong. The obvious conclusion is that the best preparation for a health emergency is tackling systemic weaknesses before a crisis arrives.

Alas, two years after the most acute phase of the pandemic, learning lessons and turning them into action is already being deprioritized on the political and societal agenda.

AJPH October 2024, Vol. 114, No. 10

While international cooperation and solidarity proved to be a key to success, we see a return to national reflexes. Promising national and international policy initiatives may remain unfinished.

THE URGENT NEED FOR MORE BOLD AND MORE RAPID REFORM

This is all the more reason, as was the main conclusion of the OECD Health Ministerial, to waste no time and move forward with reforms that improve the foundations of our systems. Even if national specificities exist, there is a clear set of common objectives for all our health systems. Pursuing them is a response to both future health emergencies and to the challenges of an aging population, increasing chronic conditions, and multimorbidity. Indeed, maximizing people's health before a crisis minimizes the health damage to the population.

Health cannot only be the responsibility of the health care system. If many countries have shown remarkable progress in treatment of illness, primary and secondary prevention remain underdeveloped in spite of all the evidence on their positive return on investment. Our first objective is to make our societies fundamentally more healthy and supportive for healthy lifestyles. Apart from achieving climate neutrality and addressing determinants of poor health, like poverty or bad housing, commercial determinants of unhealthy behavior and preventable morbidity and mortality need to be unveiled and addressed. At the individual level, we must strengthen health literacy, including digital, self-management competencies. While securing a healthy environment for all, we also have to appeal to individual responsibility, without stigmatization or exclusion.

Turning to the health care system, its organization and financing has to become more need-driven, integrated, and person-centered, supported by digitization and data sharing. The historical development of health systems led to reasoning in terms of lines of care (primary, secondary, tertiary) and types of care (somatic, mental). Primary care remains underdeveloped, highly fragmented, and underdigitized. Shortages in the health workforce are worsened by an outpaced, corporatist, often overregulated division of labor between health professionals that prevents people from working at the top of their competencies. Health care remains, in spite of many investments, an economic sector in which digital solutions are underused.

We should applaud many countries for their efforts but, at the same time, probably be more bold and hurry these transformations, taking into account the very rapidly changing economic and societal environment of health care. This is not only a matter of structures, technologies, and processes, and regulatory or financial arrangements, but equally of developing a culture of collaboration that puts the patient and their needs really at the center. That requires a strong commitment and open mind of health professionals and their representative organization: they need to be ready to shift and share tasks and rethink everyone's role within the health care organization, beyond professional interests and existing business models. Health workforce policies, covering the whole range from planning, recruiting, training, pay, working conditions, autonomy, and recognition, to continuously developing and retraining, should be at the heart of national and international health policies in the next decade.

THE VIRTUOUS CYCLE OF TARGETED INVESTMENTS

Such systemic transformation demands consistent reforms that go hand in hand with targeted investments. To boost the resilience of health systems, OECD had calculated that, relative to expenditure in 2019, investments of on average 1.4% of GDP are required. Half of these should focus on strengthening the health workforce. The other half involves protecting underlying population health through additional spending on preventive care and fortifying the foundations of health systems by investing in better health information systems and core infrastructure.[3]

In times of a difficult fiscal context and competition of other societal needs, we must not forget the virtuous cycle of social investment: strong social protection, including health systems, lead to a stronger economy and society, which in turn lead to better health and less burden for health systems. The recent Belgian presidency of the EU Council has anchored these principles in a call for action through the Declaration on the Future Social Agenda of the European Union.[4]

In many health systems, investments are mainly decided in a bottom-up, incremental, sectoral, and interest-driven way, often linked to the yearly budget process. Shifting toward a strategic, multiannual, system-wide approach, based on health and health care objectives and informed by evidence and health technology assessment, will create tensions with stakeholders and vested interests. Convincing them that this shift will, in the long term, apart from patients and populations, also serve their constituencies better requires stewardship, leadership, and dialogue.

Next to the three priority investment domains (workforce, prevention, and infrastructure, including information systems), budgets are needed for other policy challenges like improving coverage and financial protection of patients or for underinvested domains of health care like mental health. The OECD Joint Network of Senior Budget and Health Officials identifies four nonexclusive options.[5] First, overall government spending can be increased to allocate additional funds to health. Second, within the existing government budget, the focus on health can be increased. Third, the boundaries between public and private spending can be altered. Fourth, health systems can finance their needs through efficiency gains. Tax pressure is already historically high in many countries and increasing the proportion of health expenditure in the overall budget is difficult, given investment needs in the domains of climate transition, defense and other priorities. Reassessing boundaries between public and private spending is at odds with the harsh reality that out-of-pocket expenditure in many countries is already high with postponement of care and impoverishment as consequences. And even if private insurance can to a certain extent bring solutions as an additional layer of protection, it comes with risks of equity and efficiency and cannot replace a solid public health insurance.

The fourth—for most countries, the preferable option—is to improve the efficiency of health expenditure. Even if it often seems like the "Holy Grail," it is far from evident and requires strong stewardship because it challenges the already mentioned vested interests, business models, and "the way we have always done things." Investing in capacity for thematic spending reviews, policy evaluation, and building evidence, and anchoring these in concertation and decision-making processes are conditions for success.

The next decade, with all its challenges and turbulence, must be about person-centered, sustainable, and resilient health systems. Reform and investment are two sides of the same coin. Health policymakers have to train themselves to one of the most difficult disciplines in sport: the sprint marathon. Rapid responsiveness to emerging events (resilience) has to be combined with a focus on the long term (sustainability). This cannot be a solitary, strictly individual discipline. Strategic dialogue and partnership among political actors, civil servants, and stakeholders are key to transforming systems. Inspiration, support, and solidarity at the international level are equally essential: institutions like OECD, the European Union, and WHO are platforms for mutual learning, for building trust and confidence, for pushing the boundaries of our thinking, and for maximizing the effectiveness of policy action. AJPH

CORRESPONDENCE

Correspondence should be sent to Pedro Facon, RIZIV-INAMI, Avenue Galilée 5 B-1210 Saint-Josse-ten-Noode, Belgium (e-mail: pedro.facon@riziv-inami.fgov.be). Reprints can be ordered at https://www.ajph.org by clicking the "Reprints" link.

PUBLICATION INFORMATION

Full Citation: Vandenbroucke F, Facon P. Deep reform and targeted investment: essential strategies for preparing for the next health emergency in Europe and elsewhere. *Am J Public Health*. 2024;114(10):977–979.

Acceptance Date: June 22, 2024.

DOI: https://doi.org/10.2105/AJPH.2024.307779

ORCID iDs:
Frank Vandenbroucke https://orcid.org/0000-0001-9748-9567

Pedro Facon https://orcid.org/0009-0005-1344-4545

CONTRIBUTORS

F. Vandenbroucke and P. Facon equally contributed to the article.

CONFLICTS OF INTEREST

The authors report no conflicts of interest.

REFERENCES

1. *Declaration on Building Better Policies for More Resilient Health Systems*. Paris, France: Organization for Economic Cooperation and Development; January 2024.
2. LeBlanc TT. Strengthening social and economic, medical, and public health systems before disasters strike. *Am J Public Health*. 2021;111(5):842–843. https://doi.org/10.2105/AJPH.2021.306247
3. *Ready for the Next Crisis? Investing in Health System Resilience*. Paris, France: Organization for Economic Cooperation and Development; February 2023.
4. *La Hulpe Inter-institutional Declaration on the Future Social Agenda of the EU*. La Hulpe, Belgium: Belgian Presidency of the EU Council; April 2024.
5. *Fiscal Sustainability of Health Systems. How to Finance More Resilient Health Systems When Money Is Tight?* Paris, France: Organization for Economic Cooperation and Development; January 2024.

Social Media and Adolescent Health

Jon-Patrick Allem, PhD, MA

ABOUT THE AUTHOR

Jon-Patrick Allem is with the Department of Health Behavior, Society and Policy, Rutgers School of Public Health, State University of New Jersey, New Brunswick.

In December 2023, the National Academies of Sciences, Engineering, and Medicine (NASEM) released a report titled *Social Media and Adolescent Health*.[1] Reports like this are authored by a committee of experts and include findings, conclusions, and recommendations based on the extant literature gathered by the committee. NASEM is a congressionally chartered organization in the United States and appoints the experts to each committee. This editorial raises concerns over the committee's lack of experts trained in the field of public health, the evidence that was overlooked in the report, and how those from public health could have been able to improve the report by extending the scope of evidence that was considered in the report and by providing actionable policy recommendations in line with previous public health work.

PUBLIC HEALTH REPRESENTATION

Surprisingly, NASEM appointed only one expert to this committee with an appointment in a school of public health. This should be considered an oversight by the appointers of the committee because scholars have cogently argued that social media should be considered a commercial determinant of health,[2] and the field of public health has a rich history of studying "the private sector activities that affect people's health, directly or indirectly, positively or negatively."[3] Although the committee had representation from information science, communication, law, and psychology, scholars from these fields often lack the background in and knowledge of how corporations influence health and how evidence related to the commercial determinants of health can be collected, analyzed, and put into context for government action.

What is more, scholars from information science, psychology, and communication often have formal partnerships (e.g., they often have access to propriety data, receive unrestricted gifts, receive consulting fees, are paid speakers, coauthor reports) with those from social media companies. Scholars who partner with industry or come from a field where partnering with industry is normalized may view commercial determinants of health differently from scholars who are trained, and socialized, in public health.

What was equally surprising was that NASEM appointed two experts to this committee who had received funding from industry.[1,4] These conflicts of interest reduce the integrity of the committee and the report it was charged with writing. Those trained in public health, especially those in tobacco control, alcohol prevention, nutrition, and gun violence prevention, are familiar with the importance of qualifying research from industry-funded scientists. The conclusions and recommendations found in the report should be considered with these committee members' conflicts of interest in mind. For decades, industry-funded research has muddied the waters of the scientific literature,[5] casting doubt on the harms to society caused by tobacco, guns, and alcohol. Those trained in schools of public health are often taught about the lengths the tobacco, firearm, and alcohol industries have gone to discredit public health research.[6]

To accomplish this, each industry has funded research and researchers to produce studies that contradict (i.e., sow doubt about) the prevailing evidence on a topic area.[7] The ability to sow doubt has cascading effects on public opinion and agenda setting at the legislative level. Therefore, NASEM committees charged with understanding and summarizing issues of public concern, and with providing recommendations for (in)action by the government, should be free of members with conflicts of interest.

SOCIAL MEDIA CONTENT

Again, this specific committee was asked to comment on the relative risks and benefits of various forms of online media and the consequences of their use in adolescence. The committee did this, in part, by looking at systematic reviews (i.e., a synthesis of the evidence on a topic) and meta-analyses (i.e., statistical integration of evidence from the literature on a specific topic) on the association between social media and adolescent health. There were several pieces of evidence that seemed overlooked by the report. Most notably, research studying how the content found on social media platforms can affect offline attitudes and behaviors in young people.

Instead, the committee focused on the literature related to the amount of time spent on social media, which is unrelated to the content a young person could be exposed to. Time by itself is not inherently problematic. In other words, one could spend hours watching instructional videos on algebra homework, and one could spend hours watching videos glamorizing substance use. A study measuring time on social media would treat these two experiences equally. Additionally, the outcomes of interest in the selected studies were limited primarily to mental health–related outcomes, which precludes any understanding of how social media affects other areas of adolescent health.

Unfortunately, only one systematic review (of the 25 listed in Appendix C in the report) focused on the content that young people were exposed to and its association with offline behavior. In this systematic review, it was suggested that there is an association between exposure to unhealthy food content on social media and unhealthy diet in children and adolescents.[8] Had the committee tried to include similar evidence, they would have found a meta-analysis on the impacts of tobacco content on social media and offline tobacco use in adolescents.[9] An additional, similarly relevant meta-analysis exists on the effects of alcohol content on social media and offline drinking behavior in adolescents.[10] By overlooking or deemphasizing research on the content of social media platforms, the report failed to provide a comprehensive assessment of the relationship between social media and adolescent health.

WHAT TO DO IN THE FUTURE

It is unsurprising that, given the absence of research on the content of social media described in the report, the recommendations offered on what government, companies, and stakeholders should consider in fostering better online experiences for adolescents were tangentially related to the content on the platforms. For example, in the summary report and in Box 4–1 titled "Notes for Parents," a single sentence suggests, "An objective quality benchmark could be invaluable to parents who are struggling to discern various platforms' commitments to young people's privacy and safety online."[1] It was unclear from the report how a benchmark should be established or how safety should be defined.

WHAT CONTENT TO LOOK FOR

Social media companies know how toxic their platforms can be. They are the first to exclaim how much they care about, and spend money on, identifying and removing content that violates their community standards.[11] What they are less eager to tell the public is what specific content they are on the lookout for, how often that content is missed by the content moderation process,[11] who on the platform ends up viewing such content, and how this initial exposure affects the subsequent content recommended to each user while on the platform.

Social media companies should be required by law to disclose the materials that guide their content moderation process. In other words, the public should be made aware of the content that each company is on the lookout for by publishing the operational guidelines for how such content is identified and defined. Would a parent like to know that a social media platform has operational guidelines for identifying content such as human trafficking, torture, or drug use? Would this affect their decision on whether a platform is appropriate for their adolescent? If such a law were to pass, it would help establish a more disciplined way of thinking about the content on social media platforms, allowing more meaningful scrutiny. For example, to what extent does content such as torture, human trafficking, and drug use exist on each platform? Who is exposed to it? How is exposure shaping offline attitudes and behaviors?

If social media companies were required by law to disclose the materials that guide their content moderation process, public health researchers could better study the impact of exposure to such content on adolescent health. The leaders in public health with subject matter expertise in nutrition, body image, violence, sex, and substance use, to name only a few, could focus their efforts on studying and ultimately contextualizing the role that social media plays in shaping the multilayered area of adolescent health.

CONCLUSIONS

Ultimately, the committee's review of the literature, "did not support the conclusion that social media causes changes in adolescent health at the population level."[1] The question of causality is undoubtedly important, and the report goes into detail about the difficulty of establishing causality, especially where complicated social phenomena are concerned. However, in the case of the role of social media's influence on adolescents, it seems conservative to wait for this kind of evidence to accumulate before action is taken to better protect adolescents' health. Should we wait for a randomized controlled trial (i.e., the gold standard for establishing causality), assigning adolescents to social media for a period to compare their health against those who were prevented from using social media for the same period? It may be that the evidence that currently exists is sufficient for action. Until then, we need the public health community to engage in research to help us comprehensively understand how social media and adolescent health are related. Social media companies are not going to act in adolescents' best interests. AJPH

CORRESPONDENCE

Correspondence should be sent to Jon-Patrick Allem, 303 George St, Suite 500, New Brunswick, NJ 08901 (email: jon.patrick.allem@rutgers.edu). Reprints can be ordered at https://www.ajph.org by clicking the "Reprints" link.

PUBLICATION INFORMATION

Full Citation: Allem J-P. Social media and adolescent health. *Am J Public Health*. 2024;114(10):980–982.

Acceptance Date: June 26, 2024.

DOI: https://doi.org/10.2105/AJPH.2024.307784

CONFLICTS OF INTEREST

J.-P. Allem has received fees for consulting services in court cases pertaining to the content on social media platforms. He reports no other conflicts of interest.

REFERENCES

1. National Academies of Sciences, Engineering, and Medicine. *Social Media and Adolescent Health*. Washington, DC: National Academies Press; 2024. Available at: https://nap.nationalacademies.org/read/27396/chapter/1. Accessed July 9, 2024.
2. Zenone M, Kenworthy N, Maani N. The social media industry as a commercial determinant of health. *Int J Health Policy Manag*. 2023;12:6840. https://doi.org/10.34172/ijhpm.2022.6840
3. World Health Organization. Commercial determinants of health. March 21, 2023. Available at: https://www.who.int/news-room/fact-sheets/detail/commercial-determinants-of-health. Accessed April 18, 2024.
4. Choudhury MD. Curriculum vitae. November 2023. Available at: http://www.munmund.net/vitae/m-dechoudhury-CV.pdf. Accessed July 9, 2024.
5. Oreskes N, Conway EM. *Merchants of Doubt: How a Handful of Scientists Obscured the Truth on Issues From Tobacco Smoke to Global Warming*. New York, NY: Bloomsbury Publishing; 2010.
6. Freudenberg N. *Lethal but Legal: Corporations, Consumption, and Protecting Public Health*. Oxford, UK: Oxford University Press; 2014.
7. Otto SL. *The War on Science: Who's Waging It, Why It Matters, What We Can Do About It*. Minneapolis, MN: Milkweed Editions; 2016.
8. Sina E, Boakye D, Christianson L, Ahrens W, Hebestreit A. Social media and children's and adolescents' diets: a systematic review of the underlying social and physiological mechanisms. *Adv Nutr*. 2022;13(3):913–937. https://doi.org/10.1093/advances/nmac018
9. Donaldson SI, Dormanesh A, Perez C, Majmundar A, Allem JP. Association between exposure to tobacco content on social media and tobacco use: a systematic review and meta-analysis. *JAMA Pediatr*. 2022;176(9):878–885. https://doi.org/10.1001/jamapediatrics.2022.2223
10. Curtis BL, Lookatch SJ, Ramo DE, McKay JR, Feinn RS, Kranzler HR. Meta-Analysis of the association of alcohol-related social media use with alcohol consumption and alcohol-related problems in adolescents and young adults. *Alcohol Clin Exp Res*. 2018;42(6):978–986. https://doi.org/10.1111/acer.13642
11. Roberts ST. *Behind the Screen*. New Haven, CT: Yale University Press; 2021.

The Dire Need for Surveillance of Vaccine Hesitancy in the United States

David M. Higgins, MD, MPH, and Sean T. O'Leary, MD, MPH

ABOUT THE AUTHORS

David M. Higgins and Sean T. O'Leary are with the Adult and Child Center for Outcomes Research and Delivery Science (ACCORDS), University of Colorado School of Medicine/ Children's Hospital Colorado, Aurora.

See also Kapadia, p. 974.

Epidemiology is "the study of the distribution and determinants of health-related states or events in specified populations, and the application of this study to control for health problems."[1(p180)] Understanding the epidemiology of a significant health threat is the cornerstone of addressing the problem. Despite vaccine hesitancy being recognized as a top global health threat by the World Health Organization (WHO),[2] its epidemiology in the United States and worldwide is poorly understood and relies on basic or outdated data.

"Vaccines don't save lives. Vaccinations save lives." This often-quoted public health saying highlights a critical reality: even the best vaccine is ineffective when people do not accept it. If the vaccine challenge of the 20th century was the discovery of new vaccines, the challenge for the 21st century is addressing suboptimal vaccination uptake driven primarily by vaccine hesitancy.

This challenge will not be overcome without robust surveillance to understand the epidemiology of vaccine hesitancy and respond to this significant threat to health.

The last 50 years have seen an explosion of new vaccine development, technology, and improvements to distribution, saving at least an estimated 154 million lives globally.[3] However, alongside this success, vaccine hesitancy—low vaccination intention or motivation leading to a delay in acceptance or refusal of vaccines despite the availability of vaccination services—has grown.

In the United States, every year, millions of Americans forgo recommended vaccines, resulting in tens of thousands of vaccine-preventable diseases, hospitalizations, life-altering complications, and deaths.[4] Childhood school-required vaccine exemptions are at an all-time high, leading to the resurgence of outbreaks of diseases such as measles.[5] And despite Nobel Prize–winning achievements leading to the rapid development of COVID-19 vaccines, hundreds of thousands of Americans died unnecessarily from COVID-19 simply because they refused to be vaccinated.[6]

Vaccines for future potential pandemic pathogens, such as avian influenza, are being developed and stockpiled, and plans are being implemented for rapid manufacturing and distribution using the latest vaccine technology. However, given the gaps in vaccine uptake during the recent COVID-19 pandemic, will people be confident enough to accept these vaccines?

Despite the tragically high burden of vaccine-preventable morbidity and mortality in the United States, which is fueled by vaccine hesitancy, the epidemiology of vaccine hesitancy in the United States—and throughout the world, for that matter—is poorly understood. Effective interventions to address vaccine hesitancy and improve confidence exist[7]; however, a timely and actionable understanding of vaccine hesitancy within populations is critical to direct interventions. Unfortunately, leaders in vaccine delivery are often left with outdated data from small, regional studies or national surveys and polling data that do not have the granularity to apply at local community levels.

The lack of a surveillance system for vaccine hesitancy across the lifespan is a glaring omission from the repertoire of epidemiological surveillance systems in the United States. For instance, there are systems in place to understand the epidemiology of hundreds of potential threats to the health of the American public, including both common and rare infectious diseases, cancers, environmental hazards, poor oral health, insufficient sleep, tobacco use, drug use, diabetes and other chronic medical conditions, injuries, mental health conditions—the list goes on and on.[8] Yet, despite the severe threat posed by vaccine hesitancy, we have essentially no national monitoring system. This must change.

To effectively direct interventions to address vaccine hesitancy, improve confidence, and ultimately increase vaccine uptake, a vaccine hesitancy

AJPH October 2024, Vol. 114, No. 10

surveillance system must (1) use validated and reliable measures of vaccine hesitancy determinants; (2) assess a wide array of modifiable determinants of vaccine hesitancy; (3) improve vaccination equity by representing diverse populations, including historically marginalized groups; and (4) provide data that are timely and geospatially granular enough to be utilized by local public health and vaccination leaders.

Vaccine hesitancy can only be effectively measured and compared across populations using valid and reliable measurement tools. Multiple survey instruments that measure the major determinants of vaccine hesitancy have been developed.[9] However, these instruments must be studied further, continually refined, and consistently applied for effective surveillance. And these instruments must correlate with vaccination behavior, as this is the ultimate outcome of interest.

An actionable surveillance system must assess the significant underlying determinants of vaccine hesitancy—including complacency, convenience, and confidence—as defined by the WHO Strategic Advisory Group of Experts on Immunization.[10] Vaccine hesitancy is a complex issue influenced by evolving historical, sociocultural, environmental, institutional, economic, political, and individual and group determinants, which vary between communities, types of vaccines, geography, and time. Assessing these modifiable determinants of hesitancy in communities will enable the application of appropriate tailored interventions.

Vaccine hesitancy surveillance must be designed to improve vaccination equity by representing diverse populations, including historically marginalized groups. This will involve purposive sampling, using multiple languages, and adapting survey instruments for contextual differences. These vaccine hesitancy data must also be matched with vaccination uptake data to determine the main drivers of low vaccination rates in populations. Low vaccine uptake in communities may be wrongly assumed to result from vaccine hesitancy when equitable access is the primary driver, necessitating different intervention types.

Finally, vaccine hesitancy surveillance must provide real-time data that can be utilized by public health and vaccination leaders. Data are not useful if they reflect a period before particular vaccination attitudes have shifted. Data must also be accessible by local vaccination leaders who are directly responsible for vaccine delivery in communities. Additionally, data must have enough geospatial granularity to apply to the populations that local vaccination leaders serve.

Implementing vaccine hesitancy surveillance in the United States will not be a straightforward task. None of the needs discussed here are inexpensive or easy, but the technology and expertise exist. The US National Vaccine Advisory Committee (NVAC) recommends implementing vaccine hesitancy surveillance systems.[11] Among other things, NVAC calls for the US Department of Health and Human Services (HHS) to fund research and data collection, which is made publicly available, to increase the timely assessment of vaccine confidence and improve knowledge that can guide the development of tailored strategies to address vaccine hesitancy. Additionally, it calls for the HHS to fund research to improve an understanding of what works to address vaccine hesitancy. These recommendations will require the HHS, other federal agencies involved in vaccination services, and Congress to increase funding to public health and research infrastructures that assess and address vaccine hesitancy. Although these tasks are challenging, every life-altering complication or death that vaccines could have prevented is unacceptable.

In addition to substantial investment and resources, accomplishing this task will require partnerships among experts in various disciplines and industries, vaccination leaders, and policymakers. As well as traditional surveillance methods, new technologies and modernized processes, such as the collection of social media and digital data as well as artificial intelligence, can be leveraged to rapidly and efficiently gather and interpret data. Utilizing these cutting-edge technologies and methods in vaccine hesitancy epidemiological surveillance will require contributions from experts in fields not typically involved in vaccine delivery, including those in social marketing, behavioral science, information technology, and computer science.

Vaccinations save lives. To tackle the vaccine hesitancy challenge of the 21st century, robust epidemiological surveillance systems to understand and respond to vaccine hesitancy must be funded and implemented. The United States can lead in this endeavor, but, ultimately, we must collaborate with WHO and countries worldwide. As the COVID-19 pandemic painfully reminded us, pathogens care little for geopolitical borders. AJPH

CORRESPONDENCE

Correspondence should be sent to Sean T. O'Leary, Mailstop F443, 1890 North Revere Court, Aurora, CO 80045 (e-mail: sean.oleary@cuanschutz.edu). Reprints can be ordered at https://www.ajph.org by clicking the "Reprints" link.

PUBLICATION INFORMATION

Full Citation: Higgins DM, O'Leary ST. The dire need for surveillance of vaccine hesitancy in the United States. *Am J Public Health*. 2024;114(10):983–985.

Acceptance Date: July 8, 2024.
DOI: https://doi.org/10.2105/AJPH.2024.307806
ORCID iD:
David M. Higgins https://orcid.org/0000-0003-2130-7442

CONTRIBUTORS

Both authors contributed to the conceptualization and writing of this article.

CONFLICTS OF INTEREST

The authors report no potential or actual conflicts of interest.

REFERENCES

1. Last JM, ed. *A Dictionary of Epidemiology.* 3rd ed. New York, NY: Oxford University Press; 1995.
2. World Health Organization. Ten threats to global health in 2019. Available at: https://www.who.int/news-room/spotlight/ten-threats-to-global-health-in-2019. Accessed May 12, 2023.
3. Shattock AJ, Johnson HC, Sim SY, et al. Contribution of vaccination to improved survival and health: modelling 50 years of the Expanded Programme on Immunization. *Lancet.* 2024;403(10441): 2307–2316. https://doi.org/10.1016/S0140-6736(24)00850-X
4. Centers for Disease Control and Prevention. Vaccine-preventable adult diseases. Available at: https://www.cdc.gov/vaccines/adults/vpd.html. Accessed June 6, 2024.
5. Seither R, Calhoun K, Yusuf OB, et al. Vaccination coverage with selected vaccines and exemption rates among children in kindergarten—United States, 2021–22 school year. *MMWR Morb Mortal Wkly Rep.* 2023;72(2):26–32. https://doi.org/10.15585/mmwr.mm7202a2
6. Jia KM, Hanage WP, Lipsitch M, et al. Estimated preventable COVID-19-associated deaths due to non-vaccination in the United States. *Eur J Epidemiol.* 2023;38(11):1125–1128. https://doi.org/10.1007/s10654-023-01006-3
7. O'Leary ST, Opel DJ, Cataldi JR, et al. Strategies for improving vaccine communication and uptake. *Pediatrics.* 2024;153(3):e2023065483. https://doi.org/10.1542/peds.2023-065483
8. Centers for Disease Control and Prevention. Surveillance Resource Center. Available at: https://www.cdc.gov/surveillancepractice/index.html. Accessed June 15, 2024.
9. Omer SB, O'Leary S, Danchin M. Vaccine hesitancy and behavioral factors associated with vaccine uptake. In: Orenstein W, Offit P, Edwards KM, Plotkin S, eds. *Plotkin's Vaccines.* 8th ed. Philadelphia, PA: Elsevier; 2023:1696–1703.e4. https://doi.org/10.1016/B978-0-323-79058-1.00084-0
10. World Health Organization. Report of the SAGE Working Group on Vaccine Hesitancy. Available at: https://www.asset-scienceinsociety.eu/sites/default/files/sage_working_group_revised_report_vaccine_hesitancy.pdf. Accessed June 6, 2024.
11. National Vaccine Advisory Committee. Sustaining and increasing confidence in vaccination across the lifespan: recommendations from the National Vaccine Advisory Committee. Available at: https://www.hhs.gov/sites/default/files/sustaining-increasing-confidence-vaccination-across-lifespan-recommendations-national-vaccine-advisory-committee.pdf. Accessed June 19, 2024.

Reenvisioning Title X to Meet Early Pregnancy Needs

Kavita Vinekar, MD, MPH, Alice Abernathy, MD, MSHP, and Kristin L. Rising, MD, MSHP

ABOUT THE AUTHORS

Kavita Vinekar is with the Department of Obstetrics & Gynecology, Sidney Kimmel Medical College, and the College of Population Health, both at Thomas Jefferson University, Philadelphia, PA. Alice Abernathy is with the Department of Obstetrics & Gynecology, Perelman School of Medicine, and the Leonard Davis Institute of Health Economics, both at the University of Pennsylvania, Philadelphia. Kristin L. Rising is with the Department of Emergency Medicine, Sidney Kimmel Medical College, and the Jefferson Center for Connected Care, both at Thomas Jefferson University.

With widespread availability of home urine pregnancy testing, early self-diagnosis of pregnancy is increasingly common.[1] Although many people become aware of their pregnancies by around six weeks[2] and pregnancies can be reliably confirmed by ultrasound around this time, health systems rarely accommodate patients seeking to initiate prenatal care before 10 to 12 weeks. The American College of Obstetricians and Gynecologists (ACOG) recommends universal first-trimester ultrasound for pregnancy confirmation and dating, and this is most accurate prior to nine weeks.[3] For the 25% of pregnant people who experience early pregnancy complications such as bleeding or abdominal pain,[4] clinical pathways focus on rapid diagnosis and management of early pregnancy loss and ectopic pregnancy. However, most of the 75% of patients who do not experience these symptoms are told to wait weeks to establish prenatal or abortion care.[2] For many people, the one to two months between pregnancy self-diagnosis and engagement with a health care provider may be a time of uncertainty.

Without access to timely pregnancy confirmation by ultrasound, some patients decide to seek advice in online communities[5]; in crisis pregnancy centers (CPCs), which are facilities that pose as health care institutions and aim to dissuade clients from seeking abortions; or in emergency departments (EDs), which are often an inefficient use of resources and may not meet patient needs in early pregnancy.[6] CPC and ED utilization for routine pregnancy confirmation reflects a gap in the health care system—one that we believe can be filled through federally funded reproductive health clinics. To promote equitable, patient-centered, evidence-based reproductive health care, we encourage increased support for Title X programs to offer comprehensive early pregnancy confirmation services (Figure 1).

TITLE X PROGRAM

Established in 1970 and administered by the US Department of Health and Human Services Office of Population Affairs (OPA), Title X is the nation's only dedicated domestic federal family planning program. Title X services include contraceptive counseling and management, fertility services, screening and treatment of sexually transmitted infections, and reproductive preventive health interventions such as the human papillomavirus vaccination.[7] In its most recent Title X five-year program plan, OPA has prioritized health equity, expanded service access, and emphasized high-quality service delivery.[8] The program explicitly does not fund abortions, but supports nondirective pregnancy options counseling and referrals to prenatal or abortion care.[7]

"Pregnancy testing and counseling" is explicitly included within the scope of Title X.[7] Although point-of-care urine pregnancy testing is offered in Title X programs, this is insufficient to confirm the pregnancy location, gestational age, or presence of multiple gestations. Definitive pregnancy confirmation with ultrasound is within the mandate of Title X. Yet, to our knowledge, most Title X clinics do not routinely offer bedside sonographic pregnancy confirmation. This may reflect lack of funding for ultrasound equipment, a paucity of providers with the skills needed to perform ultrasounds, or merely a general perception that these services would not fall under the scope of Title X. Approximately 12% of Title X grantees are Planned Parenthoods, most of which do provide early pregnancy confirmation with pregnancy testing and ultrasound, although this does not often fall under Title X service provision.[9,10] We propose increased support for Title X clinics to provide basic pregnancy confirmation services (urine pregnancy testing and bedside ultrasound) for patients with uncomplicated early pregnancies.

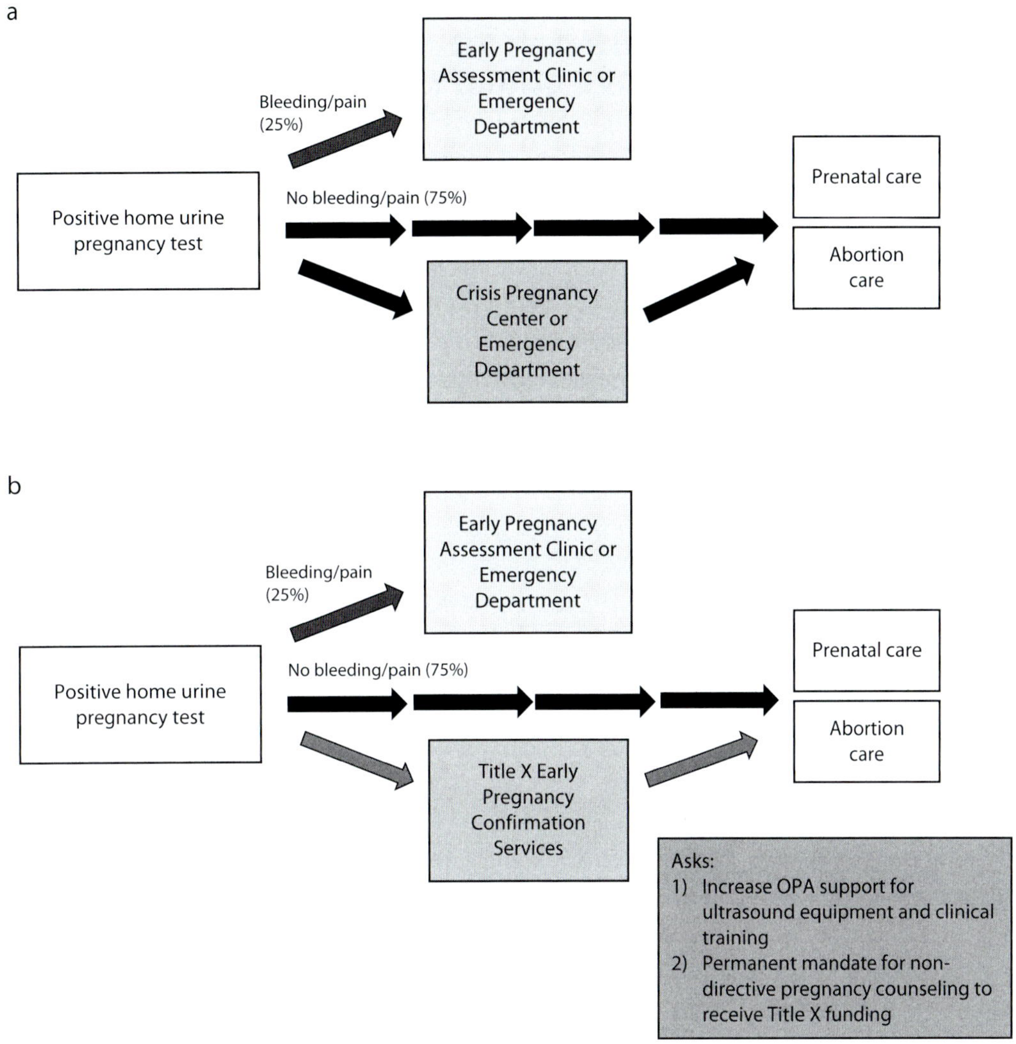

Figure 1— Routine Early Pregnancy Experience by (a) Current Experience and (b) Proposed Experience With Title X Comprehensive Pregnancy Confirmation Services: United States, 2024

Note. OPA = US Department of Health and Human Services Office of Population Affairs.

AN OPPORTUNITY FOR EQUITABLE PREGNANCY CARE

The United States has seen an astonishing rise in maternal mortality. Black and Indigenous pregnant individuals are two to three times more likely than their White counterparts to have a pregnancy-related death, reflecting deep-seated structural racism in the United States and in health care.[11] Additionally, pregnant individuals with lower incomes, those from rural communities, and adolescents suffer from diminished access to reproductive health services.[12–14] Thus, any efforts to improve health care in pregnancy must be guided by a lens of equity.

Health equity and access are cornerstones of the Title X program. In 2022, Title X funds supported a network of 4126 service sites in all 50 states and the District of Columbia, serving 2.6 million clients over 4.1 million encounters.[15] Of these clients, only 65% were insured, and of the insured clients, 66% had public insurance. Furthermore, 31% of Title X users identified as Black, Asian, Native Hawaiian/Pacific Islander, American Indian/Alaska Native, or more than one race, and 37% identified as Hispanic or Latinx. Nineteen percent had limited English proficiency.[15] Given the diversity of patients served by Title X sites, integrating early pregnancy diagnostic services into Title X programs may facilitate access to preventive, obstetric, and abortion care for minoritized communities, and result in more equitable pregnancy outcomes.

TITLE X: AN ALTERNATIVE TO CRISIS PREGNANCY CENTERS

CPCs provide free or low-cost pregnancy testing and "non-diagnostic" ultrasound, and disseminate disinformation to dissuade clients from seeking abortions.[16] Pregnancy confirmation services at CPCs are widely accessible[10] and commonly utilized,[17] and early pregnancy confirmation is a leading reason clients seek care at CPCs.[18] Despite broad availability, ultrasounds at CPCs are often conducted in the absence of any medical professionals; one large study of CPCs found that only 16% had a physician on staff, and only 25% had a registered nurse.[16]

In Pennsylvania, decades of state-funded support of CPCs ended in 2023.[19] In January 2024, funds were reallocated to existing reproductive care sites, the majority of which are Title X grantees. Such policy changes, which combat deceptive practices by CPCs and redirect funding toward essential health care, are commendable. However, it is crucial to ensure that the recipients of this redirected funding can provide the very service that often leads people to seek care at CPCs: sonographic pregnancy confirmation. Provision of early pregnancy ultrasound and evidence-based early pregnancy counseling can both meet patient needs and reduce the harms of patients seeking care in nonmedical settings such as CPCs. The continued existence of CPCs throughout the country is reflective of a void in our medical system, namely, a dearth of evidence-based, patient-centered comprehensive pregnancy confirmation. Defunding CPCs is a first step in improving care. The next step is to support equitable access to comprehensive pregnancy confirmation.

EARLY PREGNANCY ENGAGEMENT TO IMPROVE QUALITY

Regardless of whether a person plans to continue or terminate a pregnancy, earlier access to pregnancy confirmation is beneficial. For those who continue a pregnancy, sonographic pregnancy confirmation promotes more accurate pregnancy dating and early entry to prenatal care—a long-standing strategy for improved birth outcomes. This early engagement is an opportunity for earlier initiation of proven preventive interventions such as folic acid supplementation and aspirin for preeclampsia prevention, and for medication review for teratogenic drugs or expedited referrals to maternal–fetal medicine or social services as indicated. These preventive interventions improve the quality of pregnancy care and should be broadly incorporated into the Title X setting. Furthermore, for the 36% of Title X patients who are uninsured,[9] a new pregnancy diagnosis may provide qualification for Medicaid enrollment, and pregnancy confirmation in the Title X setting may help to expedite engagement with these resources.

For individuals desiring pregnancy termination, early engagement with abortion care is associated with fewer abortion complications and improved access to both medication and procedural abortion options. As patients navigate the patchwork of onerous regulations, gestational age limits, and abortion bans in the post-*Dobbs* era, early pregnancy diagnosis is critical to ensure timely health care access. Although sonographic pregnancy confirmation is not needed for safe abortion care in most cases, some individuals may desire pregnancy confirmation before proceeding with abortion care.

EXPANDING THE EARLY PREGNANCY ASSESSMENT CLINIC

Early pregnancy assessment clinics (EPACs) are an integrated model for outpatient management of the 25% of patients who experience early pregnancy complications such as vaginal bleeding or pain.[4] This model is well-established in Canada and the United Kingdom, and has been growing in the United States.[20] Most EPACs confirm pregnancy location and viability in patients with first-trimester vaginal bleeding or pelvic pain, with comparable safety and improved cost and efficiency compared with the ED setting.[21,22] EPACs ideally integrate miscarriage, ectopic management, and abortion care into a single setting. Although EPACs provide an important service to individuals with early pregnancy complications (and, in some models, to patients seeking abortion care), they often do not have the capacity to provide more routine early pregnancy care to the 75% of individuals without early pregnancy pain or bleeding, nor are they designed to do so.

The Title X program, given its vast reach across the nation, could exist as a complement to EPACs in early pregnancy. The focus of Title X early pregnancy services would be on confirmation of intrauterine pregnancy for individuals without bleeding or pain, including sonographic confirmation of pregnancy dating. Although some Title X clinics may also have the capacity to manage individuals experiencing early pregnancy complications, many would still likely refer patients with symptomatic pregnancies of unknown location, miscarriages, or ectopic pregnancies to an EPAC, ED, or outpatient general gynecological office setting as deemed appropriate. These workflows should be determined by individual clinical sites, depending on staffing and resource availability. In either scenario, patient needs are met by facilities licensed and capable of providing the evidence-based care that patients are often currently seeking outside the formal health care system.

CONSIDERATIONS AND FUTURE DIRECTIONS

In the era of broad access to high-sensitivity home pregnancy testing, for Title X clinics to operate within their scope of "pregnancy testing and counseling," capacity building for sonographic pregnancy confirmation in alignment with ACOG first-trimester recommendations is needed. For the small proportion of Title X clinical sites that are already equipped with ultrasound and trained personnel to initiate early pregnancy confirmation services, we encourage inclusion of these services within Title X programming. For most Title X clinics, OPA investment in early pregnancy service expansion through provision of ultrasound equipment and point-of-care ultrasound training of personnel may be necessary. Since 2014, there have been no increases in Title X funding and no adjustments for inflation.[9] To appropriately support the family planning needs of Title X clients, substantial funding increases are needed. We call for increased federal funding for Title X, to better equip OPA to support training Title X clinicians in early pregnancy imaging and management, to develop clinical protocols and guidelines for referral in early pregnancy, and to ensure access to appropriate equipment, including bedside ultrasound machines. This will require federal investment and institutional partnerships. Such an investment will reap long-term benefits, allowing for improved access to comprehensive early pregnancy confirmation care nationwide. Furthermore, continued advocacy around insurance reimbursement for point-of-care early pregnancy ultrasound is necessary for the sustained provision of these services within the Title X clinical setting.

Although the Title X program remains steadfast in its mission-driven provision of family planning services nationally, particularly to minoritized communities, it has historically been subject to notable disruptions and obstacles related to changes in administration. In 2019, for example, the Trump administration issued regulations prohibiting Title X programs from providing abortion referrals or from locating in spaces where abortion care was provided, resulting in many clinics withdrawing from Title X funding and a 21% reduction of Title X client volume. Some Title X funds were even redirected to CPCs during this time, further distancing patients from much-needed evidence-based pregnancy care. Although these obstructive regulations were reversed by the Biden administration in 2021, such fluctuations point to a vulnerability in the current Title X structuring. As we embark on a presidential election year, it is essential to strengthen and protect the essential reproductive health care provided by Title X sites. As a first step, to prevent CPCs from receiving Title X funds in the future, we call on the OPA to permanently mandate nondirective pregnancy options counseling as a requirement for all Title X funding recipients.

Particularly in the wake of the assault to reproductive rights brought on by *Dobbs v Jackson Women's Health Organization*, access to swift, safe, confidential, and evidence-based early pregnancy care is more important now than ever. The provision of pregnancy confirmation services in Title X clinics should never prevent nor delay a patient from seeking an abortion (in fact, ultrasound confirmation of pregnancy is often not needed for safe abortion care) but should be available for patients, including those who desire pregnancy confirmation prior to seeking an abortion. Moreover, Title X clinics provide abortion referrals and may provide patients with accurate information about accessing safe abortion care. It should also be noted that, although the mean age of pregnancy awareness in the United States is 5.5 weeks, many people—particularly younger people—do not learn of their pregnancies until later, with one in three pregnant people not knowing their pregnancy status until six weeks or later.[1] Thus, although early pregnancy services should be made available to all pregnant individuals, it is critical to acknowledge the significant number of people who do not have access to early pregnancy diagnoses, and will suffer disproportionate harm from early abortion bans.

Pregnancy confirmation services, including sonographic pregnancy confirmation, fall within the scope of Title X services, but have not historically been integrated into Title X clinical programs. In pursuance of the OPA priorities of equity, access, and quality, we call for the addition of comprehensive pregnancy confirmation services at Title X clinical sites as a means of improving and advancing the state of reproductive health care nationwide. AJPH

CORRESPONDENCE

Correspondence should be sent to Kavita Vinekar, MD, MPH, 833 Chestnut St, Philadelphia, PA 19107 (e-mail: kavita.vinekar@jefferson.edu). Reprints can be ordered at https://www.ajph.org by clicking the "Reprints" link.

PUBLICATION INFORMATION

Full Citation: Vinekar K, Abernathy A, Rising KL. Reenvisioning Title X to meet early pregnancy needs. *Am J Public Health*. 2024;114(10):986–990.

Acceptance Date: July 7, 2024.

DOI: https://doi.org/10.2105/AJPH.2024.307795

ORCID iDs:

Kavita Vinekar https://orcid.org/0000-0003-4971-7697

Alice Abernathy https://orcid.org/0000-0003-0767-8984

Kristin L. Rising https://orcid.org/0000-0003-3882-4956

CONTRIBUTORS

K. Vinekar led the conceptualization, planning, and writing of the editorial. A. Abernathy contributed to the conceptualization, planning, writing, and editing. K. L. Rising provided mentorship, editing and revision, and conceptual guidance.

ACKNOWLEDGMENTS

We thank Sonya Borrero, MD, MS, for her insights and review of this editorial.

CONFLICTS OF INTEREST

A. Abernathy is supported by a grant from the National Institutes of Health (K12-HD001265). K. L. Rising reports research grant funding from Abbott Diagnostics, DermTech, MeMed, Prenosis, Siemens Healthcare Diagnostics, PROCOVAXED (funded by NIAID 1R01AI166967), and PREVENT (funded by CDC U01CK00048) outside the submitted work.

REFERENCES

1. Ralph LJ, Foster DG, Barar R, Rocca CH. Home pregnancy test use and timing of pregnancy confirmation among people seeking health care. *Contraception*. 2022;107:10–16. https://doi.org/10.1016/j.contraception.2021.10.006
2. Branum AM, Ahrens KA. Trends in timing of pregnancy awareness among US women. *Matern Child Health J*. 2017;21(4):715–726. https://doi.org/10.1007/s10995-016-2155-1
3. American College of Obstetrics and Gynecology. Committee Opinion No. 700: methods for estimating the due date. *Obstet Gynecol*. 2017;129(5):e150–e154. https://doi.org/10.1097/AOG.0000000000002046
4. Hasan R, Baird DD, Herring AH, Olshan AF, Jonsson Funk ML, Hartmann KE. Patterns and predictors of vaginal bleeding in the first trimester of pregnancy. *Ann Epidemiol*. 2010;20(7):524–531. https://doi.org/10.1016/j.annepidem.2010.02.006
5. Wexler A, Davoudi A, Weissenbacher D, et al. Pregnancy and health in the age of the Internet: a content analysis of online "birth club" forums. *PLoS One*. 2020;15(4):e0230947. https://doi.org/10.1371/journal.pone.0230947
6. Benson LS, Holt SK, Gore JL, et al. Early pregnancy loss management in the emergency department vs outpatient setting. *JAMA Netw Open*. 2023;6(3):e232639. https://doi.org/10.1001/jamanetworkopen.2023.2639
7. Dept of Health and Human Services. 2021 Title X Final Rule. Available at: https://www.govinfo.gov/content/pkg/FR-2021-10-07/pdf/2021-21542.pdf. Accessed February 8, 2024.
8. Marcella JS. The Title X Program: setting standards for contraceptive and health equity. *Am J Public Health*. 2022;112(S5):S511–S514. https://doi.org/10.2105/AJPH.2022.306900
9. National Family Planning & Reproductive Health Association. Title X Family Planning Fact Sheet. January 2023. Available at: https://www.nationalfamilyplanning.org/file/Title-X-101-January-2023-final_2.pdf. Accessed May 1, 2024.
10. Vinekar K, Jarlenski M, Meyn L, et al. Early pregnancy confirmation availability at crisis pregnancy centers and abortion facilities in the United States. *Contraception*. 2023;117:30–35. https://doi.org/10.1016/j.contraception.2022.08.008
11. Hoyert DL. Maternal mortality rates in the United States, 2021. National Center for Health Statistics. Available at: https://www.cdc.gov/nchs/data/hestat/maternal-mortality/2021/maternal-mortality-rates-2021.pdf. Accessed April 16, 2024.
12. Wang E, Glazer KB, Howell EA, Janevic TM. Social determinants of pregnancy-related mortality and morbidity in the United States: a systematic review. *Obstet Gynecol*. 2020;135(4):896–915. https://doi.org/10.1097/AOG.0000000000003762
13. Harrington KA, Cameron NA, Culler K, Grobman WA, Khan SS. Rural–urban disparities in adverse maternal outcomes in the United States, 2016–2019. *Am J Public Health*. 2023;113(2):224–227. https://doi.org/10.2105/AJPH.2022.307134
14. Liang M, Simelane S, Fortuny Fillo G, et al. The state of adolescent sexual and reproductive health. *J Adolesc Health*. 2019;65(S6):S3–S15. https://doi.org/10.1016/j.jadohealth.2019.09.015
15. Office of Population Affairs. Title X Family Planning Annual Report—2022 National Summary. Available at: https://opa.hhs.gov/sites/default/files/2023-10/2022-FPAR-National-Summary.pdf. Accessed February 8, 2024.
16. The Alliance: State Advocates for Women's Rights and Gender Equality. Designed to Deceive: A study of the crisis pregnancy center industry in nine states. Available at: https://alliancestateadvocates.org/wp-content/uploads/sites/107/Alliance-CPC-Study-Designed-to-Deceive.pdf. Accessed April 16, 2024.
17. Rice R, Chakraborty P, Keder L, Turner AN, Gallo MF. Who attends a crisis pregnancy center in Ohio? *Contraception*. 2021;104(4):383–387. https://doi.org/10.1016/j.contraception.2021.05.011
18. Kimport K. Pregnant women's reasons for and experiences of visiting antiabortion pregnancy resource centers. *Perspect Sex Reprod Health*. 2020;52(1):49–56. https://doi.org/10.1363/psrh.12131
19. Whelan A. Shapiro administration ends contract with crisis pregnancy center funders. *Philadelphia Inquirer*. August 9, 2023. Available at: https://www.inquirer.com/health/crisis-pregnancy-center-abortion-real-alternatives-state-funding-ending-pennsylvania-20230809.html. Accessed March 25, 2024.
20. Rovner P, Stickrath E, Alston M, Lund K. An early pregnancy unit in the United States: an effective method for evaluating first-trimester pregnancy complications. *J Ultrasound Med*. 2018;37(6):1533–1538. https://doi.org/10.1002/jum.14474
21. VanArendonk SH, Rockhill K, Stickrath EH, Alston MJ. Evaluation of early pregnancy concerns in an early pregnancy unit compared with an emergency department. *Obstet Gynecol*. 2020;136(5):995–1000. https://doi.org/10.1097/AOG.0000000000004080
22. Pinnaduwage L, Honeyford J, Lackie E, Tunde-Byass M. The sustained value of an early pregnancy assessment clinic in the management of early pregnancy complications: a 10-year retrospective study. *J Obstet Gynaecol Can*. 2018;40(8):1017–1023. https://doi.org/10.1016/j.jogc.2017.12.002

Recommitting to Ventilation Standards for Healthy Indoor Air Quality

Joseph G. Allen, DSc, MPH

ABOUT THE AUTHOR

Joseph G. Allen is associate professor and director of the Healthy Buildings Program, Harvard T. H. Chan School of Public Health, Boston, MA.

The history of ventilation is fraught, indeed. We are in the sick building era, ushered in by a historic mistake in the 1970s with the promulgation of a standard that lowered ventilation rates in nearly every building we spend our time, and which represented a gross departure from earlier health-focused higher ventilation targets.

THE SICK BUILDINGS ERA

In 1859, Florence Nightingale emphasized the critical role of ventilation in medical settings to combat infections: "Cleanliness and fresh air from open windows . . . are the only defense a true nurse either asks or needs."[1(p34)] Not long after, in 1893, and motivated by tuberculosis, a physician–scientist named John Shaw Billings proposed the first health-focused ventilation rate: 30 cubic feet per minute per person (30 cfm/p).[2] In 1895, this health-focused 30 cfm/p was adopted by a standards organization, American Society of Heating and Ventilation Engineers (ASHVE). By 1925, 22 states required a minimum of 30 cfm/p. Thus, health-focused ventilation became the basis for building design in the early part of the 20th century, until a monumental and costly pivot away from health in the 1970s.

In 1973, ASHRAE, the standard-setting body that followed ASHVE, released a new standard for ventilation, ASHRAE 62. The earlier 30 cfm/p health-focused targets were lowered by half (or more), and were "based in part on the ventilation required to control odors from human bioeffluents."[3] In the 1981 version, the title of the standard was explicit that the focus was merely "acceptable" indoor air quality ("ASHRAE Standard 62-1981: Ventilation for Acceptable Indoor Air Quality"). The departure from earlier health-focused ventilation to lower "acceptable" ventilation targets based on odor control marks the birth of the sick building era, with the term "sick building syndrome" first appearing in the early 1980s.

The sick building era, unsurprisingly, caught the attention of researchers and spawned an entire field of study on indoor air quality (IAQ). In the 1980s and 1990s, the then-new field of IAQ generated research documenting that ventilation rates above this minimum standard were associated with many health benefits, and throughout the 1990s to 2000s, research efforts were also underway to evaluate—and expand—the understanding and value proposition of better indoor air quality. Research studies documented higher ventilation rates associated with better math and reading scores in students,[4] fewer missed school days for kids,[5] fewer worker absences,[6] lower risk of respiratory disease infection,[7] higher cognitive function test scores,[8] and better workplace performance.[9] Lawrence Berkeley National Laboratory estimated that there were more than $20 billion in benefits to the US economy with improvements to ventilation.[10]

The commentary by LaFay and Sampson in the August 2024 issue of *AJPH* argues that this focus on economic impacts of ventilation was a historic—and current—problem, holding back the advancement of higher ventilation standards.[11] But recent efforts by researchers to quantify the health benefits of ventilation in terms of economic benefits is in addition to—not at the expense of—the health argument. Focusing on health, and adding in an economic dimension, is good public health practice with a long history, dating back to the 1800s.[12]

Despite the accumulating research on health and economic benefits of higher ventilation rates, not much changed, and the standard for "acceptable" ventilation rates remained the basis for many building codes and industry practice. Within ASHRAE itself, there was controversy and lack of clarity that spanned two decades. There was "a membership petition in 1999 that called to restrict all ASHRAE IAQ and ventilation standards to make no claims regarding 'health, comfort or occupant acceptability,'" and, as late as 2008, the ASHRAE Board of Directors was still debating the intent of the standard.[3(p6)]

AJPH October 2024, Vol. 114, No. 10

THE BEGINNING OF A NEW HEALTHY BUILDINGS ERA

The year 2020 marked a major turning point in the history of ventilation. Severe acute respiratory syndrome coronavirus 2 (SARS-CoV-2), spread predominantly indoors, found an ally in buildings designed to minimal "acceptable" ventilation standards. As early as February 2020, researchers raised concern over airborne transmission and highlighted that enhanced ventilation and filtration were key control strategies. In April 2020, ASHRAE also made recommendations for increasing ventilation.

Yet, in all these recommendations, there was still a glaring omission—there were recommendations made to increase ventilation rates, but no standard-setting body was willing to offer a recommended target ventilation rate. This omission left many organizations grappling with how much ventilation was recommended to safeguard against the virus.

In late 2020, the ASHRAE Epidemic Task Force convened a group of experts and gave them an explicit task of making recommendations on ventilation rate targets. This team submitted their first recommendations to the ASHRAE Epidemic Task Force in 2021, but the recommendations were never released to the public.

In the fall of 2022, the *Lancet* COVID-19 Commission released a report with recommended clean air rates for reducing exposure to airborne respiratory diseases.[13] The *Lancet* Task Force used a "good/better/best" approach, and designated 30+ cfm/p as "best." This report also revealed to the public the previously unreleased recommendations made by ASHRAE's internal committee. The *Lancet* Report was timed to coincide with the first-ever White House Summit on Indoor Air Quality, and it was shared with The White House Office of Pandemic Response and The White House Office of Science and Technology Policy. Shortly thereafter, ASHRAE announced they would produce a health-focused ventilation standard within six months.[14] In June 2023, and one month after the official declaration of the end of the emergency phase of the pandemic, ASHRAE released ASHRAE Standard 241: Control of Infectious Aerosols, wherein they recommended a total "clean air" target (outdoor air + filtered/cleaned air) more in-line with historical, health-focused ventilation rates.[15] Inexplicably, the standard was tempered by the inclusion of an "on/off switch" in the guidelines (what they call "risk management mode"), which suggested that enhanced ventilation could be discretionary and that baseline levels of influenza, COVID-19, and other respiratory diseases—which, for influenza alone, the Centers for Disease Control and Prevention estimates resulted in up to 41 million illnesses, 710 000 hospitalizations, and 51 000 deaths annually since 2010[16]—were somehow not worthy of being declared a full-time risk.

We are at a precipice. The World Health Organization has declared clean indoor air a fundamental human right, and ventilation is a key component of ensuring clean indoor air. The current standards governing our ventilation rates are not based on health and have not been for decades. There does seem to be alignment forming on health-focused ventilation targets. A group of more than 40 international experts wrote a commentary in *Science* in March 2024 proposing indoor air quality standards, wherein they recommended . . . 30 cfm/p[17]; the same target recommended by The *Lancet* COVID-19 Commission,[13] and the same health-focused ventilation target used 100 years ago. The lessons from our past combined with recent experiences present an unambiguous call to action: to recommit to ventilation not as a technical standard for minimally acceptable conditions but as a cornerstone of public health. *AJPH*

CORRESPONDENCE

Correspondence should be sent to Joseph G. Allen, 401 Park Dr, 4th Floor W, Boston, MA 02215 (e-mail: jgallen@hsph.harvard.edu). Reprints can be ordered at https://www.ajph.org by clicking the "Reprints" link.

PUBLICATION INFORMATION

Full Citation: Allen JG. Recommitting to ventilation standards for healthy indoor air quality. *Am J Public Health*. 2024;114(10):991–993.

Acceptance Date: July 10, 2024.

DOI: https://doi.org/10.2105/AJPH.2024.307809

CONFLICTS OF INTEREST

The author reports no conflicts of interest.

REFERENCES

1. Nightingale F. *Notes on Nursing: What It Is and What It Is Not*. London, England: Harrison; 1859.
2. Janssen JE. The history of ventilation and temperature control. *ASHRAE Journal*. September 1999: 47–52. Available at: https://www.ashrae.org/File%20Library/About/Mission%20and%20Vision/ASHRAE%20and%20Industry%20History/The-History-of-Ventilation-and-Temperature-Control.pdf. Accessed July 30, 2024.
3. Persily A. *Challenges in Developing Ventilation and Indoor Air Quality Standards: The Story of ASHRAE Standard 62*. Gaithersburg, MD: National Institute of Standards and Technology; 2015.
4. Petersen S, Jensen KL, Pedersen AL, Rasmussen HS. The effect of increased classroom ventilation rate indicated by reduced CO_2 concentration on the performance of schoolwork by children. *Indoor Air*. 2016;26(3):366–379. https://doi.org/10.1111/ina.12210
5. Mendell MJ, Eliseeva EA, Davies MM, et al. Association of classroom ventilation with reduced illness absence: a prospective study in California elementary schools. *Indoor Air*. 2013;23(6):515–528. https://doi.org/10.1111/ina.12042
6. Myatt TA, Staudenmayer J, Adams K, Walters M, Rudnick SN, Milton DK. A study of indoor carbon dioxide levels and sick leave among office workers. *Environ Health*. 2002;1(1):3. https://doi.org/10.1186/1476-069X-1-3
7. Rudnick SN, Milton DK. Risk of indoor airborne infection transmission estimated from carbon dioxide concentration. *Indoor Air*. 2003;13(3):237–245. https://doi.org/10.1034/j.1600-0668.2003.00189.x

8. Allen JG, MacNaughton P, Satish U, Santanam S, Vallarino J, Spengler JD. Associations of cognitive function scores with carbon dioxide, ventilation, and volatile organic compound exposures in office workers: a controlled exposure study of green and conventional office environments. *Environ Health Perspect*. 2016;124(6):805–812. https://doi.org/10.1289/ehp.1510037
9. Seppanen O, Fisk WJ, Lei QH. Ventilation and work performance in office work. *Indoor Air*. 2006;16(1):28–36. https://doi.org/10.1111/j.1600-0668.2005.00394.x
10. Fisk WJ, Black D, Brunner G. Benefits and costs of improved IEQ in US offices. *Indoor Air*. 2011; 21(5):357–367. https://doi.org/10.1111/j.1600-0668.2011.00719.x
11. Lafay E, Sampson P. Ventilation and public health: a fraught history. *Am J Public Health*. 2024;114(8):798–804. https://doi.org/10.2105/AJPH.2024.307670.
12. Gounder C, Spencer C. The decline in life expectancy harms more than our health. *Los Angeles Times*. April 16, 2024. Available at: https://www.latimes.com/opinion/story/2024-04-16/united-states-economy-covid-public-health. Accessed July 30, 2024.
13. Azimi P, Keshavarz Z, Jones E, et al. Proposed non-infectious air delivery rates (NADR) for reducing exposure to airborne respiratory infectious diseases. The *Lancet* COVID-19 Commission Task Force on Safe Work, Safe School, Safe Travel. November 18, 2022. Available at: https://covid19commission.org/safe-work-travel. Accessed July 30, 2024.
14. ASHRAE commits to developing an IAQ pathogen mitigation standard. Atlanta, GA: ASHRAE; December 7, 2022.
15. ASHRAE. *ASHRAE Standard 241, Control of Infectious Aerosols*. 2024. Available at: https://www.ashrae.org/technical-resources/bookstore/ashrae-standard-241-control-of-infectious-aerosols. Accessed July 30, 2024.
16. Centers for Disease Control and Prevention. Disease burden of flu. Available at: https://www.cdc.gov/flu/about/burden/index.html. Accessed July 30, 2024.
17. Morawska L, Allen J, Bahnfleth W, et al. Mandating indoor air quality for public buildings. *Science*. 2024;383(6690):1418–1420. https://doi.org/10.1126/science.adl0677

Understanding the Post-*Dobbs* Landscape for Abortion Care in the United States

Farzana Kapadia, PhD, MPH, Laura Ferguson, PhD, SM, and Wendy E. Parmet, JD

ABOUT THE AUTHORS

Farzana Kapadia is the deputy editor of AJPH *and is with the School of Global Public Health, New York University, New York. Laura Ferguson is an* AJPH *associate editor and is with the Institute on Inequalities in Global Health, University of Southern California, Los Angeles, CA. Wendy E. Parmet is an associate editor of* AJPH *and is with Northeastern University, Boston, MA.*

See also Abortion Access 2 Years After *Dobbs v Jackson* Ruling, pp. 997–1050.

AJPH October 2024, Vol. 114, No. 10

The US Supreme Court's June 2022 *Dobbs v Jackson Women's Health Organization* decision dismantled the 50-year precedent protecting the right to abortion care, leaving the United States as one of a handful of high-income countries where that right is no longer secure. As the World Health Organization has noted, "Inaccessibility of quality abortion care risks violating a range of human rights of women and girls."[1] Restrictions on abortion care violate rights to "decisional and bodily autonomy in a way that rejects the agency, dignity, and equality of people who can become pregnant."[2] They also undermine rights to health, privacy, and freedom from cruel, inhuman, and degrading treatment.[3] Since the *Dobbs* decision, 24 states have banned or significantly restricted access to abortion care,[4] whereas 21 states have enacted further protections for abortion access.[5]

Protective states have increasingly sought to provide substantial funding to expand access to abortion services. They also aim to offer protections for health workers who provide abortions, including to residents of other states. But the legal landscape is complex, which engenders fear in providers and people who might want to access services. Traveling to a state where abortion is legally protected is a privilege that many cannot afford.

Although there are currently no federal restrictions, a new presidential administration will be able to further restrict access to abortion care even if Congress does not enact any nationwide restrictions. The articles in this issue of *AJPH* present recent evidence from across the United States on the impact of the *Dobbs* decision over the past two years. The articles review the litigation, legislative, and policy quagmire that *Dobbs* has spawned as well as the turmoil it has caused for those seeking or providing care. They also present local and global examples of how to build a movement to regain abortion care rights and reproductive justice.

PUSHING ABORTION CARE MORE OUT OF REACH

Even before the *Dobbs* ruling, the confusion caused by state-level decisions and challenges to these decisions had a chilling effect on abortion care access. This was most evident in Texas, where various waves of executive orders and abortion restrictions have curtailed abortion care. As Whitfield et al. (p. 1013) note, Governor Greg Abbott's 2020 executive order prohibiting abortion care under the premise that it is a nonessential procedure that would divert protective personal equipment from other medical procedures reduced access to timely abortion care. By 2021, the executive order was replaced by a more restrictive policy—Senate Bill 8 (SB8)—which banned abortion care for pregnancies in which a fetal heartbeat had been detected. SB8 threatened anyone with a civil lawsuit if they provided an abortion or aided someone seeking an abortion. Following the *Dobbs* decision, all facility-based abortion care providers in Texas were shut down, effectively prohibiting abortion care in the state.

An insightful geospatial analysis by Sauter et al. (p. 1024) reveals that after the passage of SB8 and the *Dobbs* decision, the distance to the nearest abortion care provider significantly increased for some Texas residents, particularly those living in neighborhoods with concentrated disadvantage and severe income inequality. New Mexico is one state that experienced a surge in people traveling from other states for abortion care. McQuade et al. (p. 1008) provide a powerful picture of the lived realities of people who went to New Mexico for abortion care between 2020 and 2023. The authors present journal entries that capture the complex emotions and medical dilemmas that surrounded the decision to seek abortion care. For those coming from Texas, the desire for autonomy and to overcome the political barriers that restricted abortion care access were powerful themes.

In Ohio, one of several states where referenda have succeeded in rolling back post-*Dobbs* restrictions, a state ban on abortion care was overturned by a ballot initiative. Smith et al. (p. 1034) examined unique data from monthly abortion care provider surveys. They sought to ascertain changes in the number of abortions provided, determine which states patients seeking abortion care were traveling from, and gather qualitative information on the clinical and socioeconomic burdens placed on out-of-state patients seeking abortion care in Ohio.

A natural next question is what happens to women, children, and families in states that have enacted strict abortion care regulations since the *Dobbs* decision. Not surprisingly, the cumulative burden of abortion bans and restrictions as well as curtailed access to timely and appropriate medical care are heaviest on women who are the most socially, economically, and geographically vulnerable. In their analytic essay, Madden et al. (p. 1043) report that states with the most stringent post-*Dobbs* abortion care restrictions are home to, on average, a greater proportion of persons of reproductive age who identify as non-Hispanic Black and are of low socioeconomic status. These states are more likely to have rejected Medicaid expansion and have less supportive medical and social safety net services for children and families.

EVOLVING RESTRICTIONS ON ABORTION CARE

Nationwide, determining *Dobbs*'s full impact is difficult because of the increasingly complex and uncertain legal and political landscape. As Ziegler (p. 997) cogently explains, after the *Dobbs* decision, litigation on abortion care has "multiplied" in both state and federal courts, deepening the uncertainty of patients and providers alike. Some of this litigation features relatively novel challenges to state abortion care bans; other cases threaten to further limit abortion care access at either the state or federal level.

Two recent Supreme Court decisions in cases that Ziegler anticipated highlight the uncertainty. In *Food and Drug Administration v Alliance for Hippocratic Medicine* (June 13, 2024), the Supreme Court, as Ziegler predicted, ruled that the plaintiffs lacked standing to challenge the US Food and Drug Administration's decision to expand access to mifepristone. Because that decision rests on standing, it leaves the door open to other challenges to mifepristone. These appear even more viable following the court's June 2024 decision in *Loper Bright Enterprises v Raimondo* to override the 40-year-old *Chevron* deference, which required lower courts to defer to regulatory agencies when they offered plausible interpretations of their statutory authority.

The Supreme Court also punted on a set of cases that Ziegler discusses concerning whether Idaho's abortion care ban conflicts with federal protections for patients in emergency departments. The court's decision to return those cases to lower courts without review means that litigation and uncertainty will persist. In the meantime, the rights and health of pregnant persons will continue to be contested politically and legally across the country.

LEARNING FROM LATIN AMERICA

Although more than 60 countries have moved to broaden access in the past 50 years, the United States is one of four countries—along with El Salvador, Nicaragua, and Poland—where legal protection of abortion rights has been reversed (https://bit.ly/4bLKa3O). However, strategies from activists across several Latin American countries may serve as a blueprint for fostering a national movement in support of reproductive justice. Roth and Jones (p. 1003) argue that a successful public health movement in the United States ought to draw inspiration and lessons learned from the Marea Verde (the Green Wave), which spread across Latin America and successfully overturned restrictive abortion care bans. Their argument calls for forging a movement that (1) prioritizes access to abortion care as central to any future legalization efforts; (2) advocates legal reform at both state and federal levels and in multiple legal contexts (e.g., legislative, judicial); and (3) supports grassroots organizations, including those that provide funds to guarantee safe, legal, and accessible abortion care. To this end, Rice et al. (p. 1000) provide examples of how local policymaking along with the establishment of a network of community-based clinics and direct-aid organizations has played a vital role in sustaining access to abortion care across the Southern US, including Texas. Their examples provide a powerful reminder that even in the face of continued attacks, the actions of committed public health advocates can help to grow a movement for reproductive justice.

CONCLUSIONS

As this period of uncertainty continues, people face significant barriers to reproductive health services, with the most vulnerable communities oftentimes the most affected. Now more than ever, public health researchers must study and report on the impact of these barriers and the complex policy landscape, and the public health community must champion the rights, dignity, and health of individuals who are, may become, or want to become pregnant. AJPH

CORRESPONDENCE

Correspondence should be sent to Farzana Kapadia, PhD, MPH, New York University, School of Global Public Health, 708 Broadway, Room 729, New York, NY 10003 (e-mail: farzana.kapadia@nyu.edu). Reprints can be ordered at https://www.ajph.org by clicking the "Reprints" link.

PUBLICATION INFORMATION

Full Citation: Kapadia F, Ferguson L, Parmet WE. Understanding the post-*Dobbs* landscape for abortion care in the United States. *Am J Public Health*. 2024;114(10):994–996.

Acceptance Date: July 22, 2024.

DOI: https://doi.org/10.2105/AJPH.2024.307827

ORCID iDs:

Farzana Kapadia https://orcid.org/0000-0003-3459-767X

Laura Ferguson https://orcid.org/0000-0002-1340-793X

Wendy E. Parmet https://orcid.org/0000-0002-5797-0863

CONTRIBUTORS

The authors conceptualized and wrote the content of this editorial equally.

CONFLICTS OF INTEREST

The authors have no conflicts of interest to disclose.

REFERENCES

1. World Health Organization. Abortion: key facts. May 17, 2024. Available at: https://www.who.int/news-room/fact-sheets/detail/abortion. Accessed August 2, 2024.
2. Human Rights Watch. Human rights crisis: abortion in the United States after *Dobbs*. Available at: https://www.hrw.org/news/2023/04/18/human-rights-crisis-abortion-united-states-after-dobbs. Accessed August 2, 2024.
3. *Committee on the Elimination of Discrimination Against Women, L.C. v Peru,* Communication No. 22/2009, UN Doc. CEDAW/C/50/D/22/2009 (2011).
4. Nash E, Guarnieri I. Six months post-Roe, 24 US states have banned abortion or are likely to do so: a roundup. January 2023. Available at: https://www.guttmacher.org/2023/01/six-months-post-roe-24-us-states-have-banned-abortion-or-are-likely-do-so-roundup. Accessed August 2, 2024.
5. New York Times. Tracking abortion bans across the country. June 25, 2024. Available at: https://www.nytimes.com/interactive/2024/us/abortion-laws-roe-v-wade.html. Accessed August 2, 2024.

The Post-*Dobbs* Legal Landscape

Mary Ziegler, JD

ABOUT THE AUTHOR

Mary Ziegler is Martin Luther King Professor at University of California, Davis School of Law.

See also Abortion Access 2 Years After *Dobbs v Jackson* Ruling, pp. 994–1050.

In 2022, in overturning *Roe v Wade*, Justice Samuel Alito suggested that the Supreme Court had returned the abortion issue—long tied up in the courts—to the people and their elected representatives. Since the *Dobbs* decision, abortion has certainly become far more salient politically, ranked as a top issue by many Democratic voters, driving results in ballot initiatives across the country, and helping stem what was expected to be a wave election for Republicans in 2022.[1]

And yet in the months since *Dobbs*, court battles around abortion have only multiplied. Well before *Dobbs*, some state supreme courts recognized key protections for abortion rights. Since the undoing of *Roe*, however, state courts have become still more central: the site of struggle over whether state guarantees of privacy, equality, or a right to life protect access to abortion, and the start of a plan to overturn *Dobbs* itself. The flood of state litigation reflects abortion-rights supporters' reticence about litigating cases that will land before the justices who reversed *Roe*. State courts offer opportunities to experiment with different constitutional strategies as part of a broader strategy to weaken and ultimately reverse *Dobbs*. And because many state supreme courts require judges to face some sort of election, state judges may be more responsive to popular will, especially in high-salience cases like those involving reproductive rights.[2]

Some of the most critical cases to date involve the adequacy of state exceptions, which tend to permit abortion in cases of threats to life or substantial and permanent impairment of a major bodily function. In *In re Texas*, Kate Cox, a woman whose fetus was diagnosed with trisomy 18, requested a court order permitting her to have an abortion; the Texas Supreme Court ultimately rejected her request.[3] Other plaintiffs in Texas, Tennessee, and Kentucky have argued that state abortion bans should be interpreted to permit abortions in cases of certain threats to health, fertility, or fetal conditions incompatible with life—and that if the law cannot be interpreted in this way, it violates the state constitution. Reproductive rights litigators have also challenged the constitutionality of entire statutory schemes, with mixed results. These strategies have offered an important opportunity to test constitutional justifications, such as those based on state theories of equality, privacy, dignity, and a pregnant patient's right to life, that might prove consequential in other states and even, eventually, in federal court.[4]

Victories (or losses) in state court can also easily disappear, with judicial retirements or other changes in court composition. In South Carolina, for example, a reconfigured state supreme court upheld a six-week ban that was virtually identical to one that the court had just struck down less than a year before.[5] There are ongoing efforts, too, to erase existing constitutional rights. In Florida, the state supreme court overturned a 1989 precedent protecting the abortion decision under the state's Privacy Clause and allowed a six-week abortion ban to go into effect.[6] After the Alabama Supreme Court recognized embryos as "children" under the state's Wrongful Death of a Minor Act, some antiabortion lawyers have called for state litigation to recognize fetuses as persons under state constitutions.[7]

But federal courts are hardly out of the picture. In November 2022, the Alliance Defending Freedom (ADF), one of the most prominent groups in the conservative Christian legal movement, filed a suit on behalf of a group of antiabortion physicians challenging the authority of the Food and Drug Administration (FDA) to approve mifepristone. The ADF also asserted that the FDA lacked the power to permit telehealth abortion—a move made permanent in 2023—because the Comstock Act, a federal obscenity law passed in 1873, made it a crime to mail anything intended, designed, or adapted for abortion.[8]

In April 2023, Judge Matthew Kacsmaryk agreed with the plaintiffs that the FDA lacked the authority to approve mifepristone or subsequently lift restrictions on it.[9] The Fifth Circuit Court of Appeals issued a somewhat more modest ruling, holding that the plaintiffs had waited too long without excuse to challenge the initial approval but concluding that the FDA had acted arbitrarily and capriciously when lifting restrictions on mifepristone.[10] In deciding the FDA's appeal in the case, *Food and Drug Administration v Alliance for Hippocratic Medicine*, the Supreme Court held that the plaintiffs do not have standing to sue. Nevertheless, the claims that the ADF brought in the case—regarding the FDA's authority to approve mifepristone and the proper interpretation of the Comstock Act—will not disappear with the disposition of the case. Indeed, Justices Clarence Thomas and Samuel Alito seemed convinced that the Comstock Act functioned as a ban on mailing anything intended, designed, or adapted for abortion. Antiabortion lawyers plan to keep those claims alive in other cases.[11]

Alliance for Hippocratic Medicine is not even the only case before the High Court this term. After *Dobbs*, the Biden Administration issued guidance concluding that the federal Emergency Medical Treatment and Labor Act (EMTALA) required physicians and hospitals to make abortion available in certain emergencies, state bans notwithstanding. Passed in 1986, EMTALA was intended to discourage hospitals from refusing to screen or treat patients with emergent conditions who could not afford the cost of care. The law requires any hospital participating in the Medicare program to screen patients for emergent conditions and provide either stabilizing treatment or transfer to a facility that can do so. As the Biden Administration interprets the law, EMTALA requires any physician who thinks that abortion is the proper stabilizing treatment of patients in medical emergencies to perform the procedure. The administration further argues that EMTALA preempts state bans that would not permit an abortion under these circumstances.

The administration later took Idaho to court, arguing that its ban conflicted with EMTALA. Texas, for its part, went on the offensive, insisting that EMTALA did not require anyone to perform an abortion—and that the statute's references to the "unborn child" mandated that physicians treat the fetus as an equal, rights-holding patient. The district court enjoined enforcement of the Idaho law but was reversed on appeal by the Ninth Circuit. After that court granted *en banc* review, the Supreme Court agreed to hear the case.[12] Texas, meanwhile, prevailed at both the district court level and in the Fifth Circuit Court of Appeals.[13]

The Supreme Court dismissed Idaho's appeal as improvidently granted, but the courts' interpretation of EMTALA will make a difference to clinicians and patients dealing with emergencies. If the court addresses the language of the statute referencing the "unborn child," the decision might set a valuable precedent for the antiabortion movement. Antiabortion groups have detailed an incremental strategy to recognize fetal rights and personhood in statutory contexts, including those involving in vitro fertilization, child support, wrongful death, fetal homicide, and child endangerment. Convincing the court to interpret EMTALA to create some fetal protections could bolster this incremental strategy.[14]

Other major questions are looming in both federal and state court. After *Dobbs*, conservative states have experimented with strategies to limit abortion-related travel. Idaho recently prohibited "abortion trafficking" through a law that makes it a crime for an adult other than a parent to help a minor arrange for an abortion out of state; a separate provision permits civil suits against abortion providers who provide services for minors, even if a physician is based in a state where abortion is legal. A challenge to the criminal provisions is under way; the plaintiffs maintain that Idaho's law violates both the right to travel and the right to freedom of speech.[15] Other plaintiffs belonging to faith traditions that frame some abortions as morally permissible or even mandatory have argued in state and federal court that abortion bans violate their exercise of religious liberty.[16]

Before *Dobbs*, the courts were certainly central to the war over abortion, as each new restriction spurred debate about the meaning of a right to choose abortion. But the end of *Roe* did not mean the end of this conflict. Constitutional battles have begun in many states, with ballot initiatives and state supreme court elections making any ruling appear less than permanent. Federal courts are poised to decide issues that might once again take the issue from voters and their elected representatives. As far as the courts and abortion are concerned, then, *Dobbs* has not resolved conflicts around reproduction. Instead, the 2022 decision has merely opened a new era in the conflict. AJPH

CORRESPONDENCE

Correspondence should be sent to Mary Ziegler (e-mail: mziegler@ucdavis.edu). Reprints can be ordered at https://www.ajph.org by clicking the "Reprints" link.

PUBLICATION INFORMATION

Full Citation: Ziegler M. The post-*Dobbs* legal landscape. *Am J Public Health*. 2024;114(10): 997–999.

Acceptance Date: June 3, 2024.

DOI: https://doi.org/10.2105/AJPH.2024.307752

ACKNOWLEDGMENTS

Thank you to the editors of the *American Journal of Public Health* for their help on this piece.

CONFLICTS OF INTEREST

The author reports no conflicts of interest.

REFERENCES

1. *Dobbs v Jackson Women's Health Organization*, 597 US 215 (2022).
2. Ballotpedia. Judicial selection in the states. Available at: https://ballotpedia.org/Judicial_selection_in_the_states. Accessed May 19, 2024.
3. *In re State*, 682 SW 3d 890 (Tex 2023).
4. Center for Reproductive Rights. State constitutions and abortion rights. Available at: https://reproductiverights.org/state-constitutions-abortion-rights. Accessed May 19, 2024.
5. *Planned Parenthood of South Atlantic v State*, 892 SE 2d 121 (SC 2023).
6. *Planned Parenthood of Southwest and Central Florida v State*, __ So. 3d __, 2024 WL 1363525 (Fl 2024).
7. *LePage v Center for Reproductive Medicine*, __ So 3d __, 2024 WL 656591 (Ala 2024).
8. Brief for the Respondents at 56-57, *FDA v Alliance for Hippocratic Medicine*, No. 23-235 (US February 22, 2024).
9. *Alliance for Hippocratic Medicine v US Food and Drug Administration*, 668 F Supp 3d 507 (ND Tex 2023).
10. *Alliance for Hippocratic Medicine v US Food and Drug Administration*, 78 F 4th 210 (5th Cir 2023).
11. *Food and Drug Administration v Alliance for Hippocratic Medicine*, 602 US 367 (2024).
12. *United States v Idaho*, 83 F 4th 1130 (9th Cir 2023).
13. *Texas v Becerra*, 89 F 4th 529 (5th Cir 2023).
14. *Moyle v United States*, 603 US __, 2024 WL 3187605 (2024).
15. *Matsumoto v Labrador*, __ F.3d __, 2023 WL 7388852 (D Id 2023).
16. Schwartzman M, Schragger R. Religious freedom and abortion. *Iowa Law Rev.* 2023;108(5):2299–2340. Available at: https://ilr.law.uiowa.edu/volume-108-issue-5/2023/07/religious-freedom-and-abortion. Accessed June 20, 2024.

Collective Persistence, Care, and Advocacy Amid Repeated Attacks on Reproductive Freedom

Whitney S. Rice, DrPH, MPH, Sophie A. Hartwig, MPH, Hayley V. McMahon, MSPH, CPH, Crista Irwin, RN, PhD, Nicole Quinones, MPH, Sara K. Redd, PhD, MSPH, and Katherine A. Singh, MSPH

ABOUT THE AUTHORS

Whitney S. Rice, Sophie A. Hartwig, Hayley V. McMahon, Sara K. Redd, and Katherine A. Singh are with the Center for Reproductive Health Research in the Southeast (RISE) and the Department of Behavioral, Social, and Health Education Sciences, Rollins School of Public Health, Emory University, Atlanta, GA. Crista Irwin is with Feminist Women's Health Center, Atlanta. Nicole Quinones is with the Division of Health Policy and Management, School of Public Health, University of Minnesota, Minneapolis.

See also Abortion Access 2 Years After *Dobbs v Jackson* Ruling, pp. 994–1050.

In recent decades, several US states have been early adopters of increasingly oppressive reproductive health policymaking. Perhaps the best example of such a "testing ground" is Texas, which first implemented two of the most restrictive abortion laws before the US Supreme Court decision to end federal protection of abortion rights in *Dobbs v Jackson Women's Health Organization* (*Dobbs*). In 2020, Texas's governor issued an executive order banning procedural abortion during the COVID-19 pandemic—the focus of the article by Whitfield et al. in this issue of *AJPH* (p. 1013)—which substantially disrupted patients' access and reduced abortions in Texas.[1] In 2021, Texas enacted Senate Bill 8 (SB8), which bans abortion past detection of embryonic cardiac activity and allows private citizens to sue certain parties involved in aiding abortion access. SB8's results were twofold: significant decreases in in-state facility-based abortions and increases in out-of-state abortions.[2] Both SB8 and the executive order serve as models for the proliferation of similar laws in other states.

Abortion laws are structural determinants of health, which "shape the distribution of power and resources across the population"[3(p231)]; accordingly, abortion access restrictions have multilevel consequences. Pregnant people must navigate systematic, costly, and at-times-insurmountable barriers to access, as well as uncertainty about how, where, and when they will get care. In turn, they bear psychological and health outcomes of state-imposed care delay and denial. Providers cannot employ the full scope of their practice without facing legal repercussions, an emotional burden that can affect their health and well-being. While many persist, some clinicians and trainees leave or avoid restrictive settings. Clinics are forced to respond to rapid policy developments that often result in inefficient practice-altering regulations, all while steadfastly connecting patients they cannot serve to care elsewhere and trying to stay open. When states pass these laws, gaps in access compound for entire communities, states, and even regions, including the South. These harms to people and communities are not equitably felt and disproportionately burden those already facing intersecting structural barriers to and inequities in health care access (e.g., Black, Indigenous, young, and undocumented people; people with fewer economic resources, living with disabilities, or in rural areas; sexual and gender minorities; low proficiency- and non-English speakers).

Despite these realities, people, communities, and organizations in restrictive abortion policy settings continue to strive for fuller realization of reproductive autonomy, and adaptably and creatively exercise collective action in its pursuit. As with other social justice movements in the South, those committed to reproductive health, rights, and justice exhibit deep community resilience and care in dire times.

PREGNANT PEOPLE

Following *Dobbs*, dozens of states banned or sharply restricted abortion access. Despite these sizeable disruptions to already strained reproductive health landscapes, abortion volume has increased as pregnant people continue to seek out and receive abortion care. Abortion rates are at their highest in more than a decade,[4] reflecting higher numbers of abortions among residents of abortion-protective states and among people traveling from abortion-restrictive states.[4,5] The number of patients crossing state lines for abortion care through the formal health care systems has doubled—highlighting the determination of pregnant people to seek care, even in this climate.[6]

Other shifts in the abortion care access landscape also reflect the persistence of pregnant people, including increases in self-managed medication abortion and telehealth medication abortion provided under shield laws (i.e., legal protections for pregnant people, supporters, and providers) in protective states. Medication abortion accounts for most abortions provided in the United States, and Southerners account for the greatest increases in self-managed medication abortion requests. Four out of the five states with the largest increases in requests per week following *Dobbs* are in the US South.[7] Estimates from the latter half of 2023 indicate that people in states with near or total abortion bans obtained an average of nearly 5000 telehealth abortions per month under shield laws, accounting for nearly 32% of all telehealth abortions provided through formal US systems.[5]

ABORTION CLINICS AND FUNDS

An interwoven network of community-based clinics and direct-aid organizations has been critical to abortion access in Texas and the broader South. Antiabortion policies have forced dozens of clinics to close since *Dobbs*; however, many independent abortion providers in restrictive states remain oases of care—some even expanding their services to meet additional demand.[8] In the face of numerous threats from policymakers and protesters alike, clinics have leveraged creative solutions to stay open and continue providing abortion care for Southerners—for instance, establishing additional facilities located just across state lines, deploying mobile clinics to meet patients near state borders, and utilizing telehealth to provide medication abortion from states with shield laws. Even within states with total bans, clinics have been unwavering in their dedication to providing essential services such as ultrasounds and post-abortion follow-up care.[9,10]

Similarly, abortion funds and practical support organizations have undertaken tremendous efforts to maintain a safety net for pregnant people. Abortion funds, often small community-based organizations, frequently serve as the last line of defense for bodily autonomy in the South. They provide lifelines to fill pivotal gaps in medical costs, travel expenses, and other support needs for those unable to afford the extensive costs of accessing abortion care. In the first 12 months after *Dobbs*, abortion funds collectively distributed a staggering $37 million to more than 100 000 abortion seekers, many of whom would not have been able to access care otherwise.[11]

POLICY ADVOCACY

Abortion-restrictive states also serve as examples of innovative local policymaking that safeguards abortion access. For example, in 2019, responding to state-level restrictions prohibiting direct funding for abortion services, the city of Austin, Texas, passed an unprecedented measure to invest in local abortion funds. This was followed by another groundbreaking investment in 2020 that reallocated money from policing to abortion support. Austin also led the way in responding to SB8 and *Dobbs* with its 2022 passage of the Guarding the Right to Abortion Care for Everyone (GRACE) Act, a municipal measure that deprioritized criminal investigation and prosecution of abortion. Austin's policymaking has served as an example for others—five Texas municipalities passed their own versions of the GRACE Act, and several cities and states nationwide have passed resolutions that invest in local abortion funds.[12] These policy efforts are the result of a robust network of advocates who have long been working at the forefront of innovative policy approaches to promote reproductive autonomy.

CONCLUSION

Dobbs resulted from decades of multilevel policymaking that chipped away at abortion access, much like the executive order referenced in Whitfield et al. Building a future where reproductive autonomy is fully realized also requires long-term investments. We highlight here exceptional efforts by pregnant people, practical support organizations, independent clinics, providers, advocates, and policymakers. While not detailed here, we are remiss to omit other vital and integral actors—for instance, developers and maintainers of education and patient navigation tools and platforms (e.g., AbortionFinder); legal organizations and lawyers that litigate restrictive abortion policies, advise abortion clinics and providers, and represent those who seek, provide, or assist in abortion care (e.g., Abortion Defense Network); researchers and evaluators of abortion policy changes and solutions; and funders of reproductive health, rights, and justice efforts. In our current highly polarized political environment, public health actors in and beyond restrictive settings may find exemplary mitigation strategies and solutions amid reproductive health access crises. AJPH

CORRESPONDENCE

Correspondence should be sent to Whitney S. Rice, 1518 Clifton Rd NE, Atlanta, GA 30322 (e-mail: whitney.s.rice@emory.edu). Reprints can be ordered at https://www.ajph.org by clicking the "Reprints" link.

PUBLICATION INFORMATION

Full Citation: Rice WS, Hartwig SA, McMahon HV, et al. Collective persistence, care, and advocacy amid repeated attacks on reproductive freedom. *Am J Public Health*. 2024;114(10):1000–1002.

Acceptance Date: July 15, 2024.

DOI: https://doi.org/10.2105/AJPH.2024.307810

ORCID iDs:
Whitney S. Rice https://orcid.org/0000-0003-1749-023X

Sophie A. Hartwig https://orcid.org/0000-0003-3044-8220

Nicole Quinones https://orcid.org/0000-0001-8055-8546

Katherine A. Singh https://orcid.org/0009-0001-8764-2000

CONTRIBUTORS

W. S. Rice conceptualized the editorial. W. S. Rice, S. A. Hartwig, H. V. McMahon, S. K. Redd, and K. A. Singh drafted the editorial. C. Irwin and N. Quinones led the application of pregnant person, provider, and clinic-centered approaches. W. S. Rice, S. A Hartwig, C. Irwin, N. Quinones, S. K. Redd, and K. A. Singh revised the editorial. All authors reviewed and approved the final version.

ACKNOWLEDGMENTS

Work on this publication was funded by RISE through support from an anonymous foundation and the Collaborative for Gender + Reproductive Equity, a sponsored project of Rockefeller Philanthropy Advisors.

CONFLICTS OF INTEREST

The authors have no conflicts of interest to disclose.

REFERENCES

1. White K, Kumar B, Goyal V, Wallace R, Roberts SCM, Grossman D. Changes in abortion in Texas following an executive order ban during the coronavirus pandemic. *JAMA*. 2021;325(7):691–693. https://doi.org/10.1001/jama.2020.24096
2. White K, Sierra G, Lerma K, et al. Association of Texas' 2021 ban on abortion in early pregnancy with the number of facility-based abortions in Texas and surrounding states. *JAMA*. 2022; 328(20):2048–2055. https://doi.org/10.1001/jama.2022.20423
3. Crear-Perry J, Correa-de-Araujo R, Lewis Johnson T, McLemore MR, Neilson E, Wallace M. Social and structural determinants of health inequities in maternal health. *J Womens Health (Larchmt)*. 2021;30(2):230–235. https://doi.org/10.1089/jwh.2020.8882
4. Maddow-Zimet I, Gibson C. Despite bans, number of abortions in the United States increased in 2023. New York, NY: Guttmacher Institute; 2024.
5. *WeCount Report: April 2022 to December 2023*. Philadelphia, PA: Society of Family Planning; 2024.
6. Forouzan K, Friedrich-Karnik, Maddow-Zimet I. The high toll of US abortion bans: nearly one in five patients now traveling out of state for abortion care. New York, NY: Guttmacher Institute; 2023.
7. Aiken ARA, Starling JE, Scott JG, Gomperts R. Requests for self-managed medication abortion provided using online telemedicine in 30 US states before and after the *Dobbs v Jackson Women's Health Organization* decision. *JAMA*. 2022;328(17):1768–1770. https://doi.org/10.1001/jama.2022.18865
8. McCann A, Schoenfeld Walker A. One year, 61 clinics: how Dobbs changed the abortion landscape. *New York Times*. 2023. Available at: https://www.nytimes.com/interactive/2023/06/22/us/abortion-clinics-dobbs-roe-wade.html?unlocked_article_code=1.6k0.UCFj.lVmBWPiv_K08&smid=url-share. Accessed July 12, 2024.
9. McMahon HV. Come hell or high water: a patchwork of community care in Appalachia. In: Littlejohn KE, Solinger R, eds. *Fighting Mad: Resisting the End of Roe v. Wade*. Berkeley, CA: University of California Press Books; 2024. https://doi.org/10.1525/9780520396784-007
10. McPhillips D. Post-Dobbs, abortion clinics find new ways to serve patients in states with bans. *CNN*. 2024. Available at: https://www.cnn.com/2024/06/19/health/abortion-clinics-in-banned-states-pivot/index.html. Accessed July 9, 2024.
11. National Network of Abortion Funds. Critical role of abortion funds post-*Roe*. May 30, 2024. Available at: https://abortionfunds.org/abortion-funds-post-roe. Accessed July 9, 2024.
12. Tuma M. How one progressive city is fighting to decriminalize abortion. *The Nation*. 2022. Available at: https://www.thenation.com/article/society/austin-texas-decriminalize-abortion. Accessed July 12, 2024.

Latin American Nations Once Lagged on Abortion Rights: Now Some Present Role Models for the United States

Cassia Roth, PhD, MPH, and Marian Moser Jones, PhD, MPH

ABOUT THE AUTHORS

Cassia Roth is with the Department of Society, Environment, and Health Equity at the University of California, Riverside. Marian Moser Jones is with The Ohio State University College of Public Health, Columbus.

See also Abortion Access 2 Years After *Dobbs v Jackson* Ruling, pp. 994–1050.

The Supreme Court's 1973 decision in *Roe v Wade* seemed to make the United States a hemispheric role model. It was the first country in the Americas to guarantee the constitutional right to abortion at a time when abortion remained criminalized throughout most of Latin America and the Caribbean—and much of the world. The limits of the US model soon became apparent with Congress's 1976 passage of the Hyde Amendment, which barred the use of federal funds for abortion. In the ensuing years, federal and state laws and Supreme Court decisions further chipped away at the availability of abortion care. Still, even in the early 2000s, abortion remained legal, if restricted, in all US states, while most Latin American countries, except for Cuba, had restrictive bans.

In the 20 years since, Uruguay, Mexico, Argentina, and Colombia have legalized abortion and made it more accessible. Meanwhile, the Supreme Court's decision in *Dobbs v Jackson Women's Health Organization* (2022) has transformed the United States into a volatile patchwork of access and legality. As of June 2024, 14 states ban abortion outright, three ban it after six weeks' gestation, and four others ban it after 12 to 18 weeks, even as other states have enshrined abortion rights in their constitutions and enacted measures to expand access.[1,2] Recent research indicates that this situation has forced US residents to travel across state lines to access abortion care, to pursue medication abortion via telehealth with an out-of-state provider, or to forgo abortion altogether.[2]

In this editorial, we review the historical developments that have led to our current predicament. The Appendix (available as a supplement to the online version of this article at https://ajph.org) provides more references for interested readers. We argue that US advocates for legal and accessible abortion should elevate the country's own strong tradition of reproductive justice advocacy coming from communities of color and expand our vision to include successful outcomes from Latin American countries such as Mexico, Argentina, Colombia, and Uruguay. Specifically, we urge activists to center access in any future legalization efforts, to push for legal changes at multiple levels (local, state, federal) and arenas (legislative, judicial, and administrative), and to uplift grassroots organizers who are working on the ground to fund and support those seeking abortions.

1965–1992: UNITED STATES LEADS, THEN RECEDES

In 1965, Cuba became the first country in the Americas to decriminalize aspects of its abortion laws.[3] Canada followed suit in 1968.[4] Meanwhile, between 1966 and 1972, many US states also reformed abortion laws. In 1970, Hawaii, Washington, Alaska, and New York became the first four states to legalize abortion without prior approval from a hospital committee. This trend culminated in 1973, when *Roe* made the United States the first country in the Americas to declare abortion a constitutional right. But the Court's reasoning in *Roe*, based on an imputed right to privacy rather than gender equality rooted in the 14th Amendment's equal protection clause, provided what some scholars increasingly viewed as a shaky constitutional basis for guaranteeing abortion access.[5]

The Hyde Amendment became the first major curb on access by barring Medicaid funds for abortion care except in cases of child endangerment, rape, or incest. The net effect was immediate and stark. In 1978, the first full year in which the law was in effect, the number of Medicaid-funded abortions dropped by one third.[6] Moreover, after the Amendment's passage,

AJPH October 2024, Vol. 114, No. 10

antiabortion extremists initiated a longstanding if erratic pattern of violence toward abortion clinics and providers.[7] And from the 1980 presidential election forward, the antiabortion movement gained growing influence in US politics.[8] Abortion opponents in Congress passed laws preventing coverage by federal employees' health insurance, the Indian Health Service, military health plans, and for federal prison inmates and publicly insured residents of the District of Columbia.[9] State legislatures created many restrictions, from bans on insurance coverage to laws requiring spousal or parental consent to mandatory waiting periods. The Supreme Court's 1992 decision in *Planned Parenthood of Southeastern Pennsylvania v Casey* upheld these state restrictions as constitutional under *Roe*.[10]

1980S AND 1990S: ACCESS AND RESTRICTIONS DURING THE COLD WAR

In 1979, Cuba became the region's second country to legalize abortion without restrictions when it reformed its criminal code. This full liberalization broadened a 1965 decision to permit abortions up to 10 weeks' gestation by redefining a threat to a woman's "life" as a threat to her general health. Crucially, the national health care system provided the procedure for free. Thus, although Cuba's legal shift occurred six years after *Roe*, the country began guaranteeing access to early abortions just as abortion access was eroding in the United States. Later abortions remain legal, just not on request.[4] In 1988, Canada's Supreme Court declared that legal restrictions on abortion violated a personal right to security. Depending on the province, abortions are available on request from 12 to 24 weeks' gestation although funding and access further depend on provincial laws.[5]

But in most of the region, abortion rights remained stagnant, partly attributable to Cold War politics. In the 1980s and 1990s, Southern Cone countries, including Chile, Argentina, and Brazil, were emerging from decades-long violent military dictatorships, often directly funded and supported by the United States, in which governments perpetrated human rights violations including the mass murder of citizens. Under these dictatorships, women-led movements relied on reproductive justice principles, even if they did not use that phrase, to fight for the bodily autonomy of their families and children, many of whom had been "disappeared." During redemocratization, feminist activists built on these previous human rights–based claims for bodily autonomy to push for the decriminalization of abortion.[11] They set the stage for 21st century, cross-class movements that have centered abortion within larger calls for health equity, social and economic justice, and bodily autonomy in the face of state violence.[12]

In Central America, the United States also supported violently repressive right-wing regimes that destabilized countries and perpetrated massive human rights abuses. In the 1990s, as many countries emerged from their civil wars, they subsequently enacted highly restrictive abortion laws. In El Salvador, a strong antiabortion movement succeeded in criminalizing the procedure under any circumstance in 1997 and enshrining life as beginning at conception in 1999. Since then, the judicial system has taken an activist stance, investigating and prosecuting miscarriages and stillbirths as possible crimes.[13] And in 2006, Nicaraguan president Daniel Ortega, once a leftist revolutionary, allied with a conservative Catholic establishment, which exerts strong influence across the region, to criminalize abortion under all circumstances.[14] In the 1990s then, the United States' broad provision for pre-viability abortions—even with the post-*Casey* retrenchment—contrasted sharply with the situation in these Central American countries.

In the 1990s, US activists also radically reframed abortion activism, even if mainstream feminists and the media overlooked their actions. The predominantly White, middle-class, prochoice movement persisted with its narrow, individual rights–based case for legal abortion in the face of restrictions. In response, a group of US Black feminists convened in 1994 to articulate a broader "reproductive justice" framework that situated abortion among the social, economic, and political inequities that prevented many people from accessing all forms of reproductive health care specifically and health care and economic opportunities in general.[15] The framework focuses attention on addressing the structural barriers to health and well-being: it asserts that "all fertile persons and persons who reproduce and become parents require a safe and dignified context for these most fundamental human experiences."[15(p9)] In essence, all people have "the right *not* to have a child; the right to *have* a child; and the right to *parent* children in safe and healthy environments [italics in original source]."[15(p9)]

THE 21ST CENTURY SCRIPT FLIP

In the 21st century, the momentum for widening abortion rights has shifted south from the United States. Mexico (2007, 2023), Uruguay (2012), Argentina (2020), and Colombia (2022) have all taken steps to legalize abortion. Coalitions of feminist networks and health professionals have won legislative and judicial successes using strategic combinations of human rights- and public health–based approaches that adhere to reproductive justice principles of social, political, and economic equity. Although different countries and movements have made specific claims and used varied tactics, generally feminists in Latin America have argued that restrictions on abortion are a form of gender-based violence and, thus, a violation of pregnant people's human rights, as well as their bodily autonomy—a position that stemmed from opposition to state authoritarianism in the late 20th century.[11] Illegal or inaccessible abortion restricts women, girls, and pregnant people from full participation in social, political, and economic life.

In Mexico, where abortion is regulated at the state level, the first change came in 2007 when Mexico City legalized abortion up to 12 weeks' gestation and legally required that the Ministry of Health provide free services. But in subsequent years, surrounding Mexican states further criminalized abortion.[16] A broad coalition, including the feminist human rights advocacy organization *Grupo de Información en Reproducción Elegida* (GIRE), persistently organized around the issue, using federal constitutional actions (*amparos*) to press for full legalization nationwide.[17] In 2019, the state of Oaxaca became the first to legalize abortion after Mexico City. In 2023, the Mexican Supreme Court decided that the criminalization of abortion was unconstitutional as it violated pregnant people's human rights, removing it from the federal criminal code. The court further declared that defining legal personhood as beginning from conception was unconstitutional.[18] As of June 2024, 12 out of 32 Mexican states had legalized abortion.[17] Nonetheless, criminal penalties are still in effect in at least 20 states. Although people pursuing abortions no longer face criminal charges, local criminal laws restrict abortion access.[18]

In 2012, Uruguay legalized the procedure up to 12 weeks' gestation. This result represented a consensus middle ground between feminist rights-based arguments and public health harm-reduction approaches that emphasized the potential to alleviate morbidity and mortality from unsafe illegal abortions.[19,20]

Other Latin American countries also responded to a groundswell of feminist activism, marked by the transnational *Marea Verde* or Green Tide movement, in which millions of women, wearing *pañuelos verdes* (green scarves), have taken to the streets to protest against restrictive abortion laws since the mid-2010s.[11,12,19] When Argentina's legislature legalized abortion up to 14 weeks' gestation in 2020, it resulted from a decades-long fight in which a broad coalition of activists incorporated demands for legal abortion within social justice petitions and focused on the health inequities of abortion restrictions on the health and lives of poor communities.[11,19] The 2020 Argentine law further stipulates that public hospitals must provide the service free of charge.[12]

Colombian reproductive justice advocates engaged in strategic litigation, arguing that a statute criminalizing abortion with narrow exceptions constituted gender-based discrimination. In 2022, the Colombian Supreme Court legalized abortion without restrictions up to 24 weeks' gestation.[21] Other countries have made smaller steps toward decriminalization in certain circumstances. Judicial rulings in Brazil (2012) and Ecuador (2021) created more exceptions for legal abortions.[14] A senate vote in Chile (2017) passed three exemptions to the previous full ban on abortion.[19]

Alongside these successful efforts to decriminalize or legalize abortion, separate but connected grassroots "accompaniment networks" have provided information, support, and sometimes access to safe self-managed abortions in restrictive contexts. These activists have operationalized cross-regional networks to provide information on self-managing abortions and, to a lesser extent, to send medication abortion through the mail.[22] This approach draws on Latin America's pioneering role in self-managed abortion care. In the 1980s, long before the ulcer drug misoprostol was approved for abortion, women in Brazil began accessing this drug off-label in pharmacies to terminate their pregnancies.[23]

Importantly, the arguments that abortion advocates have successfully mobilized have hinged on bodily autonomy from within a human rights framework; on gender rights to ensure equal social, political, and economic participation; and on public health interests in mitigating adverse health outcomes. These arguments, while distinct and context-specific, overlap with the US-based reproductive justice framework, especially in their attention to the broader structural context that shapes access to reproductive health care.

CAUTIONARY TALES REMAIN

These advances in abortion rights have not escaped backlash. In a Catholic region—with a growing vocal and widespread evangelical movement—many antiabortion activists, politicians, and publics also rely on rights-based claims, those of the fetus.[24] Yet, broad-based pluralistic abortion rights coalitions (including *Católicas por el derecho a decidir*—a Catholic reproductive justice organization) have sought to counter this ongoing backlash by seeking to remove the discussion from a binary that pits the life of the fetus against that of the pregnant person and centering it in a framework that situates gender rights as human rights.[25]

We can also look to some Latin American countries as cautionary tales. The complete bans on abortion in El Salvador, Nicaragua, and Honduras (and the Dominican Republic, Jamaica, and Suriname) have been detrimental to reproductive health.[14] Outside of sub-Saharan Africa, Latin America and the Caribbean is one of the only regions in the world where multiple countries outlaw abortion under all circumstances.[14] In these countries, fetal rights take precedence, much like in some states within the United States—to the detriment of pregnant people.

Our hope is that the United States follows Colombia, the liberalizing Mexican states, and Argentina, and not El Salvador or Nicaragua. Currently, the country is doing both.[14] While many in the US feminist movement have historically relegated poor and minoritized women to the margins of the debate and have failed to squarely embrace reproductive justice–oriented approaches that center access and equity, success of the *Marea Verde* and other movements suggests that we have much to learn from more inclusive approaches.

Specifically, we first urge political leaders and established prochoice groups to center access in any future legalization efforts. This does not mean a return to *Roe* but, rather, thinking expansively about how the right to an abortion must go far beyond "choice." Second, we must be relentless and pragmatic when pushing for legal change, operating at multiple levels (local, state, federal) as organizers did in Mexico; in multiple arenas (legislative, judicial, administrative) as lessons from Colombia, Uruguay, and Argentina show; and across strong coalitions with different goals but ultimately focused on legalization and access. Recent ballot initiatives in favor of abortion rights provide one example for action.[3] Finally, we must uplift grassroots organizers who are working on the ground to fund and support those seeking abortions right now, especially for those living in restrictive contexts. For years, abortion funds have provided crucial support and funds for underresourced people to access abortion. Their work has become even more urgent, and central, in a post-*Dobbs* landscape.

We can learn from our counterparts in the Americas how broad-based and longstanding feminist and public health alliances can reframe the abortion issue, moving it from discussions of morality and religion and, thus, fetal life, to bodily autonomy, gender rights, and public health outcomes. Success comes through decades of long-term commitment to growing a grassroots movement across different constituencies and persistence in the face of seemingly insurmountable cultural barriers and obstacles. Similar levels of dedication, shifts in mindsets, and openness to embracing a diverse coalition will be required in the United States to turn the tide. AJPH

CORRESPONDENCE

Correspondence should be sent to Cassia Roth, 900 University Ave, Riverside, CA 92521 (e-mail: cassia.roth@ucr.edu). Reprints can be ordered at https://www.ajph.org by clicking the "Reprints" link.

PUBLICATION INFORMATION

Full Citation: Roth C, Jones MM. Latin American nations once lagged on abortion rights: now some present role models for the United States. *Am J Public Health*. 2024;114(10):1003–1007.

Acceptance Date: July 19, 2024.

DOI: https://doi.org/10.2105/AJPH.2024.307821

ORCID iD:

Cassia Roth https://orcid.org/0000-0001-8084-3355

CONTRIBUTORS

Both authors had equal participation in conceptualizing, writing, revising, and approving this editorial.

ACKNOWLEDGMENTS

The authors would like to thank the anonymous reviewers for their feedback.

CONFLICTS OF INTEREST

The authors have no conflicts of interest.

REFERENCES

1. McCann A, Schoenfeld Walker A. Tracking abortion bans across the country. *New York Times*. May 24, 2022. Available at: https://www.nytimes.com/interactive/2024/us/abortion-laws-roe-v-wade.html. Accessed June 1, 2024.
2. Felix M, Sobel L, Salganicoff A. Addressing abortion access through state ballot initiatives. KFF. February 9, 2024. Available at: https://www.kff.org/womens-health-policy/issue-brief/addressing-abortion-access-through-state-ballot-initiatives. Accessed July 8, 2024.
3. Andaya E. *Conceiving Cuba: Reproduction, Women, and the State in the Post-Soviet Era*. New Brunswick, NJ: Rutgers University Press; 2014.
4. National Abortion Federation Canada. Available at: https://nafcanada.org. Accessed July 15, 2024.
5. Ginsburg RB. Some thoughts on autonomy and equality in relation to *Roe v Wade*. *North Carol Law Rev*. 1985;63(2):375–386.
6. Trussell J, Menken J, Lindheim BL, Vaughan B. The impact of restricting Medicaid financing for abortion. *Fam Plann Perspect*. 1980;12(3):120–123. https://doi.org/10.2307/2134565
7. Wirken B, Barten DG, De Cauwer H, Mortelmans L, Tin D, Ciottone G. Terrorist attacks against

health care targets that provide abortion services. *Prehosp Disaster Med.* 2023;38(3):409–414. https://doi.org/10.1017/S1049023X23000341

8. Flowers P. *The Right-to-Life Movement, the Reagan Administration, and the Politics of Abortion.* Cham, Switzerland: Palgrave Macmillan; 2018.
9. Boonstra HD. Insurance coverage of abortion: beyond the exceptions for life endangerment, rape and incest. Guttmacher Institute. September 23, 2013. Available at: https://www.guttmacher.org/gpr/2013/09/insurance-coverage-abortion-beyond-exceptions-life-endangerment-rape-and-incest. Accessed March 18, 2024.
10. Brennan Center for Justice. *Roe v Wade* and Supreme Court abortion cases. Brennan Center for Justice. October 6, 2022. Available at: https://www.brennancenter.org/our-work/research-reports/roe-v-wade-and-supreme-court-abortion-cases. Accessed March 7, 2024.
11. Fixmer-Oraiz N, Murillo LM. "The term 'life' should return to us": learning from Latin America's Green Wave. *Women Lang.* 2023;46(1):275–284. https://iro.uiowa.edu/esploro/outputs/journalArticle/The-Term-Life-Should-Return-to/9984559773702771. Accessed November 27, 2023.
12. Lopreite D. The long road to abortion rights in Argentina (1983–2020). *Bull Lat Am Res.* 2023;42(3):357–371. https://doi.org/10.1111/blar.13350
13. Viterna J, Bautista JSG. Pregnancy and the 40-year prison sentence: how "abortion is murder" became institutionalized in the Salvadoran judicial system. *Health Hum Rights.* 2017;19(1):81–93.
14. Center for Reproductive Rights. The world's abortion laws. 2023. Available at: https://reproductiverights.org/maps/worlds-abortion-laws. Accessed August 17, 2023.
15. Ross LJ, Solinger R. *Reproductive Justice: An Introduction.* Oakland, CA: University of California Press; 2017.
16. Becker D, Díaz Olavarrieta C. Decriminalization of abortion in Mexico City: the effects on women's reproductive rights. *Am J Public Health.* 2013;103(4):590–593. https://doi.org/10.2105/AJPH.2012.301202
17. Grupo de Información en Reproducción Elegida (GIRE). Abortion in the penal codes [in Spanish]. Available at: https://gire.org.mx/plataforma/causales-de-aborto-en-codigos-penales. Accessed August 17, 2023.
18. Bonifaz Alfonzo L, Mora Sierra R. Decriminalization of abortion by the Mexican Supreme Court. *Int J Gynaecol Obstet.* 2024;165(1):375–381. https://doi.org/10.1002/ijgo.15433
19. Anderson CF. *Fighting for Abortion Rights in Latin America: Social Movements, State Allies and Institutions.* New York, NY: Routledge; 2020. https://doi.org/10.4324/9780429340499
20. Wood S, Abracinskas L, Correa S, Pecheny M. Reform of abortion law in Uruguay: context, process and lessons learned. *Reprod Health Matters.* 2016;24(48):102–110. https://doi.org/10.1016/j.rhm.2016.11.006
21. González-Vélez AC, Jaramillo-Sierra IC. Abortion reform in Colombia: from total prohibition to decriminalization up to week twenty-four. *South Atl Q.* 2023;122(2):397–406. https://doi.org/10.1215/00382876-10405161
22. Calderón-Villarreal A, Carrasco BIV, Friedman J, Schiavon R. Accompaniment on the edge: what can the US learn from Latin America about contested abortion care? *PLOS Glob Public Health.* 2023;3(5):e0001922. https://doi.org/10.1371/journal.pgph.0001922
23. Löwy I, Dias Villela Corrêa MC. The "abortion pill" misoprostol in Brazil: women's empowerment in a conservative and repressive political environment. *Am J Public Health.* 2020;110(5):677–684. https://doi.org/10.2105/AJPH.2019.305562
24. de la Dehesa R, Lionço T. Imagining fetal citizens in Brazil: on the transnational circulation of reproductive technologies and the "statute of the unborn." *Signs (Chic Ill).* 2024;49(2):333–359. https://doi.org/10.1086/726642
25. Zaremberg G, de Almeida DR. *Feminisms in Latin America: Pro-Choice Nested Networks in Mexico and Brazil.* Cambridge, UK: Cambridge University Press; 2022. https://doi.org/10.1017/9781108919258

"To Anyone Reading in the Future You Are Not Alone": How Patients Seeking Abortion in a Surge State Use Their Stories to Support Each Other

Miriam McQuade, MD, MPH, Brenna Banwarth-Kuhn, Victoria Trujillo, and Amber Truehart, MD, MS

See also Abortion Access 2 Years After *Dobbs v Jackson* Ruling, pp. 994–1050.

Amid growing restrictions on reproductive health care nationwide, understanding real-time contextualization of patient experience is critical. This qualitative approach uses inductive content analysis to examine 74 anonymous journal entries from 2020 to 2023 from patients accessing abortions in New Mexico. Prompted by a journal titled, "Tell your story, it may help someone else," entries described decision-making, highlighted autonomy, and built solidarity. This analysis explains how patients contextualized their abortion and offers insight to improving experiences for patients traveling for abortion care. (*Am J Public Health*. 2024;114(10):1008–1012. https://doi.org/10.2105/AJPH.2024.307772)

AJPH October 2024, Vol. 114, No. 10

Over the past three years, abortion access in New Mexico and the surrounding states has changed drastically. In September 2021, Texas implemented Senate Bill 8, the most restrictive state-level abortion law in the United States at the time.[1] The law left abortion patients and providers confronting very limited access within Texas, as well as capacity, logistical, and financial issues in connecting patients to timely and affordable care outside of the state.[2] Subsequently, in June 2022, after a US Supreme Court decision overturned *Roe v Wade*, abortion was completely banned in Texas and Oklahoma and dramatically restricted in Arizona.[3] These changes solidified New Mexico as an abortion surge state. A *New York Times* article recently reported that there has been a 369% increase in the number of abortions in New Mexico since 2019 and that 71% of those receiving abortions were nonresidents.[4]

New Mexico is in a unique sociopolitical context, as one of the poorest states in the country with some of the most lenient abortion laws.[5,6] Being a rural state with high levels of poverty, obtaining abortion care can mean traveling many hours even for New Mexico residents. Greater distance from an abortion facility is associated with delays in obtaining abortion care and the inability to receive abortion care.[7]

STUDY OBJECTIVES

In one New Mexico health center, patients undergoing procedural abortion could choose to write entries in a journal placed in the recovery room, titled "Tell your story, it may help someone else." These journals were not initially intended for research, but to create community. Patients can read and anonymously share their abortion experiences, providing a space for expression of their thoughts and emotions. Two of the authors are abortion providers at this clinic and saw these journals as critical to better understanding our patients seeking abortion, from both within and outside the state, during this fraught period of rapid legislative changes. We used this qualitative approach for collecting patient stories and analyzed the themes from journal entries to understand how patients contextualize their experiences.

RESEARCH QUESTION

How do patients seeking abortion use their stories to reflect on the social and emotional context of their abortion in the setting of increasing state- and federal-level abortion restrictions causing patients to travel farther distances for abortion care?

PARTICIPANTS, SAMPLE, GEOGRAPHIC LOCATION, SETTING, AND YEAR OF STUDY

This is a qualitative approach reviewing patient journal entries from a single health center providing abortion care through 23 weeks, six days gestation in Albuquerque, New Mexico, from 2020 to 2023. All journal entries were in English and were spontaneous and voluntary; patients did not receive compensation for writing entries. As entries were anonymous, no demographic information was available.

METHODS

The research team, consisting of three cisgender females (M. M., an obstetrician/gynecologist providing abortion services at the clinic; B. K., a medical student; and V. T., research staff) transcribed the journal entries and coded them in Excel. Nina Wallerstein, DrPH, an expert in qualitative research from a participatory research center, was a consultant; she assisted in development of qualitative analysis. In addition, M. M., B. K., and V. T. had all been involved in data collection and development of codebooks for qualitative research previously.

First, the research team annotated five journal entries selected at random to identify themes.[8] These themes were discussed and then formalized into a codebook. This codebook was then used by all three authors to code the entries. Codes were compared and differences rectified through discussion and consensus through iterative dialogue to promote interrater reliability. The team revised the codebook to account for themes it had not adequately captured in the preliminary codebook. After agreeing on coding, we identified overarching themes using inductive content analysis; dominant themes were then further divided into subthemes through analysis of code hierarchies.[9] Given the anonymity of the journal entries, we do not know the state of residence in all cases.

These journal entries were written by patients in the postprocedure area to share with other patients receiving abortion. Although these journals were placed in a public area, the stories shared by patients may have not been intended for the general public. In discussions within the Department of Obstetrics and Gynecology at the University of New Mexico, this ethical concern was raised. After extended discussion, the decision was made to share these journals publicly as a way to amplify abortion patients' stories and for others to understand how these patients were processing their experience, with the ultimate goal being to improve experiences for patients traveling for abortion care. A few patients expressed that they would like their stories to be shared more publicly.

KEY FINDINGS

We included all 74 anonymous narrative journal entries in this qualitative approach for collecting patient stories from 2020 to 2023. Journal entries varied in length from two to three sentences to four to five paragraphs. We identified three dominant themes. Box 1 provides examples of anonymous narrative journal entries.

Theme 1: Decision-Making

Patients often started journal entries by explaining their decision-making. They wrote about the difficulty of making the decision and the complex reasons behind their choice to terminate a pregnancy. Entries included descriptions of desired pregnancies with anomalies, discussion of unhealthy relationships leading to pregnancy, current health concerns, and the desire for pregnancy in the future but lack of current readiness.

- "This baby was a miracle. He was so wanted and loved, but unfortunately, he had trisomy 18, causing heart, intestine, spine, brain, and other abnormalities."
- "I was sexually assaulted and didn't even know that happened to me until I learned of my pregnancy."
- "42 and pregnant with SLE [systemic lupus erythematosus]. All my doctors disadvised [sic] against it. Not only my health being compromised, but the child as well."
- "I just knew I wouldn't be able to give the baby the life it deserved."
- "I already have two kids and we're barely making it."

Theme 2: Autonomy

Patients valued their option to choose an abortion and the empowerment they experienced. They commented that their autonomy was sometimes compromised in their home state and spoke about the negative impact of restrictive abortion laws on their reproductive freedom:

- "It's about wanting the best for the baby that would be born to not prepared circumstances, control of my body."
- "As another young woman coming from Texas this is the first time I've felt like my body was my own and I should never feel ashamed for

BOX 1— Examples of Anonymous Narrative Journal Entries From Journals Provided to Patients in the Postprocedure Area of an Abortion Clinic in Albuquerque, New Mexico, Collected From 2020 to 2023

Themes/Subthemes	Additional Illustrative Quotes
Decision-making	
Complex decision-making	"Something as 'taboo' as abortion, something as life changing as the decision to make that choice . . . is the most difficult thing you ever have to face."
Unhealthy relationships	"Thought I met a 'man' that was going to be there for me 100%. As soon as I found out I was pregnant, everything changed. He was not who I thought he was."
Health concerns	"I knew if I continued my pregnancy my health would be at risk, and I would be on my own."
Anomalies	"On my 16-week ultrasound what should have been a gender reveal with suddenly my worst news ever. The doctors all looked at one another and immediately left. DX: Bilateral renal agenesis they said they can't do much. My heart crumbled. My tears fell, I cried and cried, but it didn't change the outcome."
Readiness for parenting	"Everyone wanted me to have this child, but the relationship and lifestyle was not the right one for me, or my baby. I want to offer more—now I have a 5-year plan"
Impact on current parenting	"A burden for my 3-year-old son long after I would die—But who cares. I am so blessed. A great husband. And amazing son. Who am I to play God and demand more?"
Autonomy	
The power to choose	"I have never felt so heard and like the decisions being made were actually mine to make."
Ownership over one's body	"I'm grateful to have access to abortion and the funds to pay for it. I'm grateful to live in a state with access. I'm grateful to all medical staff I've encountered for their empathy and not questioning my choice. I'm grateful that you're surrounded by loved ones who support me. "
Political barriers affecting autonomy	"I came from Fort Worth, TX because that barbaric law prevented me from getting the lifesaving care I needed." "So many of us had to come from Texas, because they took away our right to choose."
Solidarity	
Camaraderie	"We are all strong, wonderful, beautiful women. No matter what! No one, no laws, nothing can change how beautiful, powerful and unstoppable we are. We as women are the boss in any in every situation in life. Always remember Mamas we can do anything!!—Love yourself more and you will never be disappointed. Love, heel, learn, and grow like the beautiful flowers we are!—We are strong! Brave! Unstoppable!"
Reassurance	"Just because you feel bad about making your decision, DOES NOT mean you made the wrong one. Regardless of what anyone tells you." "Remind yourself this too shall pass."
Advice and validation	"No matter the reason for your decision, you matter, and you will be okay. Your ancestors are still by you and now you have one more looking over you. At least until you meet again—Breathe. Go dance and smile for you! P.S. May you live and walk in health and life"
Normalization	"You are still the strong amazing, extraordinary human being you are and were before all of this. You are a good person. Allow yourself to grieve, mourn, and feel loss if you need to. This is only one chapter of your story, and you have many more to go. With love" "I will be who I was before this. I'm excited for this."

being smart and doing what is best for me and my health."

- "Since there was a heartbeat, Texas did not give us the humane option of termination even with the brain malformation."

Theme 3: Solidarity

Most journal entries concluded with a statement about solidarity and support of other patients. Patients expressed camaraderie and reassurance to future patients and validation and normalization were strong themes throughout the journal entries:

- "My loves you are so powerful and strong. We face many challenges. You have made an amazing choice for you! I love you all and send many prayers."
- "You are still the strong amazing, extraordinary human being you are and were before all of this. Allow yourself to grieve, mourn, and feel loss if you need to. This is only one chapter of your story, and you have many more to go."

EVALUATION, TRANSFERABILITY, AND ADVERSE EFFECTS

The themes uncovered in the patients' stories suggest the need to initiate the development of theory in how to best support effective and compassionate reproductive health care. Even though this is a descriptive qualitative approach for collecting patient stories of a convenience sample, we would offer the following considerations. Results from our assessment demonstrate the gravity and complexity of patients' decisions and their desire to support each other through a complex emotional and political landscape. In our supportive clinic setting, patients used their stories to foster community, highlight the importance of bodily autonomy, and support others facing similar challenges by contextualizing their own abortion experience. It is likely that the results from our studies are transferrable to other populations of patients traveling for abortion care. Our patients wrote the journal entries during this time of legislative change when a large surge of patients traveled to New Mexico for abortion care. At baseline, people seeking abortion care experience fear, judgment, and interpersonal strain and stress.[10] For people who travel more than an hour for care, the psychological and physical costs increase.[11] The ability to share stories may not only have allowed patients to process their experience anonymously but also may have given them satisfaction from supporting others.

SCALABILITY

This qualitative approach to collecting patient stories may apply to patients traveling for abortion care across the United States, not just to patients traveling for abortion care to New Mexico. This analysis was done at one clinic in one state. This approach could be scaled to include clinics in multiple locations throughout the state or to include clinics in other states with similar increases in patients traveling for abortion care. Scaling in this way may pose challenges given the time-intensive approach to journal transcription and analysis.

PUBLIC HEALTH SIGNIFICANCE

People who seek abortion care are subject to significant social stigma. The narrative around abortion care has remained relatively constant even though safety of legal abortion has been proven.[12] We still often see abortion portrayed in the media as dangerous and wrong despite major advances in abortion care after *Roe v Wade* legalized US abortion rights. One of the best strategies implemented around the world to change narrative is storytelling. There are already organizations elevating the voices and expertise of patients who have had abortions, including "We Testify," "The Abortion Diary," and "#ShoutYourAbortion."[13–15] These organizations use stories to normalize abortion for patients and as a way to advocate safe abortion access. To change the narrative, people should move away from the typical numbers and medicalization of care and center the stories and the voices of abortion patients.[16]

This qualitative approach to collecting patient stories highlights how patients frame the complexity of their experiences in accessing abortion. The journals provided a space for people to contextualize their personal stories, but rather than focus solely on themselves, many respondents fostered emotional, social, and political support for others navigating their own challenges. Real-time processing highlights patients' desire to support others facing challenges in negotiating legal restrictions and other barriers. This understanding opens the door to further explore how people support each other and build community in overcoming obstacles to access reproductive health care. As we are abortion providers, this analysis allows us to better understand the needs of our patients traveling for abortion care from a social, political, and emotional context. These journals included what information abortion patients felt was important to share while processing their experience. It may be beneficial for providers to proactively offer space for these themes: decision-making, autonomy, and solidarity. Patients may yearn for support from their peers or become support systems themselves but have challenges in doing so. Patients may want to describe their decision-making during counseling even though most providers will provide abortion care for any reason. Patients may appreciate posters and bulletin boards in the clinic that highlight their personal autonomy and solidarity with staff and other patients. We can use this information to improve experiences for patients traveling for abortion care. AJPH

ABOUT THE AUTHORS

Miriam McQuade and Amber Truehart are with the Department of Obstetrics and Gynecology, Division of Complex Family Planning, University of New Mexico Medical Center, Albuquerque. Brenna Banwarth-Kuhn is with the School of Medicine, University of New Mexico, Albuquerque. Victoria Trujillo is with the Department of Obstetrics and Gynecology, University of New Mexico Medical Center.

CORRESPONDENCE

Correspondence should be sent to Miriam McQuade, MD, MPH, Department of OB/GYN, 2211 Lomas Blvd NE, Albuquerque, NM 87131 (e-mail: mmmcquade@salud.unm.edu). Reprints can be ordered at https://www.ajph.org by clicking the "Reprints" link.

PUBLICATION INFORMATION

Full Citation: McQuade M, Banwarth-Kuhn B, Trujillo V, Truehart A. "To anyone reading in the future you are not alone": how patients seeking abortion in a surge state use their stories to support each other. *Am J Public Health*. 2024;114(10):1008–1012.
Acceptance Date: June 24, 2024.

DOI: https://doi.org/10.2105/AJPH.2024.307772
ORCID iD:
Miriam McQuade https://orcid.org/0000-0001-5260-1201

CONTRIBUTORS

M. McQuade contributed to conceptualization, methodology, formal analysis, investigation, data curation, writing the original draft, and visualization. B. Banwarth-Kuhn and V. Trujillo contributed to the investigation. A. Truehart contributed to conceptualization, methodology, validation, review and editing of the article, and supervision.

ACKNOWLEDGMENTS

This research was presented at the American College of Obstetrics and Gynecology Annual Meeting and the National Abortion Federation Annual Meeting.

Nina Wallerstein, DrPH, the director of the Center for Participatory Research and an expert in qualitative research, was a consultant; she assisted in development of qualitative analysis.

CONFLICTS OF INTEREST

The authors declare that there were no conflicts of interest.

HUMAN PARTICIPANT PROTECTION

The University of New Mexico's Human Research Review Committee found this qualitative approach for collecting patient stories to be exempt. Consent was not obtained from every patient, as this was retrospective; however, we submitted the retrospective design to our Office of Human Subjects at University of New Mexico Health Science Center as an exempt study, which was approved as HRRC 23-003.

REFERENCES

1. White K, Sierra G, Dixon L, Sepper E, Moayedi G. Texas Senate Bill 8: Medical and legal implications. Texas Policy Evaluation Project, The University of Texas at Austin. July 2021. Available at: https://sites.utexas.edu/txpep/files/2021/07/TxPEP-research-brief-senate-bill-8.pdf. Accessed July 12, 2024.
2. White K, Dane'el A, Vizcarra E, et al. Out-of-state travel for abortion following implementation of Texas Senate Bill 8. Texas Policy Evaluation Project, The University of Texas at Austin. March 2022. Available at: https://sites.utexas.edu/txpep/files/2022/03/TxPEP-out-of-state-SB8.pdf. Accessed July 16, 2024.
3. Sepper E, Moayedi G, Thaxton L, Beasley A, Dixon L, White K. After *Roe*: criminal abortion bans in Texas. Texas Policy Evaluation Project, The University of Texas at Austin. June 2022. Available at: https://sites.utexas.edu/txpep/files/2022/06/TexasPostRoeCriminalAbortionBans-TxPEP-PolicyBrief_27June22.pdf. Accessed July 12, 2024.
4. Escobar MC, Walker AS, McCann A, Reinhard S, Rosales H. 171,000 traveled for abortions last year. See where they went. *New York Times*. June 13, 2024. Available at: https://www.nytimes.com/interactive/2024/06/13/us/abortion-state-laws-ban-travel.html. Accessed July 1, 2024.
5. State facts about abortion. New Mexico. New York, NY: Guttmacher Institute; 2022.
6. White K, Sierra G, Lerma K, et al. Association of Texas' 2021 ban on abortion in early pregnancy with the number of facility-based abortions in Texas and surrounding states. *JAMA*. 2022; 328(20):2048–2055. https://doi.org/10.1001/jama.2022.20423
7. Pleasants EA, Cartwright AF, Upadhyay UD. Association between distance to an abortion facility and abortion or pregnancy outcome among a prospective cohort of people seeking abortion online. *JAMA Netw Open*. 2022;5(5):e2212065. https://doi.org/10.1001/jamanetworkopen.2022.12065
8. Ryan GW, Bernard HR. Techniques to identify themes. *Field Methods*. 2003;15(1):85–109. https://doi.org/10.1177/1525822X02239569
9. Burnard P, Gill P, Stewart K, Treasure E, Chadwick B. Analysing and presenting qualitative data. *Br Dent J*. 2008;204(8):429–432. https://doi.org/10.1038/sj.bdj.2008.292
10. Kimport K, Rasidjan MP. Exploring the emotional costs of abortion travel in the United States due to legal restriction. *Contraception*. 2023;120:109956. https://doi.org/10.1016/j.contraception.2023.109956
11. Odum T, Heymann O, Turner AN, Rivlin K, Bessett D. Assessing psychosocial costs: Ohio patients' experiences seeking abortion care. *Contraception*. 2023;117:45–49. https://doi.org/10.1016/j.contraception.2022.08.007
12. Raymond EG, Grimes DA. The comparative safety of legal induced abortion and childbirth in the United States. *Obstet Gynecol*. 2012;119(2 Pt 1):215–219. https://doi.org/10.1097/AOG.0b013e31823fe923
13. The Abortion Diary. About The Abortion Diary. Available at: https://www.theabortiondiary.com/about-the-abortion-diary. Accessed June 27, 2024.
14. Shout Your Abortion. Normalizing abortion and elevating safe paths to access, regardless of legality. Available at: https://shoutyourabortion.com. Accessed June 27, 2024.
15. We Testify. We Testify. Available at: https://www.abortion.shop. Accessed June 27, 2024.
16. Hallgarten L. Abortion narratives: moving from statistics to stories. *Lancet*. 2018;391(10134):1988–1989. https://doi.org/10.1016/S0140-6736(18)31036-5

Abortion Return Rates and Wait Times Before and After Texas' Executive Order Banning Abortion During COVID-19

Brooke Whitfield, MA, Gracia Sierra, PhD, MA, Klaira Lerma, MPH, Vinita Goyal, MD, MPH, Lauren Thaxton, MD, MBA, Bhavik Kumar, MD, MPH, Allison Gilbert, MD, and Kari White, PhD, MPH

See also Abortion Access 2 Years After *Dobbs v Jackson* Ruling, pp. 994–1050.

Objectives. To assess the associations between the executive order that Texas governor Greg Abbott issued on March 22, 2020, postponing procedures deemed not immediately medically necessary, and patients' access to abortion care in Texas.

Methods. We used 17 515 individual-level patient records from 13 Texas abortion facilities for matched periods in 2019 and 2020 to examine differences in return rates for abortion after completion of a state-mandated ultrasound and median wait times between ultrasound and abortion visits for those who returned.

Results. Patients were less likely to return for an abortion if they had an ultrasound while the executive order was under effect (82.8%) than in the same period in 2019 (90.4%; adjusted odds ratio = 2.06; 95% confidence interval = 1.12, 3.81). Compared with patients at or before 10.0 weeks' gestation at ultrasound, patients at more than 10 weeks' gestation had higher odds of not returning for an abortion or, if they returned, experienced greater wait times between ultrasound and abortion visits.

Conclusions. Texas' executive order prohibiting abortion during the COVID-19 pandemic disrupted patients' access to care and disproportionately affected patients who were past 10 weeks' gestation. (*Am J Public Health*. 2024;114(10):1013–1023. https://doi.org/10.2105/AJPH.2024.307747)

AJPH October 2024, Vol. 114, No. 10

At the onset of the COVID-19 pandemic, Texas governor Greg Abbott issued a 30-day executive order that postponed procedures deemed not immediately medically necessary. The state's attorney general interpreted this to include abortion,[1] contrary to guidance from professional medical associations that abortion care not be delayed.[2] The order went into effect on March 22, 2020, leading facilities to immediately cancel appointments, and there was uncertainty about whether the order would be extended beyond the April 21, 2020 end date. During the 30-day period when the order was in effect, there was a series of legal challenges and conflicting court decisions that resulted in short windows of time when providers could temporarily offer abortion care. Moreover, 1 court ruling restored access to medication abortion during the executive order, which was offered until 10 weeks of gestation in Texas. However, most procedural abortions were still prohibited, and some facilities halted all abortions during the 30-day period owing to legal uncertainty. Pregnant Texans who were ineligible for medication abortion and unable to travel out of state were forced to delay care until the order expired, and those nearing Texas' 22-week gestational limit for abortion may have had to continue their pregnancy.

The order also compounded existing delays to abortion care in Texas stemming from state-mandated policies requiring counseling and ultrasound visits 24 hours before an abortion[3] and from the emerging pandemic.[4–6] Research indicates that both individual factors—such as financial barriers, fear of contracting COVID-19, increases in intimate partner violence—and structural factors—such as reduced clinic hours, social distancing practices that limited the number of patients who could be seen, and physician shortages—adversely affected abortion access during the pandemic.[5,6]

Delays in abortion care can have negative consequences, such as preventing patients from obtaining a preferred medication abortion[7] and increasing procedure complexity, cost, and risk.[8–12] Additionally, fewer providers perform abortions later in pregnancy,[12] limiting options for care and potentially preventing patients from obtaining a wanted abortion altogether, which can result in adverse financial and health outcomes for both pregnant people and their children.[13]

A previous study on the implications of the executive order in Texas found that in-state abortions declined by 38% during the executive order and that abortions being performed at or after 12 weeks' gestation increased after the order was lifted.[14] This study, however, used only aggregate data and was unable to assess whether patients who had a state-mandated ultrasound during the executive order period returned for an abortion and, for those who returned, how wait times were affected. Thus, our aim was to assess (1) the association of the executive order's implementation with abortion return rates and wait times, and (2) how the executive order affected patients differently by gestational duration.

METHODS

We obtained individual-level abortion patient data from 13 of the 23 abortion facilities in Texas that provided abortion care during matched time periods in 2019 (February 21–May 22, 2019) and 2020 (February 21–May 22, 2020) to assess patterns of care in the 30-day intervals before, during, and after implementation of the executive order. These 13 facilities, representing all geographic areas where abortion care was offered during the study period, accounted for 59% of the in-state annual abortion volume. The remaining 10 facilities either did not respond to our requests or were unable to provide information needed for analyses. We collected data between January and December 2021.

The study team created a REDCap database (REDCap Consortium, Nashville, TN) to collect patient age, self-reported race and ethnicity, dates of state-mandated ultrasound visit and abortion visit, gestational duration at ultrasound and abortion visits, abortion method, and patient zip code. Research staff or facility staff manually entered this information from medical record data and recorded it in REDCap at 5 sites. At the remaining 8 sites, facility staff prepared a de-identified data set from the information collected in their electronic medical record data.

Measures

Our 2 primary outcomes were whether a patient returned to the facility for their abortion after completing their state-mandated ultrasound and, among those who returned, the number of days between their ultrasound and abortion visit (i.e., "wait time"). To assess whether implementation of the executive order was associated with our primary outcomes, we divided the 2019 and 2020 observation periods into 30-day time intervals that corresponded to the time before, during, and after implementation of the executive order during which patients had their ultrasound. Including the 30-day periods before and after the executive order enabled us to control for abortion seasonality[15,16] and potential time confounders other than the executive order, such as the onset of the pandemic, which may affect abortion outcomes and wait times. Because revised legal decisions during executive order implementation allowed the provision of medication abortion and some procedural abortions, we also assessed the association between gestational duration at the ultrasound visit and our primary outcomes.

We categorized gestational duration at ultrasound as 10.0 weeks of gestation or less, 10.1 to 14.6 weeks, and 15.0 to 22.0 weeks. These categories reflect differences in abortion methods available, patients' need for cervical preparation, and visit duration for procedural abortion. Patients at 10.0 weeks of gestation or earlier were eligible for medication abortion or uterine aspiration that requires no cervical preparation. Patients between 10.1 and 14.6 weeks of gestation were eligible for only uterine aspiration, which may require cervical priming with medications such as misoprostol.[17] Patients at 15.0 to 22.0 weeks of gestation typically require a dilation and evacuation procedure that involves cervical dilation using osmotic dilators, medications (mifepristone or misoprostol), or both.[18] Abortion procedures requiring cervical preparation typically take longer.

We examined the overall distribution of our primary outcomes by sociodemographic characteristics: age in years (< 18, 18–24, 25–29, 30–34, ≥ 35), race and ethnicity (Asian, Black, Hispanic, other, White), 1-way distance to facility in miles (< 10, 10–24, 25–49, 50–100, > 100), and an indicator of economic well-being (prosperous, comfortable, midtier, at risk, distressed). We included indicators for age and race and ethnicity, as research shows that young people and people of color are disproportionately affected by abortion restrictions.[19,20] We included 1-way travel distance because greater distance from an abortion facility is associated with delays or inability to access abortion.[21] Additionally, patients living 100 miles or more from an abortion facility may have shorter wait times since they could waive Texas' mandatory 24-hour waiting period between ultrasound and abortion visits.

We calculated 1-way distance from the population-weighted centroid of patients' zip code of residence to the abortion facility where they obtained care using the georoute module in Stata version 18 (StataCorp LP, College Station, TX).[22] We also included a measure of patients' economic well-being because patients living in disadvantaged areas may take longer to return for their abortion visit because of financial barriers, such as difficulty finding enough money for the visit, transportation, childcare, or other needs. For this measure, we used patients' zip code and the 2020 Distressed Communities Index, which groups geographic areas into quintiles: prosperous, comfortable, midtier, at risk, and distressed.[23]

Missing Data

Patient data were not missing at random for race and ethnicity (8%; n = 1400) and gestational duration at ultrasound (6%; n = 1004). Most records missing race and ethnicity information were from 2 higher-volume facilities where patients opted not to indicate their race and ethnicity on their medical history form. Similarly, most records missing gestational duration were from a single high-volume facility where gestational duration at ultrasound was not recorded and was only captured in patients' electronic medical records if they went in for an abortion procedure. Because data were not missing at random, we did not impute values and instead included missing data as a separate category in each covariate.

Our analytic samples included 17 515 observations for analyses assessing the association between having an ultrasound visit during the executive order period and not returning for an abortion and 14 438 observations for analyses assessing the association between having an ultrasound visit during the executive order and the wait time interval between ultrasound and abortion visits.

Data Analysis

To assess the association between having an ultrasound visit during the executive order period and returning for an abortion visit, we ran unadjusted and multivariable-adjusted logistic regressions and clustered SEs at the facility level. The unadjusted model controlled for the 30-day observation periods. In the first multivariable-adjusted model, we also included sociodemographic characteristics to ensure that potential compositional differences of patients across facilities and periods were not biasing results. In a separate multivariable-adjusted model, we also included a composite variable containing each combination of 30-day period and gestational duration at ultrasound category. We used this to determine whether patients who were ineligible for medication abortion (i.e., were at > 10 weeks' gestation) during the executive order were less likely to return for an abortion (either during a temporary lifting of the order or after the order expired) than were patients during the same 30-day period in 2019. Comparisons of Akaike information criterion (AIC) and Bayesian information criterion (BIC) scores indicated that the inclusion of covariates and the composite variable improved model fit.

We calculated the median number of days between ultrasound and abortion visits and the interquartile range (IQR) for each 30-day period overall and by sociodemographic characteristics. We estimated Cox proportional-hazard models with SEs clustered at the facility level to assess the association between having an ultrasound during the executive order period and the wait time between ultrasound and abortion visits. We did not include patients who did not return for an abortion appointment in this analysis. We used the same approach for unadjusted and multivariable-adjusted models described previously and compared the AIC and BIC to assess model fit. We conducted all analyses using Stata 18.

RESULTS

In 2020, the number of ultrasound visits decreased following Texas' declaration of a public health emergency for COVID-19 (March 6, 2020) and reached a low of 132 ultrasound visits and 131 abortion visits during the midpoint of the executive order period. Ultrasound and abortion visits then increased to 831 and 734, respectively, the week before the executive order expired, approaching 2019 numbers (Figure 1).

The percentage of patients who did not return for an abortion after their ultrasound visit varied between 9.6% and 11.1% in 2019 and 11.0% to 17.2% in 2020 (Table 1). During the 30-day

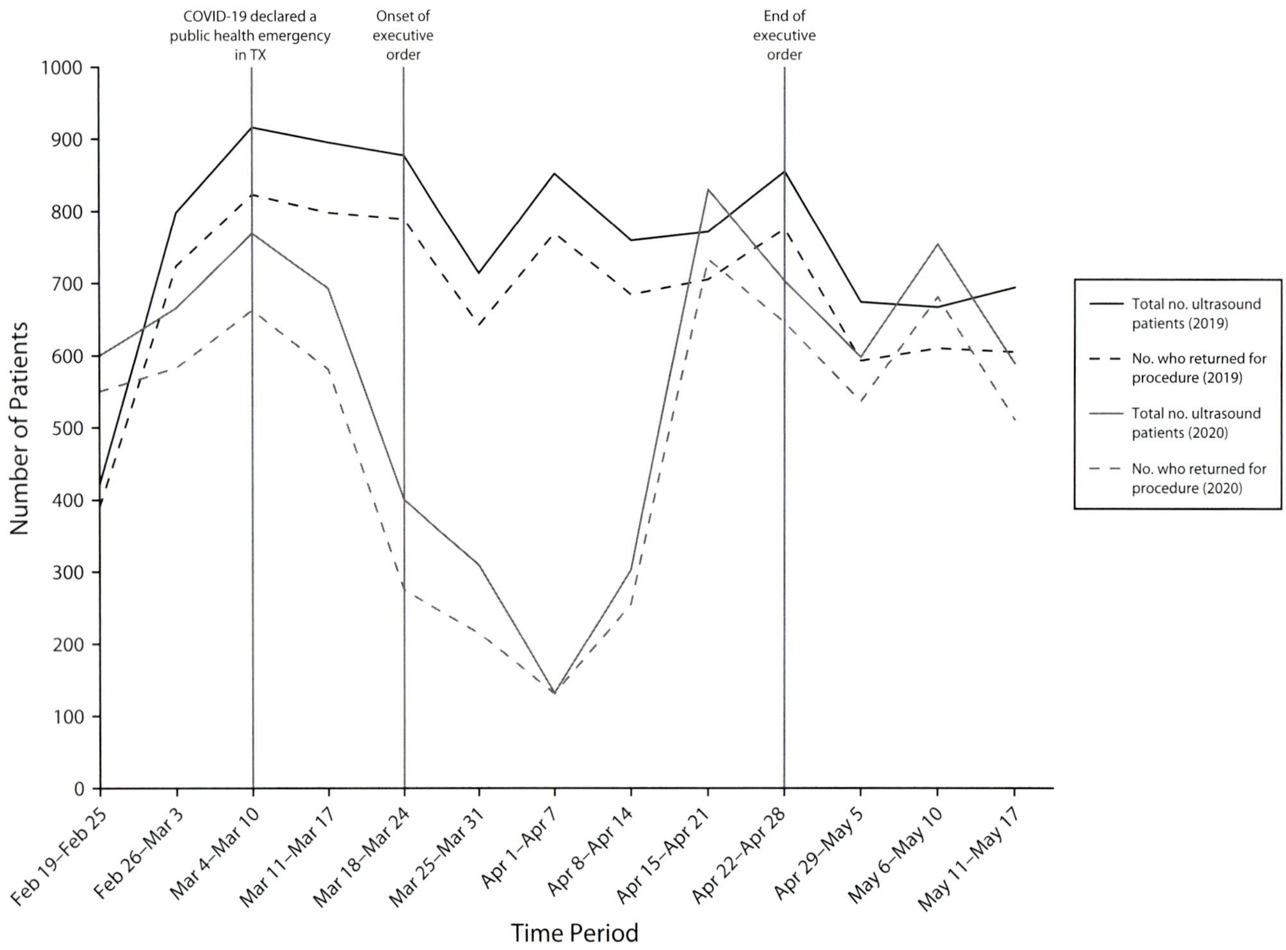

	2019		2020	
Week of:	Total No. Ultrasound Patients	No. Who Returned for Procedure	Total No. Ultrasound Patients	No. Who Returned for Procedure
Mar 4–Mar 10	916	823	769	663
Mar 18–Mar 24	877	789	400	275
Apr 22–Apr 28	855	775	703	646

FIGURE 1— Weekly Number of Texas Patients Who Completed a State-Mandated Ultrasound Visit and Who Returned for an Abortion: February 21–May 22, 2019, February 21–May 22, 2020

Note. The sample size was n = 17 515.

executive order period, 282 of the 1640 patients who had an ultrasound did not return to the facility for an abortion (17.2%) compared with 317 of the 3307 patients (9.6%) during the same 30-day period in 2019 (odds ratio [OR] = 1.96; 95% confidence interval [CI] = 1.09, 3.53; unadjusted model results not shown in table).

After multivariable adjustment, the odds of not returning for an abortion remained higher for patients who had an ultrasound visit during the executive order period (adjusted odds ratio [AOR] = 2.06; 95% CI = 1.12, 3.81) compared with patients who had an ultrasound visit during the same 30-day period in 2019. Patients who had an ultrasound visit during the 30-day period in which Texas declared COVID-19 a public health emergency but before the executive order was issued (February 21, 2020–March 21, 2020) also had higher odds of not returning for an abortion (AOR = 1.46; 95% CI = 1.20, 1.77) than did patients who had an ultrasound during the same 30-day period in 2019.

TABLE 1— Percentage of Texas Patients Who Did Not Return for an Abortion After Completing the State-Mandated Ultrasound Visit and Probability of No Return: February 21–May 22, 2019, February 21–May 22, 2020

	No. Patients	% Not Returning (No.)	AOR (95% CI)
Period			
Feb 21–Mar 21, 2019	3612	9.6 (347)	0.88 (0.71, 1.10)
Mar 22–Apr 21, 2019	3307	9.6 (317)	1 (Ref)
Apr 22–May 22, 2019	3243	11.1 (359)	1.18 (0.84, 1.65)
Feb 21–Mar 21, 2020	2913	14.8 (432)	1.46 (1.20, 1.77)
Mar 22–Apr 21, 2020[a]	1640	17.2 (282)	2.06 (1.12, 3.81)
Apr 22–May 22, 2020	2800	11.0 (307)	0.85 (0.61, 1.18)
Gestational duration at ultrasound, wk			
≤ 10	13150	5.4 (706)	1 (Ref)
10.1–14.6	2168	8.8 (191)	1.77 (1.40, 2.22)
15.0–22.0	1193	17.4 (208)	3.89 (3.07, 4.93)
Missing	1004	93.5 (939)	269 (72.4, 998)
Age, y			
< 18	468	16.5 (77)	1.67 (1.16, 2.43)
18–24	6345	11.5 (731)	1.05 (0.90, 1.21)
25–29	4920	11.0 (542)	1 (Ref)
30–34	3315	11.2 (371)	1.00 (0.87, 1.17)
≥ 35	2462	13.1 (322)	1.11 (0.90, 1.37)
Missing	5	20.0 (1)	0.47 (0.18, 1.21)
Race/ethnicity			
Asian	830	11.5 (95)	0.73 (0.50, 1.05)
Black	4166	13.3 (555)	1.13 (0.89, 1.43)
Hispanic	6374	11.1 (709)	0.94 (0.75, 1.17)
Other[b]	355	9.0 (32)	1.02 (0.64, 1.63)
White	4390	11.3 (498)	1 (Ref)
Missing	1400	11.1 (155)	0.91 (0.47, 1.77)
1-way distance to facility, miles			
< 10	2995	11.1 (332)	1 (Ref)
10–24	6854	11.9 (813)	0.98 (0.77, 1.25)
25–49	3521	13.6 (479)	1.13 (0.76, 1.67)
50–100	1862	12.2 (228)	1.19 (0.71, 2.00)
> 100	1774	6.8 (121)	0.74 (0.40, 1.38)
Missing	509	14.0 (71)	0.72 (0.15, 3.41)
Distressed Community Index score			
Prosperous	4214	11.5 (484)	1 (Ref)
Comfortable	2660	11.3 (301)	0.94 (0.73, 1.20)
Midtier	2980	12.9 (385)	1.12 (0.91, 1.37)
At risk	3563	11.3 (402)	0.91 (0.64, 1.29)
Distressed	3552	11.1 (396)	0.78 (0.48, 1.26)
Missing	546	13.9 (76)	1.66 (0.39, 7.00)

Note. AOR = adjusted odds ratio; CI = confidence interval. The sample size was n = 17 515.
[a]Denotes the 30-d executive order period.
[b]Other includes American Indian, Alaska Native, Native Hawaiian, Pacific Islander, and multiracial.

Compared with patients who were at 10.0 weeks or less of gestation at their ultrasound visit, those who were at 10.1 to 14.6 weeks of gestation (AOR = 1.77; 95% CI = 1.40, 2.22) and 15.0 to 22.0 weeks of gestation (AOR = 3.89; 95% CI = 3.07, 4.93) had higher odds of not returning for an abortion. Additionally, minors (< 18 years) had higher odds of not returning for an abortion than did patients aged 25 to 29 years (AOR = 1.67; 95% CI = 1.16, 2.43). There were no statistically significant differences in sociodemographic characteristics among patients who came in for an ultrasound across 30-day periods.

In models that included the composite variable for 30-day period and gestational duration categories, the probability of not returning for an abortion after an ultrasound visit was 25.5% for patients at 10.1 to 14.6 weeks' gestation during the executive order compared with 4.0% for patients at up to 10.0 weeks' gestation during the same 30-day period in 2019 (AOR = 8.21; 95% CI = 3.88, 17.4; Figure 2; Table A, available as a supplement to the online version of this article at http://www.ajph.org). Similarly, the probability of not returning for an abortion after an ultrasound visit was 40.0% for patients at 15.0 to 22.0 weeks' gestation during the executive order compared with 4.0% for patients at 10.0 weeks' or less gestation during the same 30-day period in 2019 (AOR = 17.0; 95% CI = 6.75, 42.7; Figure 2; Table A).

Among patients who returned for an abortion, the median wait time between ultrasound and abortion visit was 2 days (IQR = 1–6) for patients who had an ultrasound during the executive order period and 2 days (IQR = 1–6) for patients during the same 30-day period in 2019 (Table 2). There was no significant difference in wait times between these groups in unadjusted (hazard ratio [HR] = 0.99; 95% CI = 0.79, 1.25; results not shown in table) and multivariable-adjusted models (HR = 1.00; 95% CI = 0.78, 1.27).

In models that included the composite variable for 30-day period and gestational duration category, there were significant differences in wait times between the 2019 and 2020 periods that corresponded to the executive order (Table B, available as a supplement to the online version of this article at http://www.ajph.org). The median wait time between ultrasound and abortion visit was 2 days (IQR = 1–5) for patients at 10.1 to 14.6 weeks' gestation during the 30-day period in 2019 that corresponded to the executive order, compared with 9 days (IQR = 6–14) during the executive order period (Table B; Figure A, available as a supplement to the online version of this article at http://www.ajph.org). Similarly, the median wait time between ultrasound and abortion visit was 2 days (IQR = 1–6) for patients at 15.0 to 22.0 weeks' gestation in 2019 compared with 8 days (IQR = 1.5–12) during the executive order period (Table B; Figure A). Median wait time between visits for patients at 10.0 weeks' or less gestation at ultrasound was 2 days for both the 2019 (IQR = 1–7) and the 2020 (IQR = 1–4) executive order periods.

DISCUSSION

We found that the implementation of a 30-day executive order banning abortion in Texas was significantly associated with a reduction in the number of patients who returned for an abortion after their state-mandated ultrasound. Furthermore, we found that patients at more than 10 weeks' gestational duration who were ineligible for medication abortion during the executive order were disproportionately affected by the ban.

Although we do not know the pregnancy outcomes of people who did not return to the facility for an abortion, more people may have obtained an abortion than the 82.8% documented here. They may have gone to another Texas facility or traveled out of state, particularly those who were nearing the 22-week gestational duration limit for abortion procedures.[14,24] Previous research found that many Texas patients obtained out-of-state abortion care during the executive order, but they had to travel long distances, which increases financial, logistic, and emotional burdens.[25–27] Others may have self-managed their abortion, as indicated by the large increase in online requests for medication abortion during this period,[28] but many Texans were likely unaware or unwilling to access medication abortion online given the legal uncertainty.

Furthermore, some may have continued their pregnancy, as the financial, logistical, and legal barriers to obtaining an abortion may have been too difficult to overcome. Our findings indicate that patients at more than 10 weeks' gestation were more likely to experience these burdens. Additionally, our findings show that minors were less likely to return for an abortion during the executive order, supporting previous research indicating that young people are disproportionately harmed by abortion restrictions.[19]

We also found that for patients at more than 10 weeks' gestation, median wait time between ultrasound and abortion visits increased by more than 5 days during the executive order

a

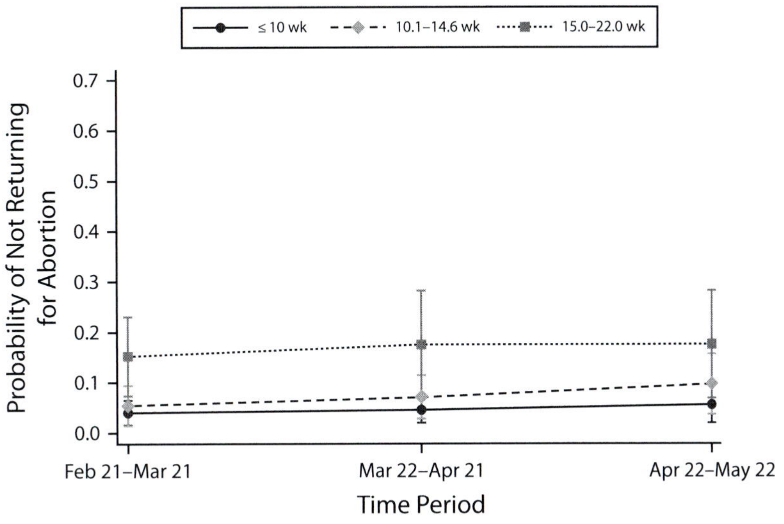

Gestation	Feb 21–Mar 21 Proportion (95% CI)	Mar 22–Apr 21 Proportion (95% CI)	Apr 22–May 22 Proportion (95% CI)
≤ 10 wk	0.04 (0.02, 0.06)	0.05 (0.02, 0.07)	0.06 (0.02, 0.09)
10.1–14.6 wk	0.05 (0.01, 0.09)	0.07 (0.03, 0.11)	0.10 (0.04, 0.16)
15.0–22.0 wk	0.16 (0.07, 0.23)	0.18 (0.07, 0.28)	0.18 (0.07, 0.28)

b

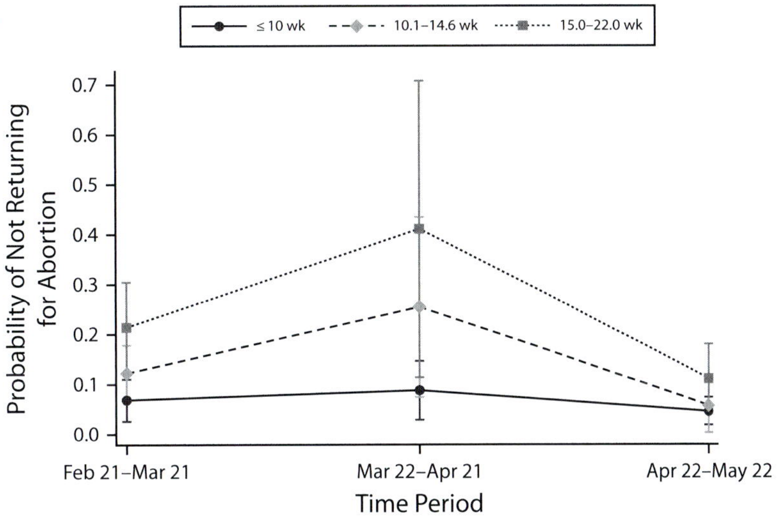

Gestation	Feb 21–Mar 21 Proportion (95% CI)	Mar 22–Apr 21 Proportion (95% CI)	Apr 22–May 22 Proportion (95% CI)
≤ 10 wk	0.07 (0.03, 0.11)	0.09 (0.03, 0.26)	0.05 (0.02, 0.07)
10.1–14.6 wk	0.13 (0.08, 0.18)	0.25 (0.07, 0.43)	0.06 (0.02, 0.11)
15.0–22.0 wk	0.22 (0.12, 0.30)	0.40 (0.11, 0.71)	0.11 (0.04, 0.18)

FIGURE 2— Proportion of Texas Patients Who Completed a State-Mandated Ultrasound but Did Not Return to the Facility for an Abortion, by Gestational Duration at Ultrasound and 30-Day Period in (a) 2019 and (b) 2020

Note. CI = confidence interval.

TABLE 2— Texas Patients' Median Number of Days ("Wait Time") Between Ultrasound and Abortion Visit and HR for Number of Days Between Visits: February 21–May 22, 2019, February 21–May 22, 2020

	No. Patients	Median No. Days Between Appointments (IQR)	HR (95% CI)
Period			
Feb 21–Mar 21, 2019	3044	2 (1–6)	0.98 (0.92, 1.04)
Mar 22–Apr 21, 2019	2764	2 (1–6)	1 (Ref)
Apr 22–May 22, 2019	2668	2 (1–7)	0.99 (0.92, 1.07)
Feb 21–Mar 21, 2020[a]	2292	2 (1–7)	1.01 (0.95, 1.08)
Mar 22–Apr 21, 2020	1323	2 (1–6)	1.00 (0.78, 1.27)
Apr 22–May 22, 2020	2347	3 (1–5)	1.10 (0.94, 1.29)
Gestational duration at ultrasound, wk			
≤ 10	11 661	2 (1–6)	1 (Ref)
10.1–14.6	1795	2 (1–7)	0.96 (0.91, 1.02)
15.0–22.0	922	3 (1–6)	1.02 (0.87, 1.20)
Missing	60	4.5 (2–14.5)	0.60 (0.42, 0.86)
Age, y			
< 18	348	3 (2–7)	0.94 (0.84, 1.05)
18–24	5216	2 (1–7)	0.92 (0.88, 0.96)
25–29	4106	2 (1–6)	1 (Ref)
30–34	2762	2 (1–6)	1.03 (0.97, 1.11)
≥ 35	2002	2 (1–5)	1.05 (1.01, 1.10)
Missing	4	3 (2–4)	1.31 (0.94, 1.84)
Race/ethnicity			
Asian	714	2 (1–5)	1.13 (1.02, 1.25)
Black	3491	3 (1–7)	0.93 (0.84, 1.02)
Hispanic	5224	2 (1–6)	1.00 (0.94, 1.07)
Other[b]	306	3 (1–7)	0.95 (0.86, 1.05)
White	3583	2 (1–7)	1 (Ref)
Missing	1120	2 (1–4)	1.14 (0.99, 1.31)
1-way distance to facility, miles			
< 10	2644	2 (1–6)	1 (Ref)
10–24	6012	2 (1–6)	0.99 (0.94, 1.05)
25–49	3031	2 (1–7)	0.94 (0.87, 1.02)
50–100	1620	2 (1–7)	0.93 (0.83, 1.04)
> 100	796	2 (1–5)	1.03 (0.92, 1.16)
Missing	335	2 (1–5)	1.36 (0.93, 1.98)
Distressed Community Index score			
Prosperous	3602	2 (1–6)	1 (Ref)
Comfortable	2252	2 (1–6)	1.01 (0.98, 1.05)
Midtier	2416	2 (1–7)	1.00 (0.93, 1.07)
At risk	2967	2 (1–6)	1.07 (0.97, 1.17)
Distressed	2843	2 (1–6)	1.02 (0.90, 1.17)
Missing	358	2 (1–5)	0.85 (0.62, 1.18)

Note. CI = confidence interval; HR = hazard ratio; IQR = interquartile range. The sample size was n = 14 438.
[a]Denotes the 30-day executive order period.
[b]Other includes American Indian, Alaska Native, Native Hawaiian, Pacific Islander, and multiracial.

compared with the same 30-day period in 2019. This increase in wait time for patients at more than 10 weeks' gestation may be because those patients were ineligible for medication abortion and unable to travel out of state and therefore were unable to obtain an abortion until after the order was lifted. Longer wait times can increase both cost and risks related to abortion[11,29] in addition to the mental and emotional toll of prolonged forced pregnancy.[13] Longer wait times may also prevent some patients from obtaining an abortion because abortion care later in pregnancy may be more difficult to access because fewer facilities provide this service.[12,13]

The executive order period shares several similarities to the current legal context. The suspension of abortion procedures during the order and changing court decisions created confusion for patients about whether and what types of abortion services were available.[30] Similarly, following the US Supreme Court's decision in *Dobbs v Jackson Women's Health Organization*, which overturned *Roe v Wade*, state-level abortion restrictions have frequently been implemented, temporarily enjoined, and later upheld or struck down. This has already occurred in Ohio, Georgia, Florida, and Iowa[31–33] and may soon occur in Arizona.[34] Changing state-level abortion policies creates confusion for patients about the legality of abortion and may lead some patients to inaccurately believe they are unable to obtain in-state care. Expanded access to health care navigators who can provide abortion seekers with timely and accurate information about their options could reduce confusion and improve abortion access in this new abortion landscape.[30]

Limitations and Strengths

There are several limitations to this study. Although our data account for more than half of all abortions provided in Texas during the study period, we were able to obtain data from only 13 of the 23 Texas abortion facilities operating at that time. The 13 facilities included in our study were located in each of the metropolitan areas where abortion care was provided; however, the 10 facilities that either did not respond to our requests or were unable to provide information needed for analyses may have served different populations, which may bias our findings. Furthermore, data on race, ethnicity, and gestational duration at ultrasound were not missing at random, so we did not impute these values. Consequently, our findings may not adequately capture the abortion experiences of people of color or those at later gestational stages.

Additionally, although we included information from 30-day time intervals before and after the executive order period in both 2019 and 2020 to control for time confounders, we could not fully disentangle the effect of the executive order from the potential effects of the onset of COVID-19. The inability of physicians who resided out of state to travel to Texas, reduction in clinic hours, financial stressors, and fear of contracting COVID-19 may have also contributed to declines in abortion return rates. However, similar patterns in ultrasound and abortion visits in the 30-day period following the executive order and the same 30-day period in 2019, despite the ongoing COVID-19 pandemic, lend credibility to the order's unique impacts.

Strengths of this study include our use of a large sample of individual-level data to examine effects of the executive order on abortion visit return rates, wait time between ultrasound and abortion visits, and disparities by gestational duration, which previous studies using aggregate data were unable to do.[14,24]

Public Health Implications

We estimate that the 83% of patients who had an ultrasound during the executive order in Texas and were able to return for their abortion spent an additional 5 to 7 days pregnant if they were not eligible for medication abortion. Moreover, nearly 1 in 6 patients were not able to return for their abortion. These patients may have traveled to another state or clinic in Texas, self-managed their abortion, or continued their pregnancy. We conclude that short-term abortion bans are associated with reduced access to timely care and disproportionately harm patients at more than 10 weeks' gestation. Expanding access to patient navigators could help mitigate the negative impacts of future and impending abortion bans by increasing patients' awareness of their options and resources. AJPH

ABOUT THE AUTHORS

Brooke Whitfield, Gracia Sierra, Klaira Lerma, Vinita Goyal, and Kari White are with the Population Research Center, University of Texas at Austin. Lauren Thaxton is with Dell Medical School, University of Texas at Austin. Bhavik Kumar is with Planned Parenthood Gulf Coast, Houston, TX. Allison Gilbert is with Southwestern Women's Surgery Center, Dallas, TX.

CORRESPONDENCE

Correspondence should be sent to Brooke Whitfield, 305 E. 23rd St, Stop G1800, RLP 2.602, Austin, TX 78712 (e-mail: bwhitfield@utexas.edu). Reprints can be ordered at https://www.ajph.org by clicking the "Reprints" link.

PUBLICATION INFORMATION

Full Citation: Whitfield B, Sierra G, Lerma K, et al. Abortion return rates and wait times before and after Texas' executive order banning abortion during COVID-19. *Am J Public Health*. 2024;114(10): 1013–1023.

Acceptance Date: May 28, 2024.
DOI: https://doi.org/10.2105/AJPH.2024.307747

ORCID iDs:
Brooke Whitfield https://orcid.org/0000-0002-3309-4205
Klaira Lerma https://orcid.org/0000-0002-3075-9814
Lauren Thaxton https://orcid.org/0000-0002-1368-0709
Allison Gilbert https://orcid.org/0000-0002-0053-2555

CONTRIBUTORS

B. Whitfield drafted the article and conducted all analyses. G. Sierra led data management and assisted with data analysis and visualization. K. Lerma, V. Goyal, L. Thaxton, B. Kumar, and A. Gilbert assisted with data collection and article conceptualization. K. White conceptualized the study and oversaw data collection. All authors interpretated the results and critically reviewed the article.

ACKNOWLEDGMENTS

This study was supported by a grant from the Susan Thompson Buffett Foundation and the National Institute of Child Health and Human Development awarded to the Population Research Center at the University of Texas at Austin (grant P2CHD042849).

This work was previously presented at the 2022 Society of Family Planning Annual Meeting in Baltimore, MD.

We acknowledge Gabriela Alvarez Pérez, Ashlyn Lafferty, and Allison Olfers for their support with data entry. We also acknowledge the facilities who provided data.

Note. Study sponsors were not involved in the study design; data collection, analysis, and interpretation; writing; or the decision to submit the article for publication.

CONFLICTS OF INTEREST

The authors have no potential or actual conflicts of interest to disclose.

HUMAN PARTICIPANT PROTECTION

The University of Texas at Austin institutional review board approved this study.

REFERENCES

1. Paxton K. Health care professionals and facilities, including abortion providers, must immediately stop all medically unnecessary surgeries and procedures to preserve resources to fight COVID-19 pandemic. March 23, 2020. Available at: https://www.texasattorneygeneral.gov/news/releases/health-care-professionals-and-facilities-including-abortion-providers-must-immediately-stop-all. Accessed March 30, 2020.
2. American College of Obstetricians and Gynecologists. Joint statement on abortion access during the COVID-19 outbreak. March 18, 2020. Available at: https://www.acog.org/news/news-releases/2020/03/joint-statement-on-abortion-access-during-the-covid-19-outbreak. Accessed July 23, 2024.
3. Guttmacher Institute. State facts about abortion: Texas. 2022. Available at: https://www.guttmacher.org/fact-sheet/state-facts-about-abortion-texas. Accessed April 20, 2022.
4. Fulcher IR, Onwuzurike C, Goldberg AB, Cottrill AA, Fortin J, Janiak E. The impact of the COVID-19 pandemic on abortion care utilization and disparities by age. *Am J Obstet Gynecol.* 2022;226(6):819.e1–819.e15. https://doi.org/10.1016/j.ajog.2022.01.025
5. Hwang CS, Kesselheim AS, Sarpatwari A, Huybrechts KF, Brill G, Rome BN. Changes in induced medical and procedural abortion rates in a commercially insured population, 2018 to 2022. *Ann Intern Med.* 2023;176(11):1508–1515. https://doi.org/10.7326/M23-1609
6. Roberts SCM, Schroeder R, Joffe C. COVID-19 and independent abortion providers: findings from a rapid-response survey. *Perspect Sex Reprod Health.* 2020;52(4):217–225. https://doi.org/10.1363/psrh.12163
7. US Food and Drug Administration. Information about mifepristone for medical termination of pregnancy through ten weeks gestation. 2023. Available at: https://www.fda.gov/drugs/postmarket-drug-safety-information-patients-and-providers/information-about-mifepristone-medical-termination-pregnancy-through-ten-weeks-gestation. Accessed August 23, 2023.
8. National Academies of Sciences, Engineering, and Medicine. *The Safety and Quality of Abortion Care in the United States.* Washington, DC: National Academies Press; 2018. https://doi.org/10.17226/24950
9. Upadhyay UD, Weitz TA, Jones RK, Barar RE, Foster DG. Denial of abortion because of provider gestational age limits in the United States. *Am J Public Health.* 2014;104(9):1687–1694. https://doi.org/10.2105/AJPH.2013.301378
10. Foster DG, Kimport K. Who seeks abortions at or after 20 weeks? *Perspect Sex Reprod Health.* 2013;45(4):210–218. [Erratum in: *Perspect Sex Reprod Health.* 2019;51(3):185. https://doi.org/10.1363/psrh.12114]. https://doi.org/10.1363/4521013
11. Upadhyay UD, Ahlbach C, Kaller S, Cook C, Muñoz I. Trends in self-pay charges and insurance acceptance for abortion in the United States, 2017–20. *Health Aff (Millwood).* 2022;41(4):507–515. https://doi.org/10.1377/hlthaff.2021.01528
12. Jones RK, Kooistra K. Abortion incidence and access to services in the United States. *Perspect Sex Reprod Health.* 2008;43(1):41–50. https://doi.org/10.1363/4304111
13. Greene Foster D. *The Turnaway Study: Ten Years, a Thousand Women and the Consequences of Having or Being Denied an Abortion.* New York, NY: Scribner; 2020.
14. White K, Kumar B, Goyal V, Wallace R, Roberts SCM, Grossman D. Changes in abortion in Texas following an executive order ban during the coronavirus pandemic. *JAMA.* 2021;325(7):691–693. https://doi.org/10.1001/jama.2020.24096
15. Stupp PW, Warren CW. Seasonal differences in pregnancy outcomes: United States, 1971–1989. *Ann N Y Acad Sci.* 1994;709(1):46–54. https://doi.org/10.1111/j.1749-6632.1994.tb30387.x
16. Franklin TE, Theisen G, Salyer CV, Pinkston C, Gunaratnam B. The seasonality of abortion in Kentucky. *Contraception.* 2017;95(2):181–185. https://doi.org/10.1016/j.contraception.2016.08.019
17. Allen RH, Goldberg AB. Cervical dilation before first-trimester surgical abortion (<14 weeks' gestation). *Contraception.* 2016;93(4):277–291. https://doi.org/10.1016/j.contraception.2015.12.001
18. Fox MC, Krajewski C. Cervical preparation for second-trimester surgical abortion prior to 20 weeks' gestation: SFP guideline #2013-4. *Contraception.* 2013;89(2):75–84. https://doi.org/10.1016/j.contraception.2013.11.001
19. Lantos H, Pliskin E, Wildsmith E, Manlove J. State-level abortion restrictions will negatively impact teens and children. October 19, 2022. Available at: https://www.childtrends.org/blog/state-level-abortion-restrictions-will-negatively-impact-teens-and-children. Accessed August 24, 2023.
20. Artiga S, Hill L, Ranji U, Gomez I. What are the implications of the overturning of *Roe v Wade* for racial disparities? Kaiser Family Foundation, 2022. Available at: https://www.iomc.org/resources/Documents/What%20are%20the%20Implications%20of%20the%20Overturning%20of%20Roe%20v.%20Wade%20for%20Racial%20Disparities_%20_%20KFF.pdf. Accessed August 24, 2023.
21. Pleasants EA, Cartwright AF, Upadhyay UD. Association between distance to an abortion facility and abortion or pregnancy outcome among a prospective cohort of people seeking abortion online. *JAMA Netw Open.* 2022;5(5):e2212065. https://doi.org/10.1001/jamanetworkopen.2022.12065
22. Huber S, Rust C. Calculate travel time and distance with OpenStreetMap data using the Open Source Routing Machine (OSRM). *Stata J.* 2016;16(2):416–423. https://doi.org/10.1177/1536867X1601600209
23. Economic Innovation Group. The Distressed Communities Index. 2020. Available at: https://eig.org/distressed-communities. Accessed August 17, 2022.
24. Hill BJ, Lock L, Parks V, Anderson B, Cathey JR. Coronavirus disease 2019 (COVID-19) and access to abortion. *Obstet Gynecol.* 2021;138(3):475–477. https://doi.org/10.1097/AOG.0000000000004516
25. Carpenter E, Burke KL, Vizcarra E, Dane'el A, Goyal V, White K. Texas' executive order during COVID-19 increased barriers for patients seeking abortion care. Available at: http://sites.utexas.edu/txpep/files/2020/12/TxPEP-research-brief-COVID-abortion-patients.pdf. Accessed July 23, 2024.
26. Carpenter E, Gyuras H, Burke KL, et al. Seeking abortion care in Ohio and Texas during the COVID-19 pandemic. *Contraception.* 2023;118:109896. https://doi.org/10.1016/j.contraception.2022.09.134
27. White K, Dane'el A, Vizcarra E, et al. Out-of-State travel for abortion following implementation of Texas Senate Bill 8. 2022. Available at: http://sites.utexas.edu/txpep/files/2022/03/TxPEP-out-of-state-SB8.pdf. Accessed April 28, 2022.
28. Aiken ARA, Starling JE, Gomperts R, Tec M, Scott JG, Aiken CE. Demand for self-managed online telemedicine abortion in the United States during the coronavirus disease 2019 (COVID-19) pandemic. *Obstet Gynecol.* 2020;136(4):835–837. https://doi.org/10.1097/AOG.0000000000004081
29. Bartlett LA, Berg CJ, Shulman HB, et al. Risk factors for legal induced abortion-related mortality in the United States. *Obstet Gynecol.* 2004;103(4):729–737. https://doi.org/10.1097/01.AOG.0000116260.81570.60

30. White K, Leyser-Whalen O, Whitfield B, et al. Abortion assistance fund staff and volunteers as patient navigators following an abortion ban in Texas. *Perspect Sex Reprod Health*. 2023; Epub ahead of print. https://doi.org/10.1363/psrh.12240

31. Hendrickson S. Ohio law banning nearly all abortions now invalid after referendum, attorney general says. April 1, 2024. Available at: https://apnews.com/article/abortion-amendment-ohio-attorney-general-e6586d27b115372ede261c41d3ce2346. Accessed April 14, 2024.

32. Thanawala S. Georgia Supreme Court sends abortion law challenge back to lower court, leaving access unchanged. October 24, 2023. Available at: https://apnews.com/article/abortion-ban-georgia-six-weeks-5faf4cc7d311cafc56b735825d515760. Accessed April 14, 2024.

33. Farrington B. Florida Supreme Court upholds state's 15-week abortion ban, but voters will soon have a say. April 1, 2024. Available at: https://apnews.com/article/florida-abortion-ban-supreme-court-ruling-6a4949fc7459afe9b5e298086a793126. Accessed April 14, 2024.

34. Billeaud J, Lee M. What to know about the near-total 1864 ban. Available at: https://apnews.com/article/arizona-abortion-ban-what-to-know-797a4bbbc738497fe2284d6870c5be24. Accessed April 14, 2024.

Unequal Spatial Consequences of Abortion Restrictions in Texas, 2021–2023

Sydney R. Sauter, MPH, Maeve E. Wallace, PhD, and Julie H. Hernandez, PhD

See also Abortion Access 2 Years After *Dobbs v Jackson* Ruling, pp. 994–1050.

Objectives. To demonstrate the spatially uneven effects of abortion restriction laws in Texas.

Methods. We used network analysis to determine the change in distance to the nearest surgical abortion provider for 5253 Texas neighborhoods after the passing of Texas Senate Bill 8 (SB8; 2021) and the US Supreme Court's *Dobbs v Jackson Women's Health Organization* (2022) decision. We identified associations between key measures of neighborhood socioeconomic context and change in distance to providers using multivariable linear regression models.

Results. After the *Dobbs* decision, Texas residents experienced an average change in distance to the nearest provider of 457 miles (SD = 179). Neighborhoods of concentrated disadvantage experienced the greatest increase in distance to abortion providers after SB8's passing, and neighborhoods with high levels of income inequality experienced the greatest increase in distance after the *Dobbs* decision.

Conclusions. We document the rapidly changing abortion landscape in a highly restrictive state and show that women living in more disadvantaged and unequal areas are most affected by the increasing distance to providers.

Public Health Implications. Our methods and findings will continue to be relevant in understanding the burden placed on women in areas where medical abortion has been restricted because of the *Dobbs* decision. (*Am J Public Health*. 2024;114(10):1024–1033. https://doi.org/10.2105/AJPH.2024.307652)

AJPH October 2024, Vol. 114, No. 10

On June 24, 2022, the US Supreme Court's ruling in *Dobbs v Jackson Women's Health Organization* (142 S. Ct. 2228 [*Dobbs*]) overturned the court's 1973 ruling in *Roe v Wade* (93 S. Ct. 705 [*Roe*]), thereby ending the constitutional right to abortion services in the United States. This decision allows states to restrict access to the procedure on an individual basis. As of May 2024, 14 states have total abortion bans in place, and another 7 have enforced strict gestational age limits.[1]

Since before the *Dobbs* decision, the national abortion rate has been slowly increasing.[2] This trend masks large disparities between states, however. Although states with abortion bans experienced a 100% decrease in abortions since the *Dobbs* decision, states without abortion bans have seen an increase in caseload.[3] These data suggest an increase in the need for abortion services, as well as the possibility that pregnant people needing abortion services in states with abortion bans are traveling to receive care in states where the procedure is legally allowed.

Texas has historically been one of the most hostile toward abortion services, with several pieces of legislation that limit the availability of medical abortion over the decade before the *Dobbs* decision. One such law was House Bill 2, implemented in 2014. This law forced nearly half of the state's clinics to close, resulting in increased mean distance to providers, greater congestion at remaining clinics, and a large reduction in the abortion rate.[4,5]

In 2021, the state enacted Senate Bill 8 (SB8). This law prohibited medical abortion after 6 weeks' gestation, making it one of the first near bans in the country.[6] As a result, Texas clinics were required to cease services related to abortion services or close their doors altogether. The number of facility abortions in the state fell by half in the month after SB8 implementation, whereas the proportion of Texas women receiving abortion services in the neighboring states increased from 12% to 30% over the same period, indicating that women were leaving the state to receive services.[7] With the *Dobbs* decision, Texas enacted a total abortion ban in 2022, resulting in the closure of the remaining facility-based abortion providers. Although pregnant people may previously have been able to seek abortion services in bordering states, Oklahoma, Arkansas, and Louisiana also enacted total abortion bans after the *Dobbs* decision.[1]

Given the impact of previous legislation on the abortion landscape in Texas and the surrounding region, it is important to understand the effect of both SB8 and the state's trigger ban on the residents who are now forced to seek medical abortion services elsewhere. Geographic information systems (GISs) allow a greater understanding of the distance people must travel to obtain a medical abortion across state lines, while also pinpointing the populations most affected. Although various pathways to abortion after the *Dobbs* decision have been documented, such as self-managed abortion, abortion by mail, and telehealth, recent court proceedings have challenged the legality of medication abortion by mail, and in-clinic visits may be required to obtain any abortion medication in the future.[8] Thus, distance to the nearest provider is increasingly important as abortion restrictions continue across the country.

Legislation aimed at restricting or banning abortion services has disproportionately affected socioeconomically disadvantaged pregnant people, as they are less likely to have the means to seek a new provider or travel long distances to obtain care outside their state of residence. Additionally, people of color and lower socioeconomic status have been documented to experience abortion later in pregnancy and therefore more often require surgical abortion over medication abortion, which further warrants our focus on facility-based surgical abortion.[9]

Although existing research focuses on spatial effects at the state and county levels,[10] a more detailed analysis at the neighborhood level is useful considering the spatially segregated nature of poverty and exclusion in most Southern states.[11,12] We identified the degree to which Texas neighborhoods were affected by abortion bans in 2021 and 2022 in terms of the change in the distance to the nearest facility-based surgical abortion provider. Moreover, we aimed to highlight the uneven impact of these bans by exploring the profile of the most affected neighborhoods. We hypothesized that socially and economically disadvantaged neighborhoods would have the largest increase in distance to care.

METHODS

We obtained data for this project using the National Historical GIS Data Finder and 5-year census estimates from the US Census Bureau American Community Survey (2015–2019).[13] Although the use of census tracts to approximate neighborhoods has limitations,[14] we chose to use them as our unit of analysis for data availability reasons, as is common in the public health literature.[15–17] We operationalized variables pertaining to the sociodemographic characteristics of the tract population at the individual and household levels as area-based composite measures for analysis. Census data are limited to binary definitions of gender; consequently, we exploited the category of women of reproductive age (15–49 years) to approximate the population with a capacity for pregnancy. We acknowledge that not all people with a capacity for pregnancy are captured in this definition.

We used area-based composite measures of disadvantage and inequality to characterize Texas neighborhoods. These included indices of socioeconomic position (SEP), concentrated disadvantage (CD),[18] income inequality, and concentration at the extremes (ICE).[19]

The SEP index combined the mean standardized *z* scores for the proportion of individuals in a census tract who were working class, were living in poverty, and had less than a high school education and the median household income of the tract (reverse-coded). Operationalization of CD included the proportion of households receiving public assistance, households without a vehicle available, woman-headed households, families below the poverty threshold, individuals in the labor force who were unemployed, and individuals younger than 18 years. We *z* score transformed all variables to create a measure of the mean score, and we used a confirmatory factor analysis to ensure the validity of the final composite measures. We then converted the SEP index and CD variables into quintiles to meaningfully represent the constructs and avoid assumptions of a linear trend in change in distance.

We evaluated income inequality with the Gini index, a commonly used measure ranging from 0 to 1, with 0 representing total equality of incomes and 1 representing total inequality.[20] For this analysis, we further constructed the value into a categorical variable to represent low and high income inequality relative to the rest of the sample.

Finally, we estimated the ICE to measure racial and economic spatial polarization across census tracts. The ICE value measures the degree to which the tract population is concentrated into extremes of racial and economic privilege (White and high income) and deprivation (non-White and low income). It is calculated by taking the number of White householders with more than $100 000 annual income (the 80th percentile) and subtracting the number of householders who are people of color with less than $25 000 annual income (the 20th percentile), divided by the total population with data on income in each census tract. Possible values ranged from +1 (concentrated privilege so that 100% of the neighborhood are affluent White households) to −1 (concentrated deprivation so that 100% of the neighborhood are low-income households of people of color). An advantage of the ICE over other measures of inequality is that it uniquely identifies the directionality of inequality (e.g., both a neighborhood of 100% low-income residents and a neighborhood of 100% high-income residents would have the same Gini value). It also simultaneously captures multiple dimensions of inequalities (both economic and racial), which is of particular importance for understanding the processes that underly population health inequities.

Surgical Abortion Clinic Location

We included only clinics performing surgical abortions, rather than those that provide medication abortions, to ensure that comprehensive abortion care was available at each clinic. Because each state included in the analysis has different laws and regulations for medication abortion, this restriction simplified the analysis and is likely a valid indicator given that surgical abortions constitute roughly half of induced medical abortions.[21] We compiled data pertaining to the location of surgical abortion clinics using Google Earth software and the Advancing New Standards in Reproductive Health Abortion Facilities Database.[22] We located surgical abortion clinics on a state-by-state basis using the database, and we further investigated each individual clinic using publicly available Web sites to confirm the current availability of surgical abortion procedures. We used the Google Earth Pro address locator tool to georeference these clinics and obtain their geographic coordinates (latitude and longitude). We mapped operating clinics in 3 waves: clinics open before SB8 was passed, after SB8 was passed (i.e., after August 2021), and after *Dobbs* was decided (i.e., after June 2022).

Changes in Distance-to-Care Analysis

We obtained census tract shapefiles for the 48 contiguous US states and imported them into QGIS3.21.[23] We obtained primary and secondary road network shapefiles from the US Census Bureau portal. We reprojected all data for both the basemap and abortion clinic points using ESRI 102003 (Environmental Systems Research Institute, Redlands, CA) for the US contiguous Albers equal area conic projection. The resulting maps can be found in Figures A–C (available as a supplement to the online version of this article at http://www.ajph.org/). We then created a new layer showing the centroid of each census tract in Texas and then used ESRI's OD matrix tool to complete a network analysis using the roads shapefile. The resulting database included the calculated distance between the centroid of each Texas census tract and the nearest abortion clinic using the primary and secondary road network. We allowed a topological tolerance of 6 miles for entry and exit costs.

We repeated the analysis so that each census tract received a separate distance value for each wave of analysis. We then extracted the data from QGIS for further analysis.

Outcome

The study outcome generated from the spatial analysis is the change in distance from the closest surgical abortion provider in 2 phases: after (1) the implementation of SB8, and (2) the overturning of *Roe*. We calculated the change in distance as the difference in distance (in miles) before SB8 implementation and the distance directly after each legislative wave. We then examined the change in the distance as a continuous outcome in 2 separate regression analyses.

Analytic Methods

After data exporting and merging by the GISJOIN identifier, 5253 of the 5265 census tracts in Texas were available for analysis. We carried out all statistical analyses using SAS version 9.4 (SAS Institute, Cary, NC). We ran descriptive statistics to evaluate central tendency and normality of census tract measures. Then we fit crude and adjusted linear regression models with cluster-robust SEs to estimate the associations between each neighborhood's (census tract) characteristics and the 2 change in distance outcomes, after SB8 implementation and after the *Roe* decision, controlling for all other measures of socioeconomic position and disadvantage. Given the unique advantages of each neighborhood measure we used, we present both crude and mutually adjusted models to account for the various dimensions of neighborhood (dis)-advantage we analyzed. We weighted the models by the proportion of women of reproductive age (15–49 years) in each census tract.

RESULTS

Results from the descriptive analysis are displayed in Table 1. On average, neighborhoods in Texas experienced a change in distance of 213 miles (SD = 121) to the nearest provider after the implementation of SB8. After *Roe* reversal, the mean distance change was 457 miles (SD = 179). The resulting maps appear in Figure 1. Almost all Texas census tracts were affected by both waves of legislation, with 4886 (92.8%) census tracts experiencing an increased distance change (> 0 miles) after SB8 implementation and 5207 (98.9%) census tracts experiencing a distance change after the overturning of *Roe*. We also explored additional travel days, with 1 full additional day of travel time by car calculated as an increase of 490 miles (7 hours driving at 70 miles per hour—the average speed limit on Texas highways—excluding breaks). At this threshold, roughly 48.8% of census tracts experienced at least a full additional travel day after the overturning of *Roe*, representing roughly 3.6 million women of reproductive age (not shown).

TABLE 1— Characteristics of Texas Census Tracts: American Community Survey 5-Year Estimates, 2015–2019

Characteristic	Mean ±SD or No. (%)
Change in distance to provider after SB8,[a] miles	213.7 ±121.3
Change in distance to provider after the *Roe* decision, miles	457.0 ±178.8
Affected by SB8 (change in mileage > 0)	4886 ±92.8
Affected by *Roe* reversal (change in mileage > 0)	5207 ±98.9
Additional driving day (> 490 miles change in mileage)	2571 ±48.8
SEP index (n = 5228)[b,c]	
Highest	−1.2 (0.4)
High	−0.4 (0.2)
Middle	−0.01 (0.1)
Low	0.5 (0.2)
Lowest	1.2 (0.4)
CD; standardized mean score (n = 5228)[d]	
Lowest	−0.8 (0.2)
Low	−0.5 (0.2)
Middle	−0.2 (0.1)
High	0.3 (0.2)
Highest	1.1 (0.5)
ICE (n = 5212)[b]	
Highest deprivation	−0.3 (0.1)
High deprivation	−0.2 (0.02)
Middle	−0.1 (0.02)
High privilege	−0.1 (0.02)
Highest privilege	0.1 (0.1)
Gini index (n = 5207),[b] inequality	
Lowest	0.3 (0.03)
Low	0.4 (0.01)
Middle	0.4 (0.01)
High	0.5 (0.01)
Highest	0.5 (0.04)

Note. CD = concentrated disadvantage; ICE = index of concentration; SB8 = Texas Senate Bill 8; SEP = socioeconomic position. The study population size was n = 5253.
[a]SB8 banned abortion after roughly 6 wk gestational age and was implemented August 2021.
[b]Indices categorized by quintiles.
[c]SEP index variable (mean *z* scored) composed of % individuals with less than 12 y education, % individuals living below the poverty threshold, % individuals employed in primarily working-class jobs, median household income (reverse-coded).
[d]CD variable (mean *z* scored) composed of % non-White individuals, % unemployed individuals in labor force, % woman-headed households, % households receiving public assistance, % households with no vehicle available, and % families living below poverty threshold.

The median Gini coefficient for Texas census tracts was 0.42 (SD = 0.06; not shown). Neighborhoods in the highest quintile of income inequality had Gini values at or above 0.52. Finally, the ICE value in the sample was skewed toward deprivation, with a mean value of −0.13 (SD = 0.14; not shown). Neighborhoods in the quintile of highest privilege had an ICE value of only 0.05 (SD = 0.08).

Detailed descriptive results for the remaining census tract characteristics, as well as those used to construct the contextual variables, can be found

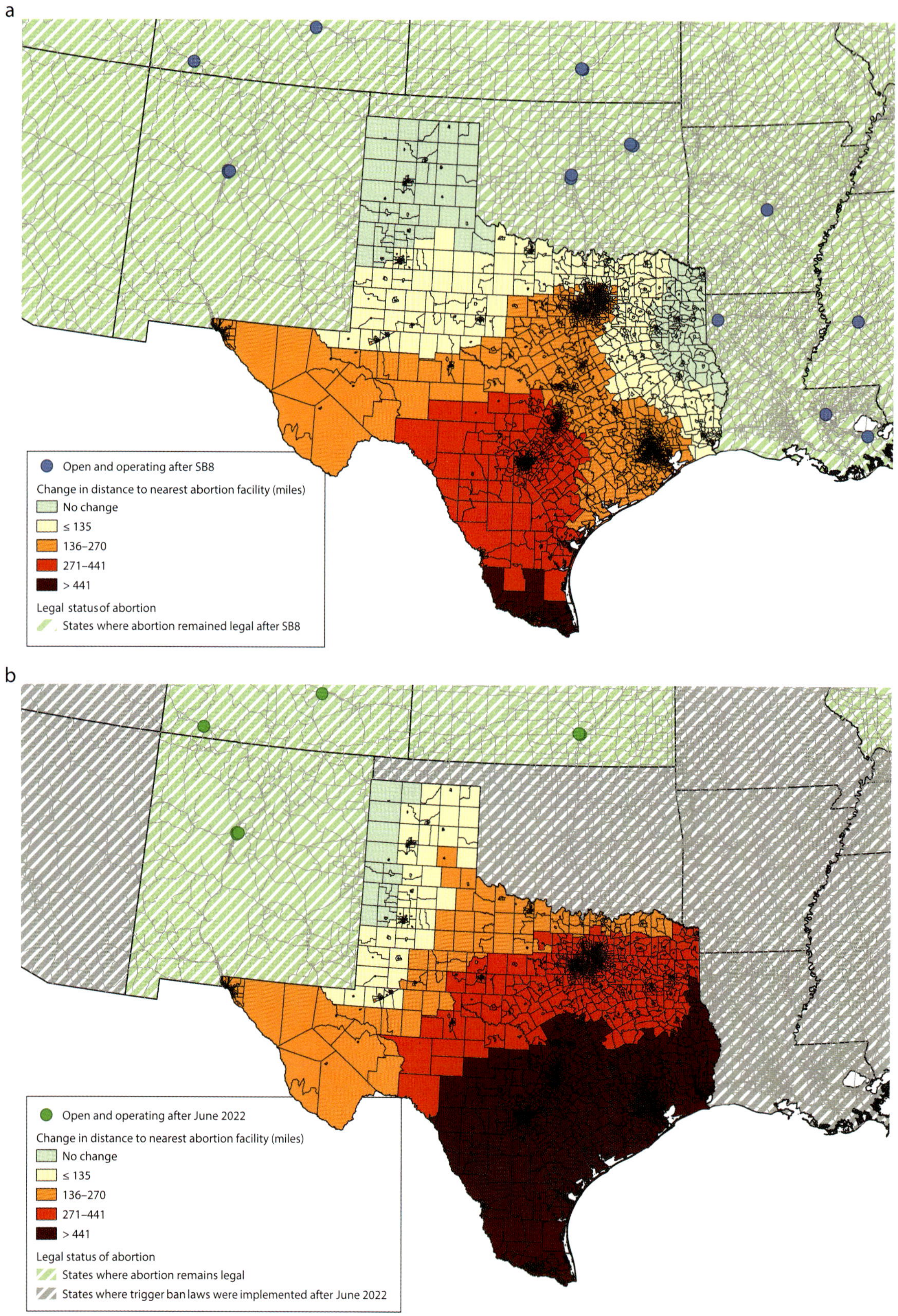

FIGURE 1— **Changes in Distance (in Miles) to Nearest Abortion Provider After (a) Texas Senate Bill 8 (SB8) Passed and (b) *Dobbs v Jackson* Decision: Texas, August 2021–July 2022**

in Appendix Table A (available as a supplement to the online version of this article at http://www.ajph.org).

Regression Analysis for SB8

Results from the generalized linear regression analysis for the change in distance after the implementation of SB8 can be found in Table 2. Model 1 demonstrates the crude, unadjusted relationship of each individual predictor with the outcome, and model 2 demonstrates the full regression model with all predictors included.

After the implementation of SB8, census tracts in the lowest SEP quintile had a significantly ($P<.001$) larger change in distance to the closest provider than did those in the highest SEP quintile. Interestingly, this relationship did not remain consistent once other predictors were controlled for in model 2. In the fully adjusted model, all lower levels of SEP experienced a significant ($P<.001$) negative change in distance compared with the highest SEP.

Census tracts with the highest levels of CD were significantly farther from providers than were those with less CD in both models, showing a clear dose–response relationship. In the fully adjusted model, census tracts with the highest levels of CD were roughly 69 additional miles (95% confidence interval [CI] = 51.66, 85.34; $P<.001$) farther from a provider than were those with the lowest levels of CD.

Both those in the highest deprivation and those in the highest privilege quintiles were significantly ($P<.001$) farther from a provider than were those in the middle quintile in model 1 (B = 79 miles; 95% CI = 67.26, 91.42 and 15 miles; 95% CI = 7.49, 22.32, respectively) although this relationship was attenuated in model 2, and only the highest deprivation census tracts were significantly ($P<.001$) farther from a provider (B = 70.5 miles; 95% CI = 58.03, 82.92). The Gini coefficient for income inequality did not demonstrate a clear significant relationship between levels in either model.

TABLE 2— Multiple Linear Regression for Change in Distance (in Miles) to Provider After Senate Bill 8 Passed in Texas: August 2021–September 2021

	Model 1 (Unadjusted), B (95% CI)	Model 2 (Adjusted),[a] B (95% CI)
SEP index[b]		
Highest (Ref)	0	0
High	−12.22 (−20.16, −4.28)	−16.58 (−25.62, −7.54)
Middle	−27.53 (−36.04, −19.00)	−47.11 (−58.66, −35.55)
Low	−12.90 (−21.94, −3.87)	−63.85 (−78.27, −49.44)
Lowest	41.46 (31.26, 51.66)	−51.92 (−69.87, −33.97)
CD[c]		
Lowest (Ref)	0	0
Low	−11.36 (−19,49, −3.24)	−3.18 (−12.02, 5.64)
Middle	−16.91 (−25.68, −8.15)	7.4 (−8.85, 18.66)
High	1.18 (−7.77, 10.14)	28.32 (14.86, 41.77)
Highest	53.77 (43.21, 64.32)	68.50 (51.66, 85.34)
ICE		
Highest deprivation	79.34 (67.26, 91.42)	70.48 (58.03, 82.92)
High deprivation	4.2 (−5.71, 14.45)	9.97 (−0.22, 20.15)
Middle (Ref)	0	0
High privilege	18.36 (10.13, 26.59)	6.04 (−2.66, 14.74)
Highest privilege	14.91 (7.49, 22.32)	−3.86 (−12.04, 4.31)
Gini Index, inequality		
Lowest (Ref)	0	0
Low	−7.95 (−16.56, 0.66)	−14.27 (−22.90, −5.64)
Middle	−7.24 (−16.40, 1.92)	−20.77 (−29.81, −11.73)
High	6.63 (−3.61, 16.86)	−17.04 (−26.99, −7.08)
Highest	4.95 (−7.56, 11.87)	−24.61 (−34.46, −14.77)
Intercept	. . .	229.83 (219.03, 224.64)

Note. CD = concentrated disadvantage; CI = confidence interval; ICE = index of concentration; SEP = socioeconomic position. The study population size was n = 5207.
[a]Adjusted model includes all covariates related to socioeconomic status (SEP, CD, ICE, and Gini).
[b]SEP Index variable (mean *z* scored) composed of % individuals with < 12 y education, % individuals living below the poverty threshold, % individuals employed in primarily working-class jobs, median household income (reverse-coded).
[c]CD variable (mean *z* scored) composed of % non-White individuals, % unemployed individuals in labor force, % female-headed households, % households receiving public assistance, % households with no vehicle available, and % families living below poverty threshold.

Regression Analysis for *Roe* Reversal

Results from the generalized linear regression analysis for the change in distance after Texas's trigger ban are displayed in Table 3. Model 1 presents the crude, unadjusted relationship of each individual predictor with the

TABLE 3— Multiple Linear Regression for Change in Distance (in Miles) to Abortion Provider After *Roe* Reversal in Texas: August 2021–July 2022

	Model 1 (Unadjusted), B (95% CI)	Model 2 (Adjusted),[a] B (95% CI)
SEP index[b]		
Highest (Ref)	0	0
High	−20.48 (−33.68, −7.28)	−28.14 (−42.79, −13.49)
Middle	−30.86 (−44.54, −17.17)	−55.67 (−73.89, −37.46)
Low	−12.12 (−26.47, −2.22)	−73.13 (−95.73, −37.46)
Lowest	47.09 (31.87, 62.31)	−56.76 (−84.56, −28.96)
CD[c]		
Lowest (Ref)	0	0
Low	−4.41 (−17.83, 9.02)	16.14 (2.00, 30.29)
Middle	−7.94 (−22.07, 6.20)	38.66 (21.29, 56.03)
High	19.11 (4.80, 33.41)	73.87 (53.10, 94.64)
Highest	81.22 (66.10, 96.32)	125.12 (99.65, 150.59)
ICE		
Highest deprivation	65.22 (47.50, 82.93)	23.37 (4.57, 42.17)
High deprivation	−0.41 (−14.89, 15.71)	−6.64 (−22.13, 8.83)
Middle (Ref)	0	0
High privilege	27.61 (14.23, 40.98)	24.03 (9.89, 38.17)
Highest privilege	30.08 (17.27, 42.89)	21.72 (7.73, 35.71)
Gini index, inequality		
Lowest (Ref)	0	0
Low	−0.08 (−14.26, 14.10)	2.47 (−11.73, 16.67)
Middle	8.92 (−5.40, 23.24)	8.42 (−6.12, 22.97)
High	31.78 (16.68, 46.88)	25.01 (9.54, 40.47)
Highest	30.98 (16.26, 45.71)	22.92 (7.47, 38.38)
Intercept	. . .	425.34 (407.56, 443.11)

Note. CD = concentrated disadvantage; CI = confidence interval; ICE = index of concentration; SEP = socioeconomic position. The study population size was n = 5207.

[a]Adjusted model includes all covariates related to socioeconomic status (SEP, CD, ICE and Gini).

[b]SEP Index variable (mean *z* scored) composed of % individuals with < 12 y education, % individuals living below the poverty threshold, % individuals employed in primarily working-class jobs, median household income (reverse-coded).

[c]CD variable (mean *z* scored) composed of % non-White individuals, % unemployed individuals in labor force, % female-headed households, % households receiving public assistance, % households with no vehicle available, and % families living below poverty threshold.

outcome, and model 2 demonstrates the full regression model with all predictors included.

The lowest SEP quintile census tracts were significantly ($P < .01$) farther from a provider than were those in the highest SEP quintile (B = 47.1 miles; 95% CI = 31.87, 62.31) in the crude model, although this finding was inconsistent in the adjusted model. Census tracts with higher levels of CD were also significantly farther from the nearest provider, again after a dose–response relationship with increasing change in distance as CD increased. Census tracts with the highest CD were roughly 125 miles (95% CI = 99.65, 150.59; $P < .001$) farther from a provider than were those with low levels of CD in the adjusted model.

Interestingly, the ICE value demonstrated a significant positive relationship with change in distance for census tracts in both the highest deprivation and highest privileged groups, reflecting that census tracts with higher deprivation and census tracts with higher privilege were significantly farther from a provider than were those in the middle ICE category (a 23-mile [95% CI = 4.57, 42.17; $P < .001$] and 21-mile [95% CI = 4.57, 42.17] difference in the adjusted model, respectively).

Finally, the Gini coefficient was significant in the crude model at $P < .001$ for those in the highest inequality group (30 miles; 95% CI = 16.26, 45.71). The increase in mileage for those with high income inequality in the tracts was slightly attenuated in the fully adjusted model to represent an average change in distance of 23 miles (95% CI = 0.47, 38.38; $P < .01$).

DISCUSSION

People in the South and Gulf Coast regions of Texas were most affected by SB8 and *Roe* reversal in terms of change in distance to nearest provider after each legislative wave. As abortion clinics in Central and West Texas had been forced to close by a previous regulation (House Bill 2, passed in 2014[24]), residents in these areas appeared less affected because they were already forced to travel out of state to seek abortion services at clinics in New Mexico before SB8 implementation.

The results estimate that pregnant Texans seeking abortion services will have to drive an additional 457 miles to obtain services out of state after the state's abortion ban. Previous research has noted that increasing distance to provider lowers a person's likelihood of obtaining an abortion.[25,26] Long-distance travel presents an additional burden beyond the cost of the procedure itself, including transportation costs, lodging costs, lost wages, childcare arrangements, and overall time lost to travel.[24] We found that roughly 48% of people in Texas census tracts now have an additional full day of driving to obtain services, meaning that these additional costs are compounded over several days of travel for pregnant people seeking abortions out of state. Furthermore, roughly 88% of the sample's nearest provider after *Roe* reversal was in Kansas, where mandatory waiting periods are enforced for a full 24 hours before the procedure.[27] Thus, many pregnant people in Texas who travel out of state to the closest provider will be faced with further time and cost burdens associated with other states' abortion restrictions, as well as increased congestion.

To the best of our knowledge, this study is the first of its kind to note the relationship between distance to abortion provider and indicators of neighborhood conditions after the overturning of *Roe v. Wade*. The study notes strikingly uneven patterns in the place-based effects of these abortion restrictions, with people in neighborhoods at the highest levels of CD and the poorest socioeconomic conditions having to travel farther after both SB8 implementation and *Roe* reversal. Most pregnant people who obtain a surgical abortion are economically disadvantaged, so the additional travel distance to the nearest provider imposed by legislation that bans abortions may present a compounding barrier for women that prevents them from obtaining services entirely.[28] This study adds to previous evidence of profound racial and socioeconomic inequities in abortion access and their contributions to racial and socioeconomic inequities in reproductive health and well-being.[29] Additionally, this study documents a unique method of examining the impact of abortion restriction among subgroups.

Despite the study's strengths, there are inherent limitations in using GIS methods. Census tracts and other administrative boundaries may not adequately capture the various social dimensions and lived experiences through which residents may define their "neighborhoods." Disadvantaged communities are also not randomly distributed across the state, as confirmed by global Moran's I analysis conducted on CD and SEP variables (results not shown). The concentration of poorer communities in the south and southeastern portion of Texas may have led to their overrepresentation among those most affected by increased travel distances.

We used centroids to estimate the distance from each census tract to the nearest provider, which may introduce some inaccuracies in distance for larger tracts in the western part of Texas. We used only primary and secondary road networks to perform the network analysis, which is also limiting, as many smaller state highways exist in this region and may be used instead. In addition, we chose to focus on distance rather than travel time for feasibility and comparability reasons, as the latter might be affected by road network, speed limit, and traffic conditions, which are likely to vary across urban and rural tracts as well as seasonally throughout the state. Moreover, the analysis does not account for other modes of transportation (e.g., flying, which would entail further direct costs to pregnant people seeking services). Previous research notes that some pregnant people prefer to drive to an abortion provider over flying for privacy and convenience, so the use of road networks is likely a valid choice.[30]

Furthermore, many pathways to abortion exist, including self-managed abortion, and thus distance to provider is not the only indicator for abortion access. Relatedly, as we did not consider congestion at remaining clinics, we likely underestimated distance to provider, as pregnant people may be forced to seek appointments farther away because of long wait times at the nearest clinics. Finally, given the restrictions and rapidly changing abortion landscape after *Roe* was overturned, abortion clinics are frequently changing their operations, and thus the nearest provider may change from day to day in a given area.

Vulnerable subpopulations may not be included in the census (e.g., undocumented individuals) or may be unidentifiable in census data (e.g., gender-nonconforming people). This consideration is especially important in the Texas context, as many towns along the US–Mexico border also have the farthest distance to the nearest domestic abortion provider. Without information on undocumented individuals or gender-nonconforming people who face greater social barriers to abortion access,[31] our measures of neighborhood social and economic inequality may be conservative. Additionally, it is unclear what additional barriers undocumented people may face. Crossing international borders was beyond the scope of the project because of the lack of robust data sources regarding facility operations in Mexican border counties; however, anecdotal evidence shows that medication abortion is available in

Mexico, illustrating some variety in abortion pathways that pregnant people in Texas may consider.[32] AJPH

ABOUT THE AUTHORS

Sydney R. Sauter and Julie H. Hernandez are with the Department of International Health and Sustainable Development, Tulane School of Public Health and Tropical Medicine, New Orleans, LA. Maeve E. Wallace is with the Department of Social, Behavioral, and Population Sciences, Tulane School of Public Health and Tropical Medicine.

CORRESPONDENCE

Correspondence should be sent to Sydney R. Sauter, MPH, Tulane University School of Public Health and Tropical Medicine, 1440 Canal St, Suite 2200, New Orleans, LA 70112 (e-mail: ssauter@tulane.edu). Reprints can be ordered at http://www.ajph.org by clicking the "Reprints" link.

PUBLICATION INFORMATION

Full Citation: Sauter SR, Wallace ME, Hernandez JH. Unequal spatial consequences of abortion restrictions in Texas, 2021–2023. *Am J Public Health*. 2024;114(10):1024–1033.

Acceptance Date: March 4, 2024.

DOI: https://doi.org/10.2105/AJPH.2024.307652

ORCID iDs:

Sydney R. Sauter https://orcid.org/0000-0003-4102-3543

Julie H. Hernandez https://orcid.org/0000-0002-0868-0958

CONTRIBUTORS

S. R. Sauter conceptualized and designed the study, conducted the statistical analysis, and produced the initial draft of the article. M. E. Wallace provided analytic support and feedback for the article. J. H. Hernandez conducted the network analysis and produced the corresponding maps. All authors were involved in the article development process and approved the final submission.

ACKNOWLEDGMENTS

This work was supported, in whole or in part, by the Bill & Melinda Gates Foundation (grant INV-033621). M. E. Wallace is supported by the National Institute of Child Health and Human Development (grant R01HD096070).

An earlier version of this work was presented at the American Public Health Association Annual Meeting, Boston, MA, November 2022.

Note. The research presented in this article is that of the authors. It does not reflect the official policy or opinions of the Bill & Melinda Gates Foundation or the National Institutes of Health.

CONFLICTS OF INTEREST

The authors have no conflicts of interest to report.

HUMAN PARTICIPANT PROTECTION

No protocol approval was needed for this study as no human participants were involved.

REFERENCES

1. Nash E, Guarnieri I. Six months post-*Roe*, 24 US states have banned abortion or are likely to do so: a roundup. January 9, 2023. Available at: https://www.guttmacher.org/2023/01/six-months-post-roe-24-us-states-have-banned-abortion-or-are-likely-do-so-roundup. Accessed May 1, 2023.
2. Jones RK, Philbin J, Kirstein M, Nash E, Lufkin K. Long-term decline in US abortions reverses, showing rising need for abortion as Supreme Court is poised to overturn *Roe v. Wade*. December 1, 2022. Available at: https://www.guttmacher.org/article/2022/06/long-term-decline-us-abortions-reverses-showing-rising-need-abortion-supreme-court. Accessed October 31, 2022.
3. Society of Family Planning. #WeCount report April 2022 to June 2023. October 24, 2023. Available at: https://doi.org/10.46621/218569qkgmbl. Accessed May 1, 2024.
4. Gerdts C, Fuentes L, Grossman D, et al. Impact of clinic closures on women obtaining abortion services after implementation of a restrictive law in Texas. *Am J Public Health*. 2022;112(9):1297–1304. https://doi.org/10.2105/AJPH.2016.303134
5. Lindo JM, Myers CK, Schlosser A, Cunningham S. How far is too far? New evidence on abortion clinic closures, access, and abortions. *J Hum Resour*. 2020;55(4):1137–1160. https://doi.org/10.3368/jhr.55.4.1217-9254R3
6. Cohen IG, Adashi EY, Gostin LO. The Supreme Court, the Texas abortion law (SB8), and the beginning of the end of *Roe v Wade*? *JAMA*. 2021;326(15):1473–1474. https://doi.org/10.1001/jama.2021.17639
7. White K, Sierra G, Lerma K, et al. Association of Texas' 2021 ban on abortion in early pregnancy with the number of facility-based abortions in Texas and surrounding states. *JAMA*. 2022;328(20):2048–2055. https://doi.org/10.1001/jama.2022.20423
8. Baker CN. History and politics of medication abortion in the United States and the rise of telemedicine and self-managed abortion. *J Health Polit Policy Law*. 2023;48(4):485–510. https://doi.org/10.1215/03616878-10449941
9. Solazzo AL. Different and not equal: the uneven association of race, poverty, and abortion laws on abortion timing. *Soc Probl*. 2019;66(4):519–547. https://doi.org/10.1093/socpro/spy015
10. Kelly BC, Brewer SC, Hanson HA. Disparities in distance to abortion care under reversal of *Roe v. Wade. Utah Women and Reproductive Health*. May 9, 2022. https://doi.org/10.26054/0d-4zt7-ts67
11. Baker RS. The historical racial regime and racial inequality in poverty in the American South. *Am J Sociol*. 2022;127(6):1721–1781. https://doi.org/10.1086/719653
12. Hattery A, Smith E. Social stratification in the new/old South: the Influences of racial segregation on social class in the Deep South. *J Poverty*. 2007;11(1):55–81. https://doi.org/10.1300/J134v11n01_03
13. Manson S, Schroeder J, Van Riper D, Kugler T, Ruggles S. IPUMS national historical geographic information system: version 16.0.
14. Sperling J. The tyranny of census geography: small-area data and neighborhood statistics. *Cityscape (Wash, DC)*. 2012;14(2):219–223. Available at: https://www.huduser.gov/portal/periodicals/cityscpe/vol14num2/Cityscape_July2012_tyranny_census.pdf. Accessed May 1, 2024.
15. Chen JT, Rehkopf DH, Waterman PD, et al. Mapping and measuring social disparities in premature mortality: the impact of census tract poverty within and across Boston neighborhoods, 1999–2001. *J Urban Health*. 2006;83(6):1063–1084. https://doi.org/10.1007/s11524-006-9089-7
16. Bureau of the Census. Census tracts and block numbering areas. In *Geographic Areas Reference Manual*. US Department of Commerce, Economics and Statistics Administration; 1994. Available at: https://catalog.lib.uchicago.edu/vufind/Record/6507215. Accessed January 10, 2024.
17. Krieger N. A century of census tracts: health & the body politic (1906–2006). *J Urban Health*. 2006;83(3):355–361. https://doi.org/10.1007/s11524-006-9040-y
18. Sampson RJ, Raudenbush SW, Earls F. Neighborhoods and violent crime: a multilevel study of collective efficacy. *Science*. 1997;277(5328):918–924. https://doi.org/10.1126/science.277.5328.918
19. Krieger N, Waterman PD, Spasojevic J, Li W, Maduro G, Van Wye G. Public health monitoring of privilege and deprivation with the index of concentration at the extremes. *Am J Public Health*. 2016;106(2):256–263. https://doi.org/10.2105/AJPH.2015.302955
20. Gini C. Measurement of inequality of incomes. *Econ J (Lond)*. 1921;31(121):124–125. https://doi.org/10.2307/2223319
21. Jones R, Nash E, Cross L, Philbin J, Kirstein M. Medication abortion now accounts for more than half of all US abortions. February 22, 2022. Available at: https://www.guttmacher.org/article/2022/02/medication-abortion-now-accounts-more-half-all-us-abortions. Accessed May 1, 2023.
22. US Abortion Clinic Locator. Power to decide. Where can I get an abortion? Available at: https://www.abortionfinder.org. Accessed October 31, 2022.
23. QGIS Development Team. QGIS geographic information system. May 2024. Available at: http://www.qgis.org. Accessed May 1, 2024.
24. Bearak JM, Burke KL, Jones RK. Disparities and change over time in distance women would need to travel to have an abortion in the USA: a spatial analysis. *Lancet Public Health*. 2017;2(11):e493–e500. https://doi.org/10.1016/S2468-2667(17)30158-5
25. Shelton JD, Brann EA, Schulz KF. Abortion utilization: does travel distance matter? *Fam Plann Perspect*. 1976;8(6):260–262. https://doi.org/10.2307/2134397

26. Joyce T, Tan R, Zhang Y. *Back to the future? Abortion before & after* Roe. Cambridge, MA: National Bureau of Economic Research; 2012. NBER working paper 18338. https://doi.org/10.3386/w18338
27. KFF. Mandatory waiting periods for women seeking abortions. May 13, 2022. Available at: https://www.kff.org/womens-health-policy/state-indicator/mandatory-waiting-periods. Accessed May 1, 2023.
28. Jerman J, Jones RK, Onda T. Characteristics of US abortion patients in 2014 and changes since 2008. May 10, 2016. Available at: https://www.guttmacher.org/report/characteristics-us-abortion-patients-2014. Accessed May 1, 2023.
29. Kozhimannil KB, Hassan A, Hardeman RR. Abortion access as a racial justice issue. *N Engl J Med.* 2022;387(17):1537–1539. https://doi.org/10.1056/NEJMp2209737
30. Makleff S, Blaylock R, Ruggiero S, Key K, Chandrasekaran S, Gerdts C. Travel for later abortion in the USA: lived experiences, structural contributors and abortion fund support. *Cult Health Sex.* 2023;25(12):1741–1757. https://doi.org/10.1080/13691058.2023.2179666
31. Moseson H, Fix L, Ragosta S, et al. Abortion experiences and preferences of transgender, nonbinary, and gender-expansive people in the United States. *Am J Obstet Gynecol.* 2021;224(4):376.e1–376.e11. https://doi.org/10.1016/j.ajog.2020.09.035
32. Eckholm E. A pill available in Mexico is a Texas option for abortion. *New York Times.* July 13, 2013. Available at: https://www.nytimes.com/2013/07/14/us/in-mexican-pill-a-texas-option-for-an-abortion.html. Accessed January 10, 2024.

Longitudinal Impact of *Dobbs v Jackson Women's Health Organization* on Abortion Service Delivery in Ohio, 2022–2023

Mikaela H. Smith, PhD, Michelle L. McGowan, PhD, Courtney Kerestes, MD, Danielle Bessett, PhD, and Alison H. Norris, MD, PhD

See also Abortion Access 2 Years After *Dobbs v Jackson* Ruling, pp. 994–1050.

Objectives. To assess the impact of Ohio's abortion policy changes on abortion provision following *Dobbs v Jackson Women's Health Organization*.

Methods. We analyzed quantitative and write-in responses from an ongoing survey of 6 abortion facilities in Ohio for 3 time periods: January–June 2022 (pre-*Dobbs*), July–September 2022 (6-week ban in effect), and October 2022–June 2023 (post-*Dobbs*, ban blocked). We disaggregated counts by method, gestation, and state of residence.

Results. Following *Dobbs*, Ohio banned abortions after detection of embryonic cardiac activity, and monthly abortion provision decreased 56%. Several months after the ban was lifted, monthly abortion means exceeded pre-*Dobbs* means. The percentage of patients from out of state increased over time.

Conclusions. The post-*Dobbs* enactment of a restrictive abortion ban drastically reduced availability of reproductive health care in Ohio. Nevertheless, Ohio remained an important destination for patients from surrounding states with abortion restrictions.

Public Health Implications. Gestational bans decrease access to necessary health care; instead, states like Ohio should work to eliminate barriers to abortion care to support the health and well-being of people in their own and surrounding states. (*Am J Public Health*. 2024;114(10):1034–1042. https://doi.org/10.2105/AJPH.2024.307775)

AJPH October 2024, Vol. 114, No. 10

On June 24, 2022, the US Supreme Court overturned 50 years of legal precedent set by *Roe v Wade* and *Planned Parenthood v Casey* in its decision on *Dobbs v Jackson Women's Health Organization*.[1] The decision returned the right to regulate abortion to the states, and many states were poised to instantly ban or severely restrict abortion.[2] One such state, Ohio, immediately enacted a ban on abortion after detection of embryonic cardiac activity, which typically takes place around 6 weeks' gestation. This ban was in place for almost 3 months before being blocked by a judge, creating a window of time during which Ohioans, and those seeking care in Ohio from other states, had severely limited access to abortion. Experts anticipated that allowing states to severely restrict abortion would lead to decreased utilization of abortion,[3,4] and, indeed, abortion numbers have dropped sharply in states with severe restrictions.[5] State restrictions were anticipated to disproportionately impact people of color and those with low incomes.[6–9]

National data tracking abortion utilization in the months surrounding *Dobbs* showed, overall, 9% fewer abortions in September 2022 versus April 2022, though there was much regional variation.[5] In this study, we outlined the legal and political changes in Ohio that accompanied the *Dobbs* decision and assessed how changes in state policy in Ohio, and surrounding states, impacted abortion availability and utilization in Ohio.

BACKGROUND

Ohio has long been an "abortion-hostile" state,[10] where policy changes reflect the dramatic increase in abortion restrictions in the past 2 decades.[11] Ohio legislators have passed more than 15 abortion restrictions, including limitations on dilation and evacuation procedures, banning abortions after 20 weeks (22 weeks from last menstrual period), requiring in-person preabortion counseling and consent followed by a 24-hour waiting period before the abortion can proceed, eliminating insurance coverage for abortion in nearly all cases for Medicaid insurance and insurance for state employees, and requiring abortion facilities to have written transfer agreements with hospitals.[12] Restrictive laws were accompanied by abortion facility closures and care churn,[13] with abortion rates falling particularly steeply for Ohioans in rural counties.[12] Overall, abortion rates in both Ohio and the United States have steadily dropped since the early 1990s.[14] Yet, after 2 decades of decreases, rates of abortion began increasing again in 2020 in Ohio, mirroring national trends and showing a continued need for abortion care in the state.[15]

Nevertheless, immediately after *Dobbs*, Ohio enacted a previously enjoined ban on abortion after detection of embryonic cardiac activity, also referred to as a "6-week" ban, because detection of such activity usually occurs around that time.[16] This ban was initially passed by the Ohio legislature in 2019 via Senate Bill 23, but did not go into effect at that time because of *Roe*'s protections. On June 24, 2022, the day of the *Dobbs* decision, approval from a federal court judge allowed the bill to go into effect (Figure 1). The 6-week ban remained in effect until September 14, 2022, when a Hamilton County Common Pleas Court Judge granted a temporary restraining order on the ban, temporarily blocking the law.[17] While this restraining order allowed facilities to again provide abortion care beyond 6 weeks' gestation, providers faced the additional challenge of having functioned with limited capacity since June, and they were unsure how long the law would stay blocked.[18] Within this same timeframe, nearby Indiana, Kentucky, and West Virginia also experienced fluctuations in abortion policy leading to diminished abortion availability in the region.[5,19]

On October 7, 2022, the county judge confirmed the ban's suspension through the end of the court case with a preliminary injunction, allowing facilities greater certainty about their ability

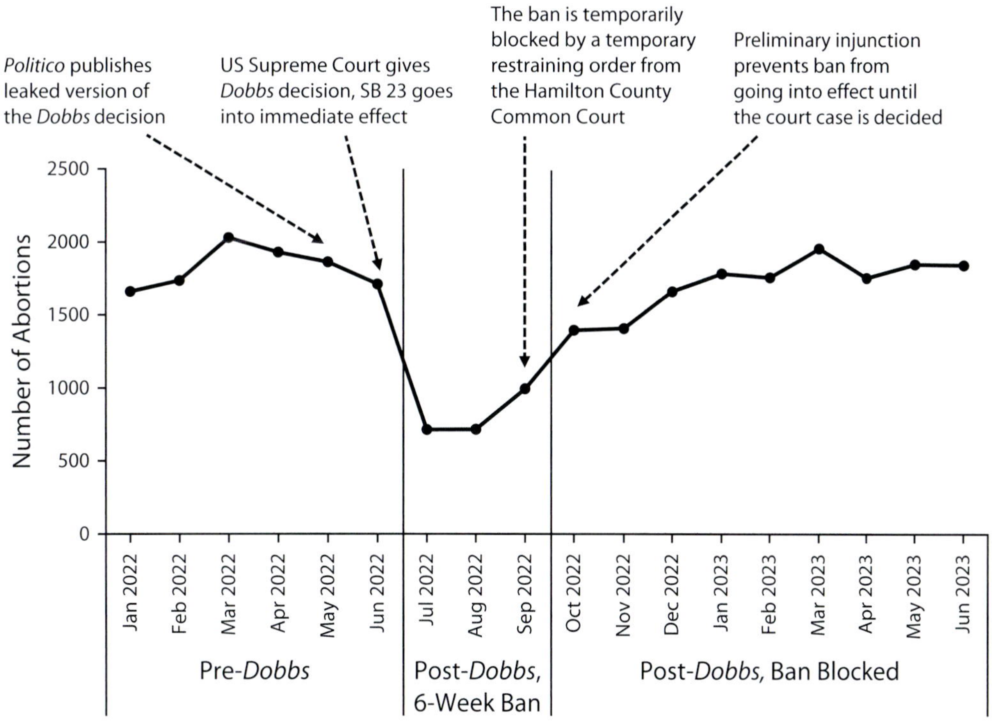

FIGURE 1— Policy Timeline and Monthly Number of Abortions at 6 Abortion Facilities for 3 Time Periods in Ohio: Pre-*Dobbs* (January–June 2022), Post-*Dobbs*, 6-Week Ban Enacted (July–September 2022), and Post-*Dobbs*, Ban Blocked (October 2022–June 2023)

to provide abortion care up to the previous state-imposed limit of 22 weeks' gestation.[20] On November 7, 2023 (outside the study period), Ohioans voted to amend the state constitution to protect abortion access through fetal viability.[21] The 6-week ban remains blocked as of time of writing; most other restrictions remain in effect in Ohio.[22]

To assess the impact of the 3-month enactment of Ohio's 6-week abortion ban, we drew on monthly data from an ongoing survey of abortion facilities to analyze changes in number of abortions pre- versus post-*Dobbs*, changes in gestation and method of abortion, and changes in patients' state of residence. In addition, we captured abortion facility staff perspectives regarding their experiences adapting to these changes. In doing so, we offer a case study of how the interplay between federal and state law created real impacts on availability of necessary health care within a tumultuous abortion ecosystem.

METHODS

Data came from an ongoing monthly survey of abortion facilities in Ohio that began in March 2020. Any abortion facility in Ohio that provided abortions for any portion of the study period was eligible to participate. We included 8 abortion facilities, some of which were operated by the same parent organization, in the present analysis (Table A, available as a supplement to the online version of this article at https://ajph.org). The abortions included in our totals represent approximately 95% of all abortions provided in Ohio during this time. One additional facility that offered medication-only abortion care during the study period was not included in this study because of nonresponse to our survey. Respondents included abortion facility owners, managers, and research staff. We administered the survey online through Qualtrics (Qualtrics, Provo, UT) and REDCap (Research Electronic Data Capture)[23,24] hosted at the lead author's institution.

We analyzed data from January 2022 to June 2023, broken into 3 time periods: pre-*Dobbs* (6 months; January 2022–June 2022); post-*Dobbs*, 6-week ban enacted (3 months; July 2022–September 2022); and post-*Dobbs*, 6-week ban blocked (9 months; October 2022–June 2023). We note that the ban went into effect in late June 2022 and was blocked mid-September, and, thus, there was small misclassification in our monthly counts, in that some abortions that took place when the 6-week ban was in effect were counted as "pre-*Dobbs*" and some without the 6-week ban in effect that were counted as "post-*Dobbs*, 6-week ban enacted."

For each period, we compared the number of abortions provided monthly, and by method (medication vs procedural), gestation (among procedural abortions, < 14 weeks vs ≥ 14 weeks), and patient state of residence (in-state vs out-of-state). We also calculated the total number of abortions by each state of patient residence for these periods. One facility (Facility B; Table A) that provides medication abortion only did not report any state-of-residence data, and, thus, we excluded them from the residence analyses. We analyzed data with Stata version 16 (StataCorp LP, College Station, TX).

We contextualized our findings with quotes from free-text survey responses from facility staff. The survey asked several open-ended questions related to service delivery, policy changes, recent challenges, and protestor presence. We invited staff to respond to the survey each month; responses to open-ended questions were not required to submit abortion count data. All facilities included in this study responded to open-ended questions at some point during the study period. Two authors (M. M. and M. S.) reviewed responses and extracted quotes referring to *Dobbs* and state court decisions.

RESULTS

From January to June 2022 (pre-*Dobbs*), 10 968 abortions took place at the 8 facilities included in our study for a monthly mean of 1828 (Table 1, Figure 1). Monthly totals peaked at 2036 in March 2022. From July to September 2022 (post-*Dobbs*, 6-week ban enacted), there were a total of 2436 abortions, for a monthly mean of 812, a 56% decrease from the pre-*Dobbs* monthly mean.

From October 2022 to June 2023 (post-*Dobbs*, ban blocked), there were a total of 15 451 abortions for a monthly mean of 1717. This represents a 6% decrease from the pre-*Dobbs* mean, and an 111% increase from the 6-week ban mean. These changes reflect a slow rise in the number of abortions beginning in September 2022, after the ban was blocked, through December 2022, when counts began to approximate pre-*Dobbs* levels. By January through June 2023, facilities were experiencing a monthly mean of 1829 abortions, slightly higher than the pre-*Dobbs* mean.

Changes by Method and Gestation

Considering breakdown by method (Table 1, Figure 2a), pre-*Dobbs*, 4848 out of 10 968 abortions were medication

TABLE 1— Monthly Abortions at 8 Abortion Facilities in Ohio—Overall and by Method, Gestation, and State of Residence—for 3 Time Periods: Pre-*Dobbs* (January–June 2022); Post-*Dobbs*, 6-Week Ban Enacted (July–September 2022); and Post-*Dobbs*, Ban Blocked (October 2022–June 2023)

	Total Abortions, No.	Total Medication, No. (%)	Procedural			In-State, No. (%)	Out-of-State, No. (%)
			Total, No. (%)	< 14 Weeks, No. (%)	≥ 14 Weeks, No. (%)		
Pre-*Dobbs*							
Jan 2022	1667	756 (45)	911 (55)	743 (82)	179 (20)	1434 (96)	59 (4)
Feb 2022	1743	739 (42)	1004 (58)	782 (78)	226 (23)	1411 (95)	80 (5)
Mar 2022	2036	895 (44)	1141 (56)	888 (78)	260 (23)	1653 (94)	103 (6)
Apr 2022	1936	828 (43)	1107 (57)	906 (82)	204 (18)	1584 (94)	98 (6)
May 2022	1869	848 (45)	1021 (55)	870 (85)	152 (15)	1552 (94)	102 (6)
Jun 2022	1718	782 (46)	936 (54)	795 (85)	145 (15)	1408 (95)	81 (5)
Monthly mean	1828	808	1020	831	194	1507	87
Post-*Dobbs*, 6-wk ban							
Jul 2022	718	374 (52)	344 (48)	348 (101)	0 (0)	619 (96)	26 (4)
Aug 2022	720	410 (57)	310 (43)	314 (101)	0 (0)	613 (92)	50 (8)
Sep 2022	998	505 (51)	493 (49)	452 (92)	43 (9)	767 (88)	106 (12)
Monthly mean	812	430	382	371	14	666	61
Post-*Dobbs*, ban blocked							
Oct 2022	1399	675 (48)	724 (52)	632 (87)	92 (13)	1067 (87)	156 (13)
Nov 2022	1411	656 (46)	755 (54)	647 (86)	115 (15)	1060 (88)	150 (12)
Dec 2022	1666	784 (47)	882 (53)	750 (85)	139 (16)	1277 (89)	165 (11)
Jan 2023	1789	805 (45)	984 (55)	883 (90)	198 (20)	1369 (89)	174 (11)
Feb 2023	1763	781 (44)	982 (56)	797 (81)	211 (21)	1365 (87)	211 (13)
Mar 2023	1961	861 (44)	1100 (56)	841 (76)	256 (23)	1455 (87)	211 (13)
Apr 2023	1760	681 (39)	1079 (61)	880 (82)	201 (19)	1397 (89)	180 (11)
May 2023	1854	785 (42)	1069 (58)	867 (81)	208 (19)	1479 (89)	187 (11)
Jun 2023	1848	811 (44)	1037 (56)	838 (81)	202 (19)	1397 (86)	223 (14)
Monthly mean	1717	760	957	793	180	1318	184

Note. Percentage of abortions is out of total number of abortions for that month; gestation breakdown is out of total number of procedural abortions.

(44%; monthly mean, 808). Under the ban, 1289 out of 2436 were medication (53%; monthly mean, 430). In the post-*Dobbs*, ban blocked period, 6839 out of 15 451 abortions were medication (44%; monthly mean, 760).

Examining gestation among procedural abortions (Table 1, Figure 2b), pre-*Dobbs*, 4984 out of 6120 procedural abortions were under 14 weeks (81%; monthly mean, 831). Under the 6-week ban, 1114 out of 1147 procedural abortions were under 14 weeks (97%; monthly mean, 371); we note again that our data captured abortions for the whole month of September, and, thus, the 43 procedural abortions that were at 14 weeks or later would have occurred after the 6-week ban was blocked or under a medical exception to the 6-week ban. In the post-*Dobbs*, ban-blocked period, 7135 out of 8612 abortions were under 14 weeks (83%; monthly mean, 793).

State of Residence

At the 7 facilities for which state of residence data were available, the majority of abortions provided in Ohio were for Ohioans, a proportion that decreased slightly over time (Table 1, Figure 2c). Pre-*Dobbs*, 9042 patients were from Ohio, out of 9565 abortions for which state of residence was known (95%; monthly mean, 1507). Under the 6-week ban, 1999 out of 2181 abortions were for Ohioans (92%; monthly mean, 666). After the 6-week ban was blocked, 11 866 out of 13 523 abortions were for Ohioans (88%; monthly mean, 1318).

The largest proportion of out-of-state patients were from Kentucky and Indiana (Table 2). Pre-*Dobbs*, patients

AJPH October 2024, Vol. 114, No. 10

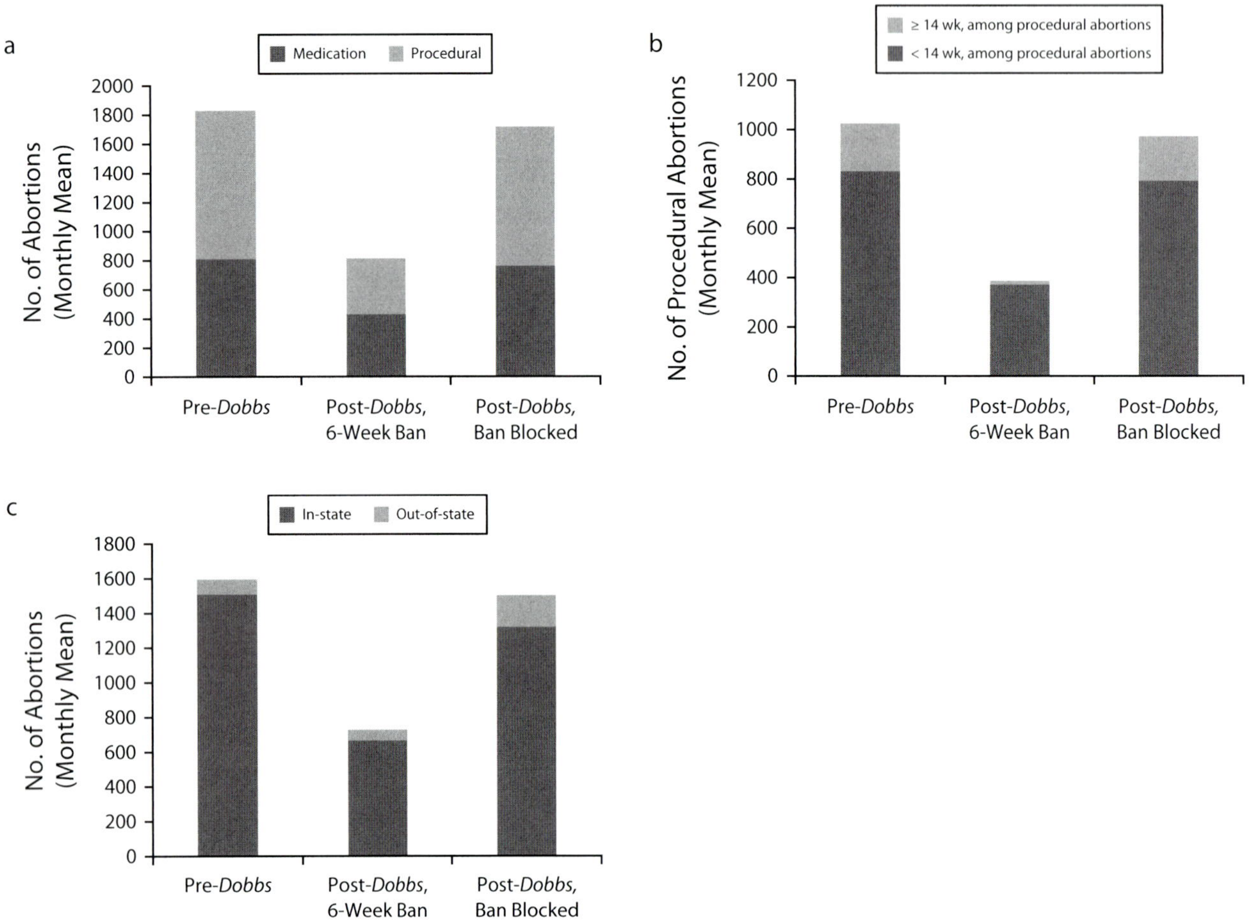

FIGURE 2— The Monthly Mean Number of Abortions That Were (a) Medication vs Procedural; (b) Among Procedural Abortions, < 14 Weeks Gestation vs ≥ 14 Weeks; and (c) Among Abortions for Known State of Residence, In-State vs Out-of-State, for 3 Time Periods in Ohio: Pre-*Dobbs* (January–June 2022), Post-*Dobbs*, 6-Week Ban Enacted (July–September 2022), and Post-*Dobbs*, Ban Blocked (October 2022–June 2023)

came from 16 states; 338 out of 9565 out-of-state patients were from Kentucky (65%), and 119 were from Indiana (23%). Under the 6-week ban, patients came from 7 states; 136 out of 2181 patients were from Kentucky (75%), and 29 were from Indiana (16%). After the ban was blocked, patients came from 24 states; 1241 out of 13 523 patients were from Kentucky (75%), and 223 were from Indiana (14%). When the 6-week ban was blocked, Ohio saw more patients coming from southern states such as Alabama, Florida, Georgia, Tennessee, Texas, and West Viriginia, where total or restrictive gestational abortion bans were implemented following *Dobbs*.

Staff Reactions and Adaptations

Throughout the study period, facility staff members described a variety of challenges to providing abortion care in Ohio, including difficulties providing care under physician and staff shortages, low morale among staff, delays in scheduling and caring for patients, medical supply chain–related shortages, and ongoing protestor presence.

Pre-**Dobbs *(January–June 2022).*** Pre-*Dobbs*, staff members noted the burden of managing patient confusion over abortion legality given various state efforts to restrict abortion, particularly in Ohio, Kentucky, and Texas. Staff at Facility A, for example, reported seeing some patients from Kentucky and "several folks from Texas, related to law changes." In May, staff noted that the Supreme Court's *Dobbs* draft decision "leak caused severe panic with patients" and that they had "two patients stating they traveled from 2 states away—arrived after 5p—providers stayed late to help patients."

TABLE 2— The Number of Patients Coming to Ohio for Abortions for 3 Time Periods: Pre-*Dobbs* (January–June 2022), Post-*Dobbs*, 6-Week Ban Enacted (July–September 2022), and Post-*Dobbs*, Ban Blocked (October 2022–June 2023)

		Post-*Dobbs*	
State	Pre-*Dobbs*, No. (%)	6-Week Ban, No. (%)	Ban Blocked No. (%)
Alabama	0 (0.0)	0 (0.0)	7 (0.4)
Arizona	0 (0.0)	0 (0.0)	1 (0.1)
District of Columbia	0 (0.0)	0 (0.0)	1 (0.1)
Florida	0 (0.0)	0 (0.0)	8 (0.5)
Georgia	3 (0.6)	0 (0.0)	12 (0.7)
Hawaii	0 (0.0)	0 (0.0)	1 (0.1)
Illinois	3 (0.6)	0 (0.0)	2 (0.1)
Indiana	119 (22.8)	29 (15.9)	223 (13.5)
Kentucky	338 (64.6)	136 (74.7)	1241 (74.9)
Louisiana	0 (0.0)	1 (0.5)	3 (0.2)
Maryland	0 (0.0)	0 (0.0)	1 (0.1)
Michigan	3 (0.6)	0 (0.0)	3 (0.2)
Minnesota	0 (0.0)	0 (0.0)	1 (0.1)
Mississippi	1 (0.2)	0 (0.0)	3 (0.2)
Missouri	0 (0.0)	0 (0.0)	2 (0.1)
Montana	1 (0.2)	0 (0.0)	0 (0.0)
Nevada	0 (0.0)	1 (0.5)	0 (0.0)
New Hampshire	1 (0.2)	0 (0.0)	0 (0.0)
New Jersey	1 (0.2)	0 (0.0)	1 (0.1)
New York	0 (0.0)	0 (0.0)	1 (0.1)
North Carolina	1 (0.2)	0 (0.0)	0 (0.0)
Pennsylvania	29 (5.5)	6 (3.3)	12 (0.7)
South Carolina	1 (0.2)	0 (0.0)	1 (0.1)
South Dakota	0 (0.0)	0 (0.0)	1 (0.1)
Tennessee	3 (0.6)	6 (3.3)	33 (2.0)
Texas	11 (2.1)	0 (0.0)	28 (1.7)
Virginia	2 (0.4)	0 (0.0)	1 (0.1)
West Virginia	6 (1.1)	3 (1.6)	70 (4.2)

Note. The percentage represents the number of out-of-state abortions out of the number of abortions for which state of residence is known.

Simultaneously, the facility staff noted an "increase in LEP [limited English proficiency] patients (multiple per day)" with "different dialects of Spanish" while experiencing "difficulties with interpreters." Additionally, staff indicated that that the "waiting room [was] also not big enough to accommodate patient/support people volume" such that they had to refer many patients to a facility in another region of the state. Despite these challenges, the facility staff reported being able to "accommodate more patients of higher gestation" after a physician increased their provision to be through 19 weeks and 6 days, and that they added a ride share program to reduce patients' transportation-related barriers to care.

*Post-*Dobbs*, 6-week ban enacted (July–September 2022).* Following the *Dobbs* decision, abortion facility staff noted a variety of challenges to facilities and patients in the environment of rapidly adapting to the 6-week ban. Staff at Facility A noted that "the state is now requiring us to do a secondary ultrasound scan on day 2 before procedure, to reconfirm that there are no fetal heart tones." In August 2022, Facility D staff noted that "there's no time for patients to get a [judicial] bypass" under the 6-week ban. Facility A staff also noted that September 2022 was "the first time in months that we have not seen any out of state patients" at one location, and the "first time in months that we have had such a low volume of out of state patients" in another location.

The ban was a significant source of stress for facility staff. Facilities indicated that during the 3 months when the 6-week ban was in effect they referred patients to Colorado, Illinois, Michigan, New York, New Jersey, and Pennsylvania. Facility A staff noted that "patients having to be navigated out of state significantly affected the staff emotionally." Facility B staff reported that "a patient advocate quit due to the stress of [Senate Bill] 23."

*Post-*Dobbs*, 6-week ban blocked (October 2022—June 2023).* The halting of the 6-week ban in September 2022 allowed facilities to resume abortion up to the state legal limit (21 weeks, 6 days), though several facilities provided abortion care to lower gestational limits than permitted by law because of facility policies, physician training, or licensing limitations. For instance, Facility

A staff noted that they immediately returned to scheduling as many abortion patients as "the schedule allowed," though even with the 6-week ban no longer in place, "an ultrasound must be repeated . . . on [the procedure] day, the patient must be offered the opportunity to see or hear the heartbeat."

In addition, referral of patients out of state continued even after the 6-week ban was no longer in effect, with Ohio facilities referring people to Pennsylvania, Michigan, and Illinois; Facility C staff noted that their referrals to Illinois were for patients who were beyond Ohio's legal gestational limit.

From October 2022 to June 2023, facility staff repeatedly noted that time and space constrained their ability to provide abortion care to meet the demand, but that remaining open was a priority. The Facility D representative indicated struggling with the fact that "our facilit[ies are] too small for our patient volume." Facility E remarked that they were seeing patients "from all over the US" and that there were "not enough hours in the day to see all the [patients]." In reflecting on 2022 in particular, Facility E noted that the facility had "never closed. We kept the doors open through all of [the *Dobbs v*] *Jackson Women's Health Organization* [time period] and were able to pivot right after the fall [of *Roe*] and pivot to full access" immediately following the lifting of the 6-week ban.

DISCUSSION

Our investigation of the dynamic abortion ecosystem in Ohio surrounding *Dobbs* illuminates the impact of federal and state laws on facility provision and patient utilization of abortion care. The *Dobbs* decision permitted a previously enjoined 6-week ban in Ohio to be enacted, and, as a result, the number abortions in the state dropped by more than half during the months that the law was enforced, as similarly seen in other states with 6-week bans.[5] When the 6-week ban was blocked, monthly mean numbers of abortions in Ohio returned slowly to pre-*Dobbs* totals, eventually exceeding pre-*Dobbs* means, and the percentage of out-of-state patients increased throughout the study period. Overall, the enactment of the 6-week ban in Ohio, along with total or restrictive abortion bans in nearby states, had swift and meaningful impacts on the availability of abortion care in Ohio.

Qualitative responses from facility staff highlight the stress and burdens for patients and providers in needing to adapt to fast-changing state policies. Abortion care churn, the chronic uncertainty surrounding abortion care that results from a dynamic restrictive regulatory environment and abortion stigma, was present in Ohio before *Dobbs*, and we see evidence of the multiplying effect of new restrictive laws and a changing legal environment in several states simultaneously.[13] Churn makes abortion care harder to provide and harder to access. It is possible, for example, that the increased influx of out-of-state patients after the 6-week ban ended may have limited Ohioans' access to care in the state, if waiting times at facilities in the state increased. Abortion facility staff were also managing moral distress throughout this time, which occurs when individuals feel powerless to do what they think is right, including when clinicians are prevented from providing health care they deem necessary.[25,26]

Our findings reflect patterns of travel to Ohio, yet not all patients who need abortions are able to travel out of state for abortion care,[27] and being denied an abortion can lead to poorer socioeconomic and health outcomes, even years later.[28] Similarly, Ohio's requirement for 2 visits (an in-person consent visit followed by an in-person medication or procedural abortion no sooner than 24 hours after the consent visit) puts additional burden on patients obtaining care in the state, especially for those traveling long distances.

The higher percentage of medication abortions during the 6-week ban is not surprising, given that most abortions in this period of time would have been eligible for medication abortion. The increase in medication abortion also reflects the facilities' adaptation to new policies and emphasizes the importance of continued availability of mifepristone for medication abortion. Medication abortion inhabits an increasingly important place in the provision of abortion care (nationally, more than half of abortions are provided via medication),[29] and the increasing availability of medication abortion via telehealth presents an especially important option for people who cannot travel to a facility for care.[5,30] Nevertheless, Ohio's in-person counseling and consent appointment requirements mean that Ohio has a de facto restriction on telehealth for abortion, and neither patients nor facilities are able to fully benefit from the advantages of telehealth.[31]

Nationally, the Centers for Disease Control and Prevention estimates that in 2021 approximately 6% of abortions took place at 14 weeks gestation or later.[32] When medication abortion was included in our gestational breakdown, we found that approximately 10% of all abortions in Ohio took place at 14 weeks or later when the 6-week ban was not in effect. Ohio's percentage, higher than the national average, may reflect that some patients came to Ohio from states that had banned abortion at lower gestations or a lack of provider availability in other states at later gestational stages.

Our study also shows the important role that Ohio continues to play in abortion provision in the region. Even during the 6-week ban period, a higher percentage of abortion patients in Ohio were from out of state than before *Dobbs*. When the ban was blocked, the proportion of out-of-state patients increased further, driven by the ongoing inaccessibility of abortion in neighboring and more distant states. Providers' description of their need to continue to refer patients out of state even when the 6-week ban was blocked reflects the extent to which gestational bans, even those after 6 weeks, can restrict access to needed health care.

Limitations

We note that this analysis, which focuses on abortion provision in Ohio in the context of Ohio's regulatory environment, should be considered with an understanding of the regional ecosystem. For example, our data did not permit us to assess changes in provision in neighboring states, including to which other states patients from Kentucky, West Virginia, and Indiana traveled, or changes to the numbers of Ohioans traveling to other states, including Pennsylvania, Michigan, and Illinois.[18] Likewise, our data did not include information about people who needed abortion and were unable to travel or otherwise unable to obtain care in abortion facilities. In addition, because our state of residence analysis did not include data from 1 participating facility, our findings may under- or overestimate the monthly out-of-state means. Despite these limitations, this unique data set provided a critical insight to abortion provision in a state that provides more than 20 000 abortions each year,[32] that both sends and receives patients from out of state, and that experienced a multimonth 6-week abortion ban.

Public Health Implications

The 3-month enactment of Ohio's 6-week ban after *Dobbs* led to a drastic reduction in availability of abortion care in the state. Throughout the entire study period (including during the 6-week ban), Ohio remained a destination state for patients from surrounding restrictive states, pointing to the need to reinforce mechanisms to protect abortion availability, particularly in regions where abortion has and is poised to be less available in a post-*Dobbs* context.

Now that Ohio voters have passed a constitutional amendment protecting the right to abortion, any previability gestational ban would be subject to legal challenge in the state. There is also some optimism that other restrictions in Ohio may be found unconstitutional in the future, such that abortion care would become more accessible in Ohio. State courts will be important for challenging abortion regulations now that *Roe* has fallen, and state constitutions will provide the standards against which state laws will be tested. AJPH

ABOUT THE AUTHORS

Mikaela H. Smith and Alison H. Norris are with the College of Public Health, The Ohio State University, Columbus. Michelle L. McGowan is with the Biomedical Ethics Research Program, Department of Quantitative Health Sciences, Mayo Clinic, Rochester, MN, and the Department of Women's, Gender, and Sexuality Studies, University of Cincinnati, OH. Courtney Kerestes is with the Department of Obstetrics and Gynecology, College of Medicine, The Ohio State University. Danielle Bessett is with the Department of Sociology, University of Cincinnati.

CORRESPONDENCE

Correspondence should be sent to Mikaela H. Smith, 250 Cunz Hall, 1841 Neil Ave, Columbus, OH 43210 (e-mail: smith.14017@osu.edu). Reprints can be ordered at https://www.ajph.org by clicking the "Reprints" link.

PUBLICATION INFORMATION

Full Citation: Smith MH, McGowan ML, Kerestes C, Bessett D, Norris AH. Longitudinal impact of *Dobbs v Jackson Women's Health Organization* on abortion service delivery in Ohio, 2022–2023. *Am J Public Health*. 2024;114(10):1034–1042.

Acceptance Date: June 17, 2024.

DOI: https://doi.org/10.2105/AJPH.2024.307775

ORCID iDs:

Mikaela H. Smith https://orcid.org/0000-0001-5658-4808

Michelle L. McGowan https://orcid.org/0000-0002-9040-7562

Courtney Kerestes https://orcid.org/0000-0002-2243-8068

CONTRIBUTORS

M. H. Smith led the data collection, analysis, interpretation, and writing of the article. M. L. McGowan conceptualized the study and contributed to the data analysis, interpretation, and writing of the article. C. Kerestes contributed to the data analysis, interpretation, and writing of the article. D. Bessett conceptualized the study and contributed to the data interpretation and writing of the article. A. H. Norris conceptualized the study and contributed to the data collection, analysis, interpretation, and writing of the article.

ACKNOWLEDGMENTS

This study was supported by a philanthropic foundation that makes grants anonymously. The REDCap tool used for data collection was supported by the National Center for Advancing Translational Sciences (grant UL1TR001070).

CONFLICTS OF INTEREST

The authors have no conflicts of interest to disclose.

HUMAN PARTICIPANT PROTECTION

This study was approved by the institutional review boards at The Ohio State University and the University of Cincinnati.

REFERENCES

1. US Supreme Court. *Dobbs v Jackson Women's Health Organization*. 2022. Available at: https://www.supremecourt.gov/opinions/21pdf/19-1392_6j37.pdf. Accessed August 30, 2024.

2. Guttmacher Institute. Abortion after *Roe*: new comprehensive map tracks abortion policies and statistics for each state. 2022. Available at: https://www.guttmacher.org/news-release/2022/abortion-after-roe-new-comprehensive-map-tracks-abortion-policies-and-statistics. Accessed December 13, 2022.
3. Minkoff H, Gibbs RS. Preparing for a post-*Roe* world. *Am J Obstet Gynecol.* 2019;220(3):249.e1–249.e3. https://doi.org/10.1016/j.ajog.2018.11.1097
4. Harris LH. Navigating loss of abortion services—a large academic medical center prepares for the overturn of *Roe v Wade*. *N Engl J Med.* 2022;386(22):2061–2064. https://doi.org/10.1056/NEJMp2206246
5. WeCount April 2022 to September 2023. Denver, CO: Society of Family Planning; 2024. https://doi.org/10.46621/675707thmfmv
6. Gilbert KL, Sanchez GR, Busette C. *Dobbs*, another frontline for health equity. Brookings. June 30, 2022. Available at: https://www.brookings.edu/blog/how-we-rise/2022/06/30/dobbs-another-frontline-for-health-equity. Accessed February 3, 2023.
7. Hill L, Artiga S, Ranji U, Gomez I, Ndugga N. What are the implications of the *Dobbs* ruling for racial disparities? KFF. July 15, 2022. Available at: https://www.kff.org/racial-equity-and-health-policy/issue-brief/what-are-the-implications-of-the-overturning-of-roe-v-wade-for-racial-disparities. Accessed February 3, 2023.
8. Diamondstein M. The disproportionate harm of abortion bans: spotlight on *Dobbs v Jackson Women's Health*. Center for Reproductive Rights. November 29, 2021. Available at: https://reproductiverights.org/supreme-court-case-mississippi-abortion-ban-disproportionate-harm. Accessed February 3, 2023.
9. Stevenson AJ. The pregnancy-related mortality impact of a total abortion ban in the United States: a research note on increased deaths due to remaining pregnant. *Demography.* 2021;58(6):2019–2028. https://doi.org/10.1215/00703370-9585908
10. Nash E. State abortion policy landscape: from hostile to supportive. Guttmacher Institute; 2021. Available at: https://www.guttmacher.org/article/2019/08/state-abortion-policy-landscape-hostile-supportive. Accessed May 12, 2021.
11. Nash E. Ohio as a window into recent US trends on abortion access and restrictions. *Am J Public Health.* 2020;110(8):1115–1116. https://doi.org/10.2105/AJPH.2020.305799
12. Norris AH, Chakraborty P, Lang K, et al. Abortion access in Ohio's changing legislative context, 2010–2018. *Am J Public Health.* 2020;110(8):1228–1234. https://doi.org/10.2105/AJPH.2020.305706
13. McGowan ML, Norris AH, Bessett D. Care churn—why keeping clinic doors open isn't enough to ensure access to abortion. *N Engl J Med.* 2020;383(6):508–510. https://doi.org/10.1056/NEJMp2013466
14. Dreweke J. New clarity for the US abortion debate: a steep drop in unintended pregnancy is driving recent abortion declines. *Guttmacher Policy Rev.* 2016;19.
15. Jones RK, Philbin J, Kirstein M, Nash E, Lufkin K. Long-term decline in US abortions reverses, showing rising need for abortion as Supreme Court is poised to overturn *Roe v Wade*. Guttmacher Institute. 2022. Available at: https://www.guttmacher.org/article/2022/06/long-term-decline-us-abortions-reverses-showing-rising-need-abortion-supreme-court. Accessed August 26, 2022.
16. Ohio Policy Evaluation Network. Ohio's six-week abortion ban. Ohio Policy Evaluation Network. 2022. Available at: https://open.osu.edu/wp-content/uploads/2022/07/7.20.22.SixWeekBanFinal.pdf. Accessed February 2, 2023.
17. *Preterm-Cleveland, et al. v David Yost, et al.* (Court of Common Pleas, Hamilton County, OH, 2022). Available at: https://www.acluohio.org/sites/default/files/pretermclevelandetal-v-davidyostetal_decisionandentry-six-weekabortionban_2022-0914.pdf. Accessed June 26, 2023.
18. Ohio Policy Evaluation Network. Abortion in Ohio post-*Dobbs*: unpacking the numbers and stories. 2023. Available at: https://bit.ly/ohiopostdobbs. Accessed June 23, 2023.
19. McCann A, Walker AS. Tracking abortion bans across the country. *New York Times.* May 24, 2022. Available at: https://www.nytimes.com/interactive/2022/us/abortion-laws-roe-v-wade.html. Accessed November 7, 2023.
20. ACLU. Ohio lower court grants preliminary injunction; six-week abortion ban will remain blocked. October 7, 2022. Available at: https://www.aclu.org/press-releases/ohio-lower-court-grants-preliminary-injunction-six-week-abortion-ban-will-remain. Accessed January 25, 2023.
21. Tebben S, Evans N. Ohio voters pass Issue 1 constitutional amendment to protect abortion and reproductive rights. *Ohio Capital Journal.* November 8, 2023. Available at: https://ohiocapitaljournal.com/2023/11/07/ohio-voters-pass-issue-1-constitutional-amendment-to-protect-abortion-and-reproductive-rights. Accessed March 11, 2024.
22. Tebben S. Clinics ask court to declare Ohio six-week abortion ban unconstitutional after amendment passage. *Ohio Capital Journal.* March 5, 2024. Available at: https://ohiocapitaljournal.com/2024/03/05/clinics-ask-court-to-declare-ohio-six-week-abortion-ban-unconstitutional-after-amendment-passage. Accessed March 11, 2024.
23. Harris PA, Taylor R, Thielke R, Payne J, Gonzalez N, Conde JG. Research Electronic Data Capture (REDCap)—a metadata-driven methodology and workflow process for providing translational research informatics support. *J Biomed Inform.* 2009;42(2):377–381. https://doi.org/10.1016/j.jbi.2008.08.010
24. Harris PA, Taylor R, Minor BL, et al. The REDCap consortium. Building an international community of software platform partners. *J Biomed Inform.* 2019;95:103208. https://doi.org/10.1016/j.jbi.2019.103208
25. Rivlin K, Bornstein M, Tomu T, Norris AH, Howard D. State abortion policy and provider moral distress levels after *Dobbs* [ID 2683541]. *Obstet Gynecol.* 2024;143(5 suppl):78S. https://doi.org/10.1097/01.AOG.0001014016.73392.ff
26. Wascher J, Howard D, Tomu T, Bornstein M, Norris AH, Rivlin K. "Disheartened and powerless": how abortion providers discuss moral distress under *Dobbs* [ID 2683590]. *Obstet Gynecol.* 2024;143(5 suppl):25S–26S. https://doi.org/10.1097/01.AOG.0001013196.32388.2e
27. Smith MH, Muzyczka Z, Chakraborty P, et al. Abortion travel within the United States: an observational study of cross-state movement to obtain abortion care in 2017. *Lancet Reg Health Am.* 2022;10:100214. https://doi.org/10.1016/j.lana.2022.100214
28. Foster DG. *The Turnaway Study: Ten Years, a Thousand Women, and the Consequences of Having—or Being Denied—an Abortion.* New York, NY: Scribner; 2020.
29. Jones RK, Friedrich-Karnik A. Medication abortion accounted for 63% of all US abortions in 2023—an increase from 53% in 2020. Guttmacher Institute. 2024. Available at: https://www.guttmacher.org/2024/03/medication-abortion-accounted-63-all-us-abortions-2023-increase-53-2020. Accessed April 1, 2024.
30. Donovan M. Improving access to abortion via telehealth. *Guttmacher Policy Rev.* 2019;22. Available at: https://www.guttmacher.org/gpr/2019/05/improving-access-abortion-telehealth. Accessed September 28, 2021.
31. Mello K, Smith MH, Hill BJ, et al. Federal, state, and institutional barriers to the expansion of medication and telemedicine abortion services in Ohio, Kentucky, and West Virginia during the COVID-19 pandemic. *Contraception.* 2021;104(1):111–116. https://doi.org/10.1016/j.contraception.2021.04.020
32. Kortsmit K, Nguyen AT, Mandel MG, et al. Abortion surveillance—United States, 2021. *MMWR Surveill Summ.* 2023;72(SS-9):1–29. http://dx.doi.org/10.15585/mmwr.ss7209a1

Post-*Dobbs* Abortion Restrictions and the Families They Leave Behind

Nigel Madden, MD, Emma Trawick, MD, Katie Watson, JD, and Lynn M. Yee, MD, MPH

See also Abortion Access 2 Years After *Dobbs v Jackson* Ruling, pp. 994–1042.

The June 24, 2022 US Supreme Court decision in *Dobbs v Jackson Women's Health Organization* resulted in an expansive restriction on abortion access that had been constitutionally guaranteed for nearly half a century. Currently, 14 states have implemented complete bans on abortion with very limited exceptions, and an additional 7 states have implemented abortion bans at 6 to 18 weeks' gestation.

It has been well demonstrated that restrictive policies disproportionately limit abortion access for minoritized people and people of low socioeconomic status; the financial and geographic barriers of these post-*Dobbs* restrictions will only exacerbate this disparity. Proponents of abortion restrictions, who identify as pro-life, assert that these policies are essential to protect children, women, and families.

We examine whether the protection of these groups extends past conception by evaluating the association between state abortion legislation and state-based policies and programs designed to provide medical and social support for children, women, and families. We found that states with the most restrictive post-*Dobbs* abortion policies in fact have the least comprehensive and inclusive public infrastructure to support these groups. We suggest further opportunities for advocacy. (*Am J Public Health*. 2024;114(10):1043–1050. https://doi.org/10.2105/AJPH.2024.307792)

AJPH October 2024, Vol. 114, No. 10

Although the state restrictions on abortion care imposed after the June 24, 2022 US Supreme Court decision in *Dobbs v Jackson Women's Health Organization* (*Dobbs*) dramatically affect all people who are able to become pregnant, certain groups bear a greater burden. Previous research documents that people of low socioeconomic status and minoritized individuals are overrepresented in the population of people seeking abortion, and they are also less likely to be able to overcome the geographic and financial barriers imposed by abortion bans and restrictions.[1,2]

Equitable access to abortion care was a longstanding issue even before the *Dobbs* decision. For people of low socioeconomic status insured by Medicaid, the Hyde Amendment, which was first enacted in 1977 and has been renewed annually by Congress since, prohibits the use of federal funds to pay for abortion.[3] As a result of financially restrictive policies and the overrepresentation of low-income populations among people seeking abortion, more than 50% of people seeking abortion pay for their care out of pocket.[1] The average cost of a first trimester medication abortion, which accounts for more than half of abortions in the United States, is estimated to be $560.[4] For a single person with an income at the federal poverty line in 2022, even the cost of the earliest and least expensive abortion represents close to half of their monthly income.[5] New previability abortion bans are likely to increase these financial barriers because more individuals will be required to travel out of state to receive care or to delay care until a later point in pregnancy, resulting in higher procedural costs.[6]

These increased costs are often insurmountable barriers to those who are financially disadvantaged. In a 2009 review on the restrictions on Medicaid funding for abortions, the Guttmacher Institute concluded that 1 in 4 individuals who have Medicaid and seek an abortion instead continue the pregnancy and give birth because of lack of insurance coverage to fund the abortion.[7] Although this review is based on older data and Medicaid coverage for abortion has expanded in some states, it highlights the important evidence that financial barriers to abortion coverage can result in people continuing unwanted pregnancies. Since *Dobbs*, we have seen an increase in telehealth provision of medication abortion and the expansion of private "abortion funds" to overcome financial and logistical barriers to abortion care; however, these work-arounds are likely to face political challenges and are no substitute for legal accessibility.[8,9]

As abortion restrictions expand, opportunities for a safer, relatively inexpensive procedure will increasingly be replaced by forced pregnancy, which is significantly more costly, both financially and physically, particularly for minoritized people.[10,11] We also know from the Turnaway Study—a large prospective evaluation of the impact of being denied an abortion—that lack of access to abortion care can cement poverty among disadvantaged populations and have negative reverberating financial and relational ramifications that last for decades for both the person seeking the abortion and their families.[12]

As demonstrated by this previous research, post-*Dobbs* abortion restrictions are likely to have unprecedented impacts, in both the short and long terms, on the most vulnerable people in the United States. These individuals include the populations that seek abortion care the most, are least likely to be able to overcome barriers to receiving abortion care, and are most likely to experience the negative consequences of abortion denial. Proponents of previability abortion bans have described themselves as pro-life and often explicitly invoke support for women and families in arguments against abortion access, yet states with abortion bans have traditionally been more fiscally conservative and less socially supportive of their most vulnerable populations.[13,14]

Although these conflicting messages have been described in the lay press, few academic studies have systematically examined the intersection between post-*Dobbs* state abortion policies and state access to reproductive health care and family social policies and programs.[15,16] As we observe in this analysis, in the states that most severely restrict abortion, the women, children, and families that abortion proponents seek to "protect" are the populations that are left behind—with less access to health care and family social services—if pregnancy is continued.

DATA REVIEW

We compiled publicly available data published by several nonpartisan organizations as well as individual states to complete a descriptive analysis of population and policy differences between states of varying abortion restriction severity. A summary of the sources for these data is provided in the Appendix (available as a supplement to the online version of this article at http://www.ajph.org). The March of Dimes defines a "maternity care desert" as a county with no hospitals providing obstetric care, no birth centers, no obstetricians or gynecologists, and no certified nurse midwives.[17] We use the term "reproductive health care" to describe care other than abortion, including gynecologic, preconception, and pregnancy and postpartum care. We acknowledge the importance of abortion in the definition of comprehensive reproductive health care, but for the purpose of this evaluation of the differences in access to care by abortion restriction level, it is necessary to exclude this component of care from the definition. We use the term "women" in the presentation of these data to maintain the integrity of how the data were originally reported; however, we recognize that not all individuals who may become pregnant identify as women, and we advocate the use of inclusive practices.

RESTRICTION CATEGORIES AND DEMOGRAPHICS

We categorized states into 3 post-*Dobbs* abortion restriction groups based on state abortion policies as of April 2024.[18,19] These are shown in Figure 1. The most restrictive group includes 21 states where abortion is severely restricted, 14 of which have complete abortion bans with very limited exceptions and 7 of which have an early gestational age ban of 6 to 18 weeks' gestation. The moderately restrictive group includes states where abortion is legally available but Medicaid coverage of abortion is prohibited, making abortion largely inaccessible to a significant portion of the population. These states also often have additional restrictive and burdensome policies (e.g., waiting periods, mandatory parental notification for minors) in place.[18] In this group, there are states that may eventually ban abortion but hostile legislation is currently blocked by courts (Wyoming and Iowa).[20] The least restrictive group includes states where abortion is both legally available and accessible. These states either have no gestational age ban or ban abortion at 24 weeks' gestation or later and allow Medicaid funds to pay for abortion.

Table 1 shows the population characteristics by post-*Dobbs* state abortion restriction category. In 2020, almost 32 million women of reproductive age lived in the 21 states that we identified as having the most restrictive post-*Dobbs* abortion laws, representing nearly half of the total US population of women of reproductive age. Before the *Dobbs* decision, the states that are now

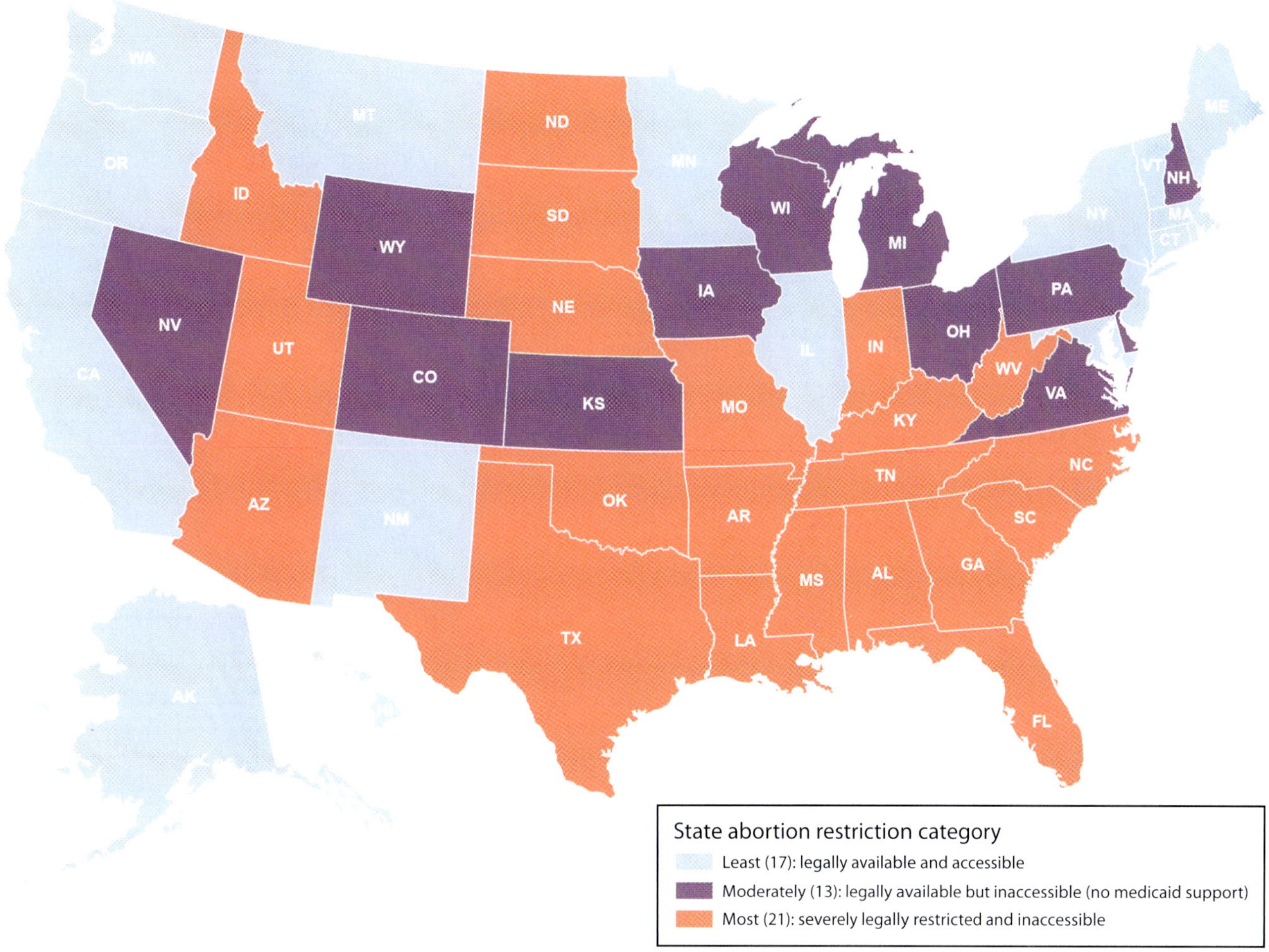

FIGURE 1— Map of the United States Showing 3 Severity Levels of Post-*Dobbs* Abortion Restrictions as of April 2024

Note. Colorado and Washington, DC, are included in the "moderately restrictive" group because despite being highly protective with no gestational age limit on abortion, they ban use of Medicaid funds to pay for abortion. The most restrictive states have complete abortion bans with the following exceptions: Florida (6-wk ban), Georgia (6-wk ban), South Carolina (6-wk ban), Nebraska (12-wk ban), North Carolina (12-wk ban), Arizona (15-wk ban), Utah (18-wk ban).
Source. Mapping created by Kelsey Rydland, Data Services Librarian at Northwestern University Libraries. Data citations are provided in the Appendix (available as a supplement to the online version of this article at http://www.ajph.org).

the most restrictive had the lowest cumulative abortion rate, but there were still close to 300 000 abortions performed in these states in 2020, which is approximately 32% of all US abortions that year.

In an analysis of the demographic characteristics of reproductive age women in the state abortion restriction groups (not shown), we found that the most restrictive states had the highest median percentage of non-Hispanic Black women, whereas the least restrictive states had the highest median percentage of women who identified as Hispanic and Asian. The most restrictive state group also had the highest percentage of reproductive age women with income less than 200% the federal poverty line (33%).

Across all 3 groups, approximately two thirds of reproductive age women had private insurance and one third had either Medicaid or were uninsured. In this one third, the most restrictive group had the lowest median percentage of women insured by Medicaid (16%) and the highest median percentage of women who were uninsured (13%), which included 5.2 million reproductive age women. By contrast to lower rates of Medicaid coverage outside pregnancy, the percentage of births paid for by Medicaid was highest in the most restrictive states (44%), likely reflecting the higher proportions of their populations that are uninsured if not pregnant who then qualify for Medicaid because of pregnancy. The most restrictive states also had the highest median percentage of births in which there was no insurance payor

AJPH October 2024, Vol. 114, No. 10

TABLE 1— Population Characteristics by Post-*Dobbs* State Abortion Restriction Category: United States, 2020

Characteristic	Least Restrictive (n = 17)	Moderately Restrictive (n = 13)	Most Restrictive (n = 21)
Total population of girls and women of reproductive age combined, no.	28 037 000	15 186 000	31 615 000
Range of girls and women of reproductive age per state	131 000–9 200 000	120 000–2 800 000	168 000–7 000 000
Total no. of abortions combined	480 850	159 990	289 360
Range of abortions before *Dobbs* per state	1 230–154 060	100–32 370	130–77 400
Abortion rate per 1000 girls and women of reproductive age	17.2	10.5	9.2
Total no. of births combined	1 312 000	731 178	1 620 000
Range of births per state	5 400–420 600	6 200–132 600	10 100–373 600
Birth rate per 1000 girls and women of reproductive age	46.8	48.1	51.2

Note. Data citations are provided in the Appendix (available as a supplement to the online version of this article at http://www.ajph.org). Figure 1 shows the states included in each abortion restriction category.

(4%), including close to 83 000 births in 2021.

As shown by these data, states with the most severe post-*Dobbs* abortion restrictions include nearly half of the total US population of women of reproductive age and, on average, have the highest percentages of individuals of reproductive age and birthing people who identify as non-Hispanic Black and who are of low socioeconomic status. As discussed previously, these are the populations that seek abortion care the most, and given their higher representation in states with more severe abortion restrictions, once again, these groups will disproportionately bear the burden of legislative limitations on access to care.[1,2]

ACCESS TO CARE AND SOCIAL SERVICES

One might hope that states with the most restrictive abortion policies—which advocate banning abortion on the grounds of protecting children and families and have the highest preexisting rates of socioeconomically disadvantaged reproductive age and birthing people—would have a highly developed public infrastructure to support access to reproductive health care and maternal and family social services. As we observe here, that is not the case. In fact, the inverse relationship is identified in several metrics.

Table 2 shows the relative access to reproductive health care and maternal and family social services by abortion restriction group. In general, states with more severe abortion restrictions are more likely to have limitations on access to reproductive health care, are less likely to implement policies that support families, have lower enrollment in state-funded assistance programs, and require that women and families be poorer to qualify for these programs compared with the least restrictive state group.

In our measures of access to general health care, the most restrictive states are less likely to implement policies that promote this access for reproductive age women. There are still 10 states that have not accepted Affordable Care Act funds to expand their Medicaid eligibility criteria, including 3 states in the moderately restrictive group and 7 states in the most restrictive group. In comparison, there are no states in the least restrictive group that have chosen to go against implementation of this expansion. This pattern is consistent with data demonstrating that the most restrictive states have the highest percentages of women of reproductive age who are uninsured. Notably, Medicaid expansion pursuant to the Affordable Care Act has been associated with a significant increase in the use of contraception, including long-acting reversible contraception, with the greatest gains in adolescents, which decreases the rate of unintended pregnancy.[21] The most restrictive states are also less likely to have policies that allow pharmacists to prescribe contraception (42.9% vs 82.4% of the least restrictive states), another barrier to access to general reproductive health care and reproductive autonomy.

People with reproductive potential continue to face restrictions to access to care in these states when they become pregnant. Of states in the most restrictive group, 10 (47.6%) have a Medicaid income eligibility level for pregnancy of less than 200% of the

TABLE 2— Access to Reproductive Health Care and Maternal and Family Social Services by Abortion Restriction Category: United States, April 2024

Measure of Access to Reproductive Health Care and Social Services	Least Restrictive (n = 17), No. (%) or Median (IQR)	Moderately Restrictive (n = 13), No. (%) or Median (IQR)	Most Restrictive (n = 21), No. (%) or Median (IQR)
Access to general preconception/gynecologic health care			
ACA Medicaid expansion	17 (100)	10 (76.9)	14 (66.7)
Pharmacists allowed to prescribe contraception	14 (82.4)	7 (53.9)	9 (42.9)
Access to prenatal and postpartum health care			
Medicaid income eligibility limit for pregnancy, % of FPL[a]	213 (205–258)	205 (200–263)	202 (162–214)
States with Medicaid income eligibility for pregnancy < 200% of FPL	4 (23.5)	3 (23.1)	10 (47.6)
Individuals of reproductive age that live in maternity care deserts	0.3 (0–3.3)	3.0 (0.7–5.4)	9.8 (4.5–16.3)
States with higher than average % of individuals of reproductive age living in maternity care deserts	2 (11.8)	3 (23.1)	14 (66.7)
WIC enrollment for pregnant and postpartum people, % of those eligible	56.3 (50.9–61.2)	52.7 (50.8–55.1)	52.0 (49.0–59.0)
States with WIC enrollment for pregnant and postpartum people < the national rate	11 (64.7)	10 (76.9)	14 (66.7)
Medicaid expansion for 1 y postpartum	17 (100)	11 (84.6)	18 (85.7)
Access to state-run family social services			
Paid family and medical leave	11 (64.7)	3 (23.1)	0
WIC enrollment for infants, % of those eligible	78.9 (72.3–85.7)	79.5 (71.8–88.2)	78.4 (75.1–85.5)
States with WIC enrollment for infants < the national rate	10 (58.8)	9 (69.2)	13 (61.9)
WIC enrollment for children, % of those eligible	43.3 (36.3–50.5)	38.5 (35.0–41.8)	37.5 (28.9–42.4)
States with WIC enrollment for children < the national rate	6 (35.3)	8 (61.5)	15 (71.4)
Maximum monthly income eligibility for TANF for a family of 3, $	1018 (908–1618)	818 (519–1061)	673 (401–908)
Maximum monthly income eligibility for TANF, % of FPL	56 (50–88)	45 (28–58)	37 (22–50)
Maximum monthly TANF benefit for a family of 3, $	632 (588–727)	508 (426–608)	292 (272–387)
States with income eligibility for childcare assistance < 200% of FPL	1 (5.9)	6 (46.2)	9 (42.9)

Note. ACA = Affordable Care Act; FPL = federal poverty level (according to the Department of Health and Human Services[5]); IQR = interquartile range; TANF = Temporary Assistance for Needy Families; WIC = Special Supplemental Nutrition Program for Women, Infants, and Children. Data citations are provided in the Appendix (available as a supplement to the online version of this article at http://www.ajph.org). Figure 1 shows the states included in each abortion restriction category.

[a]For reference, in 2022, 200% of the FPL was $27 180 for an individual, $36 620 for a family of 2, and $46 060 for a family of 3.

federal poverty line compared with only 4 (23.5%) states in the least restrictive group. Additionally, the most restrictive states have a higher median percentage of the population of reproductive age living in a maternity care desert: 9.8% versus just 0.3% in the least restrictive group. In the most restrictive states, this amounts to almost 1.1 million people of reproductive age who live in an area with no access to a hospital or birth center offering obstetric care or an obstetric provider.

Median WIC (the federally sponsored and locally administered Special Supplemental Nutrition Program for Women, Infants, and Children) enrollment for eligible pregnant and postpartum people was slightly higher in the least restrictive group but was notably barely greater than 50% across all 3 state groups. Finally, although Medicaid expansion to 12 months postpartum has become widely implemented in the past several years, there are still 3 states in the most restrictive group and 2 states in the moderately restrictive group that have not yet implemented this vital policy, compared with no remaining states in the least restrictive group.

Even after pregnancy, families and children living in the most restrictive states receive less support than those in the least restrictive states. One of the most important findings of our analysis concerns state policies mandating paid family and medical leave. Although the federal Family and Medical Leave Act

TABLE 3— Most Restrictive States and Access to Reproductive Health Care and Maternal and Family Social Services: United States, April 2024

State	No ACA Expansion	Medicaid Income Eligibility for Pregnancy <200% FPL	Higher Than Average % of Reproductive Age People Living in Maternity Care Deserts	WIC Enrollment for Pregnant and PP People Less Than the National Rate	No PP Medicaid Expansion	No Paid Family and Medical Leave	WIC Enrollment for Infants < the National Rate	WIC Enrollment for Children < the National Rate	Lowest Third of TANF Income Eligibility	Lowest Third of TANF Benefits	Income Eligibility for Childcare Assistance <200% of FPL
NC						X				X	
KY			X			X				X	
OK			X			X		X		X	
IN			X			X			X	X	X
NE			X	X		X	X				X
SD		X	X	X		X	X				
TX	X					X		X	X	X	
ND		X	X	X		X	X	X			
TN	X		X	X		X	X	X			
WV			X	X		X	X	X			X
AZ		X		X		X	X		X	X	X
LA		X	X	X		X		X	X	X	
SC	X	X		X		X	X	X		X	
UT		X		X	X	X	X	X	X		
AL	X	X	X			X		X	X	X	X
AR			X	X	X	X	X	X	X	X	
FL	X	X				X	X	X	X	X	X
GA	X			X		X	X	X	X	X	X
MS	X	X	X	X		X		X	X	X	
MO			X	X		X	X	X	X	X	X
ID		X	X	X	X	X	X	X		X	X

Note. ACA = Affordable Care Act; FPL = federal poverty level (according to the Department of Health and Human Services[5]); PP = postpartum; TANF = Temporary Assistance for Needy Families; WIC = Special Supplemental Nutrition Program for Women, Infants, and Children. Data are provided in the Appendix (available as a supplement to the online version of this article at http://www.ajph.org).

(1993) guarantees most workers access to unpaid, job-protected parental, family caregiver, and personal medical leave, it does not require employers to continue to pay their employees during this time. Despite the American College of Obstetricians and Gynecologists' endorsement of paid parental leave after childbirth, more than 50% of postpartum people do not have access to paid leave.[22] Notably, the United States is one of the only high-income countries without a national paid family caregiving or medical leave policy and, as of the writing of this essay, only 14 states have passed state-mandated paid family and medical leave policies.[23,24] Of these 14 states, 11 (78%) are in the least restrictive state group. Of the states with the most restrictive abortion bans, none has a mandatory paid family and medical leave policy.

Many states with the most severe abortion restrictions also make it harder for people with children to qualify for state-funded assistance programs, and they provide less support for those who do qualify. In 2020, the national percentage of eligible children enrolled in WIC was 40.6%. The group of most restrictive states included the highest number of states with WIC enrollment for eligible children below the national average (71% vs 35% in the least restrictive group). Additionally, in the most restrictive state group, on average, families of 3 need to make less than $673 per month to qualify for the TANF (Temporary Assistance for Needy Families) program and receive an average benefit of $292 per month. By contrast, families in the least restrictive states can make almost twice as much and still qualify, and they receive twice the benefit. Similarly, families need to be poorer to qualify for childcare assistance in the most restrictive states.

Table 3 summarizes these outcomes in each of the 21 most restrictive states. We selected 11 of these metrics of access to reproductive health care and maternal and family social services that we feel are most relevant and representative to visually compare these restrictive states. The states are ordered by the number of items they score poorly on from least to most. Some states, such as North Carolina and Kentucky, score poorly on only a few of these metrics, whereas others, such as Idaho, Alabama, Arkansas, Florida, Georgia, Mississippi, and Missouri, fail to support children, women, and families on most of these metrics. By presenting these data, we sought to highlight individual state-specific areas and policies for future advocacy efforts and research endeavors.

CONCLUSIONS

The creation and funding of state-based programs and policies that support access to care for disadvantaged pregnant persons and their children and families clearly demonstrate the importance these states place on these populations' well-being. The data presented here highlight the noticeable absence of participation in such value statements by states with the most severe abortion restrictions. Abortion opponents often assert that they are motivated by an ethical issue of fetal personhood and that by banning or significantly restricting abortion access, they are acting to protect children, women, and families.[13,14] In our analysis, states with the most severe abortion restrictions have the least comprehensive and least inclusive public infrastructure to support access to reproductive health care and family social services. It would seem in these states that the abortion opponent, pro-life attitude not only begins at conception but ends there as well.

Although it may not be surprising that the most politically conservative states with the most restrictive post-*Dobbs* abortion policies are also the most socially and financially conservative with regards to reproductive health, the degree to which these states fail to support their most disadvantaged populations warrants immediate attention and action. Although we maintain that abortion is essential health care and advocate continued efforts to eliminate restrictive abortion policies, our results also highlight an opportunity to use the child protection arguments of conservative policymakers and encourage them to "put their money where their mouth is" by advocating the implementation and improvement of policies that support individual and family well-being.

We highlight several policies and programs throughout this essay that advocates may choose to target in their own state, and Table 3 outlines these opportunities for the 21 most restrictive states. Such advocacy campaigns may target adding new policies (e.g., postpartum Medicaid expansion or paid family and medical leave), expansion of existing policies (e.g., increasing eligibility for state-based assistance programs such as WIC and TANF), or the creation of new programs (e.g., mobile health clinics to serve pregnant people in maternity care deserts).

Improvements in policies and programs designed to support vulnerable populations during pregnancy and beyond can never justify a lack of access to abortion care; however, if policymakers insist on restricting reproductive autonomy on the grounds of protection, then we believe they must also ensure that pregnancy and family building are safe, supported, and equitable. AJPH

ABOUT THE AUTHORS

At the time of this study, all authors were with the Department of Obstetrics and Gynecology, Division of Maternal-Fetal Medicine, Northwestern University Feinberg School of Medicine, Chicago, IL. Katie Watson is also with Medical Social Sciences, Northwestern University Feinberg School of Medicine.

CORRESPONDENCE

Correspondence should be sent to Nigel Madden, MD, Department of Obstetrics and Gynecology, Northwestern University Feinberg School of Medicine, Prentice Women's Hospital, 250 E. Superior St, 5th Floor, Chicago, IL 60611 (e-mail: nigelmadden@gmail.com). Reprints can be ordered at https://www.ajph.org by clicking the "Reprints" link.

PUBLICATION INFORMATION

Full Citation: Madden N, Trawick E, Watson K, Yee LM. Post-*Dobbs* abortion restrictions and the families they leave behind. *Am J Public Health*. 2024;114(10):1043–1050.

Acceptance Date: July 2, 2024.

DOI: https://doi.org/10.2105/AJPH.2024.307792

ORCID iD:

Lynn M. Yee https://orcid.org/0000-0002-6274-0544

CONTRIBUTORS

N. Madden conceptualized the project, collected and analyzed the data, and led the writing of the essay. E. Trawick assisted in writing the essay. K Watson assisted with framing the project and the essay. L. M. Yee assisted with conceptualization and supervision of the project and with writing the essay.

ACKNOWLEDGMENTS

We would like to thank Kelsey Rydland, data services librarian at Northwestern University Libraries, for assistance in creation of the map showing the post-*Dobbs* abortion restrictions categories.

CONFLICTS OF INTEREST

The authors report no conflicts of interest.

HUMAN PARTICIPANT PROTECTION

This study is exempt from institutional review board review, as all data used in the analysis were publicly available. No human participants were involved.

REFERENCES

1. Jerman J, Jones RK, Onda T. Characteristics of US abortion patients in 2014 and changes since 2008. Available at: https://www.guttmacher.org/report/characteristics-us-abortion-patients-2014. Accessed March 21, 2023.
2. Williams DR, Mohammed SA, Leavell J, Collins C. Race, socioeconomic status, and health: complexities, ongoing challenges, and research opportunities. *Ann N Y Acad Sci*. 2010;1186:69–101. https://doi.org/10.1111/j.1749-6632.2009.05339.x
3. Liu E, Shen W. The Hyde Amendment: an overview. 2022. Available at: https://crsreports.congress.gov/product/details?prodcode=IF12167. Accessed October 25, 2023.
4. Upadhyay UD, Ahlbach C, Kaller S, Cook C, Muñoz I. Trends in self-pay charges and insurance acceptance for abortion in the United States, 2017–20. *Health Aff (Millwood)*. 2022;41(4): 507–515. https://doi.org/10.1377/hlthaff.2021.01528
5. Department of Health and Human Services. 2022 Poverty guidelines: 48 contiguous states (all states except Alaska and Hawaii). Available at: https://aspe.hhs.gov/sites/default/files/documents/4b515876c4674466423975826ac57583/Guidelines-2022.pdf. Accessed August 1, 2024.
6. McDonnell J, Jarlenski M, Borrero S, Vinekar K. Association of availability of state Medicaid coverage for abortion with abortion access in the United States. *Obstet Gynecol*. 2022;140(4): 623–630. https://doi.org/10.1097/AOG.0000000000004933
7. Henshaw SK, Joyce TJ, Dennis A, Finer LB, Blanchard K. Restrictions on Medicaid funding for abortions: a literature review. June 2009. Available at: https://www.guttmacher.org/sites/default/files/report_pdf/medicaidlitreview.pdf. Accessed August 1, 2024.
8. Society of Family Planning. #WeCount Public Report. April 2022 to September 2023. Available at: https://doi.org/10.46621/675707thmfmv. Accessed August 1, 2024.
9. Aiken ARA, Starling JE, Scott JG, Gomperts R. Requests for self-managed medication abortion provided using online telemedicine in 30 US states before and after the *Dobbs v Jackson Women's Health Organization* decision. *JAMA*. 2022;328(17):1768–1770. https://doi.org/10.1001/jama.2022.18865
10. Centers for Disease Control and Prevention. Racial/Ethnic disparities in pregnancy-related deaths—United States, 2007–2016. *MMWR Morb Mortal Wkly Rep*. 2019;68(35):762–765. https://doi.org/10.15585/mmwr.mm6835a3
11. Holdt Somer SJ, Sinkey RG, Bryant AS. Epidemiology of racial/ethnic disparities in severe maternal morbidity and mortality. *Semin Perinatol*. 2017;41(5): 258–265. https://doi.org/10.1053/j.semperi.2017.04.001
12. Foster DG. *The Turnaway Study*. New York, NY: Simon & Schuster; 2020.
13. National Right to Life. *The State of Abortion in the United States*. 11th ed. February 2024. Available at: https://www.nrlc.org/wp-content/uploads/StateofAbortion2024.pdf. Accessed August 1, 2024.
14. Students for Life of America. Save babies. Empower women. Abolish abortion. 2023. Available at: https://studentsforlife.org. Accessed August 1, 2024.
15. Miller CC, Sanger-Katz M. States with abortion bans are among least supportive for mothers and children. *New York Times*. July 22, 2022. Available at: https://www.nytimes.com/2022/07/28/upshot/abortion-bans-states-social-services.html. Accessed August 1, 2024.
16. Treisman R. States with the toughest abortion laws have the weakest maternal supports, data shows. August 18, 2022. Available at: https://www.npr.org/2022/08/18/1111344810/abortion-ban-states-social-safety-net-health-outcomes. Accessed August 1, 2024.
17. Deloitte. March of Dimes maternity care desert dashboard. Available at: https://www2.deloitte.com/us/en/pages/life-sciences-and-health-care/articles/march-of-dimes-maternity-care-deserts-dashboard.html. Accessed August 1, 2024.
18. Guttmacher Institute. Interactive map: US abortion policies and access after *Roe*. July 29, 2024. Available at: https://states.guttmacher.org/policies. Accessed August 1, 2024.
19. Kitchener C, Schaul K, Kirkpatrick N, Santamarina D, Tierney L. States where abortion is legal, banned or under threat. *Washington Post*. February 22, 2023. Available at: https://www.washingtonpost.com/politics/2022/06/24/abortion-state-laws-criminalization-roe. Accessed August 1, 2024.
20. Nash E, Guarnieri I. Six months post-*Roe*, 24 US states have banned abortion or are likely to do so: a roundup. January 2023. Available at: https://www.guttmacher.org/2023/01/six-months-post-roe-24-us-states-have-banned-abortion-or-are-likely-do-so-roundup. Accessed August 1, 2024.
21. Darney BG, Jacob RL, Hoopes M, et al. Evaluation of Medicaid expansion under the Affordable Care Act and contraceptive care in US community health centers. *JAMA Netw Open*. 2020;3(6): e206874. https://doi.org/10.1001/jamanetworkopen.2020.6874
22. ACOG Committee opinion no. 733: employment considerations during pregnancy and the postpartum period. *Obstet Gynecol*. 2018;131(4):e115–e123. https://doi.org/10.1097/AOG.0000000000002589
23. Bipartisan Policy Center. State paid family leave laws across the US. January 16, 2023. Available at: https://bipartisanpolicy.org/explainer/state-paid-family-leave-laws-across-the-u-s. Accessed August 1, 2024.
24. Bipartisan Policy Center. Paid family leave across OECD countries. March 1, 2022. Available at: https://bipartisanpolicy.org/explainer/paid-family-leave-across-oecd-countries. Accessed August 1, 2024.

Navigating the Labyrinth of Pregnancy-Related Coverage for Undocumented Immigrants: An Assessment of Current State and Federal Policies

Amanda DiMeo, MSc, Rasheca Logendran, BA, Benjamin D. Sommers, MD, PhD, Alexandra Beecroft, BS, Yessamin Pazos Herencia, BS, Maria Bazan, MD, MPH, Carrie Wade, MLIS, Jeffrey Sprankle, BS, Margaret M. Sullivan, DrPH, FNP, and Rose L. Molina, MD, MPH

Insurance coverage for prenatal care, labor and delivery care, and postpartum care for undocumented immigrants consists of a patchwork of state and federal policies, which varies widely by state. According to federal law, states must provide coverage for labor and delivery through Emergency Medicaid. Various states have additional prenatal and postpartum coverage for undocumented immigrants through policy mechanisms such as the Children's Health Insurance Program's "unborn child" option, expansion of Medicaid, and independent state-level mechanisms.

Using a search of state Medicaid and federal government websites, we found that 27 states and the District of Columbia provide additional coverage for prenatal care, postpartum care, or both, while 23 states do not. Twelve states include any postpartum coverage; 7 provide coverage for 12 months postpartum.

Although information regarding coverage is available publicly online, there exist many barriers to access, such as lack of transparency, lack of availability of information in multiple languages, and incorrect information. More inclusive and easily accessible policies are needed as the first step toward improving maternal health among undocumented immigrants, a population trapped in a complicated web of immigration policy and a maternal health crisis. (*Am J Public Health*. 2024;114(10):1051–1060. https://doi.org/10.2105/AJPH.2024.307750)

AJPH October 2024, Vol. 114, No. 10

The patchwork policy landscape of pregnancy coverage for people who are undocumented across the United States is difficult to navigate. Immigration law is complex, dynamic, and regulated at the federal level, while policies determining health care coverage are regulated at both the federal and state levels, leading to variable coverage across and within states. Pregnant people who are undocumented are thus left with the extremely challenging experience of navigating the labyrinths of the immigration and health care systems while living at an intersection of divisive anti-immigration rhetoric and policy[1] and a devastating maternal health crisis.[2]

The United States continues to have poor—and worsening—maternal health outcomes, including dramatic inequities in pregnancy outcomes by race and ethnicity[2] with limited understanding of intersectional structural barriers, such as immigration and language. People who are undocumented remain at increased vulnerability because of gaps in access and quality of pregnancy care.[3] Prenatal care is a valued preventive health service with associated improvements in maternal and infant health outcomes and reduced risk of pregnancy complications.[4]

Few studies investigating pregnancy outcomes collect immigration status, and those that do are hampered by nonstandardized, inaccurate proxies for undocumented populations.[5]

Little is known about health outcomes for pregnant people who are undocumented.[6] Research is limited by the inherent challenge of understanding a population that holds valid concerns about disclosure of immigration status for fear of discrimination, job loss, deportation, and family separation.[7] In addition, there are multiple barriers that undocumented patients face in accessing pregnancy care, including fear of procedures or disclosure of pregnancy, long wait times, distant location, clinic hours that interfere with childcare or work obligations, lack of language access, implicit bias of staff, and cost of services.[7]

This analytic essay provides an overview of current federal and state-level mechanisms providing coverage for pregnant people who are undocumented and presents a cross-sectional analysis of state policies based on publicly available information. These findings can help inform policymakers and facilitate future research on the impact of these policies. The essay concludes with policy recommendations to improve care for this population at the crossroads of 2 highly complex systems.

FEDERAL PREGNANCY COVERAGE

Immigrants with authorized status include naturalized US citizens, lawful permanent residents (green card holders), or individuals who have been granted temporary lawful resident status, such as students from another country.[8] For example, the Deferred Action for Childhood Arrivals (DACA) program allows people who arrived in the United States as children a temporary status that may be renewed every 2 years and may allow them to live and work in the United States.[9] However, DACA itself does not offer citizenship. The US Department of Homeland Security also has power to grant "parole" to some noncitizens, allowing them to enter or remain in the United States if there are urgent humanitarian or public health benefits for someone to be in the United States.[10] This leads to a complex, "in-between" zone for some individuals and further complicates understanding of authorized status in this country.

The term "undocumented" fails to capture the dynamic complexity of all different authorized and unauthorized immigration statuses yet remains an umbrella term for those who are present in the United States without the permission of the US government. Many individuals have a status that may offer temporary reprieve but does not put them on the pathway toward permanent residence or citizenship. The Pew Research Center estimated that 77% of immigrants held an authorized status and approximately 23% were undocumented in 2017[8] or unauthorized, meaning they did not have sufficient documentation to remain in the country.[11] In 2017, there were an estimated 10.5 million unauthorized immigrants in the United States, making up about 3.2% of the US population.[8] For example, they may have an expired visa or a pending or denied application for asylum, or they may have entered the country outside of an official entry point. Notably, 6% of all children born in the United States have an undocumented parent.[12]

Historically, major federal public benefits programs have excluded undocumented immigrants and some immigrants on temporary stay.[13] Before immigration policy changed in 1996, some immigrants were eligible for certain benefits based on a category (not an immigration status) called "permanently resided in the U.S. under color of law," which has been interpreted differently depending on region and program.[13] Generally, it meant that the US Department of Homeland Security was aware of the person's presence in the United States and had no plans to deport them from the country. A few states continue to use this definition.[14]

In 1996, the Personal Responsibility and Work Opportunity Reconciliation Act was enacted and created 2 categories of immigrants for the purpose of benefits eligibility: "qualified" and "not qualified." The "qualified" category includes lawful permanent residents (green card holders), refugees, and other specific inclusion criteria, such as country of origin.[14] All other immigrants, including those who are undocumented, and many others who are lawfully present, are considered "not qualified." This law also created time requirements of 5 years or longer for lawfully residing qualified immigrants to become eligible for benefits coverage.[14] This is colloquially referred to as a "5-year bar." As of now, there do exist exceptions to the 5-year waiting period, including for refugees, asylees, or lawful permanent residents who were formerly refugees or asylees.[15] States also have the option to remove the 5-year waiting period to cover children or pregnant people under Medicaid or Children's Health Insurance Program (CHIP). This 5-year bar does not apply to unqualified immigrants, including those who are unauthorized or undocumented, who are not eligible for full Medicaid benefits even after 5 years.

The law itself does not specify which programs are covered as "federal public benefits programs." In 1998, the Department of Health and Human Services published a notice of which programs fall under this definition, including Medicaid, CHIP, and Medicare, among others. Importantly, the law includes some exceptions.[14] Nonqualified immigrants, including undocumented immigrants, are eligible for Emergency Medicaid if they otherwise meet income requirements and other eligibility criteria for their state's Medicaid program.[14]

All states must provide Emergency Medicaid to people who would otherwise qualify for Medicaid with the exception of their immigration status. Emergency Medicaid provides limited coverage during pregnancy, usually for childbirth only, and is essentially a payment mechanism to cover health care costs for individuals who have been diagnosed with an emergency medical condition as defined by each state, such as a heart attack or kidney failure requiring dialysis. Emergency Medicaid may cover prenatal care in the case of high-risk pregnancies only and postpartum care in cases of severe morbidity, both covering conditions that may be life-threatening. There is a federal statutory definition of "emergency medical condition" that allows states some flexibility for interpretation; however, states cannot create a new or different definition of an emergency medical condition.[16,17]

In 2010, the Affordable Care Act (ACA) catalyzed sweeping health care reform and improved access, except for people who are undocumented. The ACA does allow lawfully present people with status of less than 5 years to purchase insurance on the health care exchange, even if they may not meet income requirements.[15] People who were undocumented were excluded from state insurance exchanges, ineligible for tax credits and lower copayments, and exempt from the individual mandate to hold health care coverage; they remained eligible for Emergency Medicaid services only.[18] Notably, as of May 2024, the Biden–Harris administration removed the prohibition on DACA recipient's eligibility for ACA coverage, allowing more than 100 000 individuals to access health insurance.[19]

The public charge ruling is a federal policy that has had a chilling effect on immigrant communities, including those who are undocumented, even though it does not directly pertain to those who are undocumented.[19,20] In 2022, the US Department of Homeland Security issued a final rule clarifying public charge as a method to determine whether someone applying for lawful permanent residence (green card) or another specific visa would be likely to depend on the government as their primary means of support.[21] This did not apply to naturalized citizens, people who already have green cards, individuals with DACA, those with Temporary Protected Status, undocumented individuals without authorized status, or people with humanitarian status. However, because an earlier 2020 ruling included several additional factors in the determination of likelihood of becoming a "public charge" (including some uses of Medicaid, nutritional assistance, cash assistance, and housing with federal funding), many immigrants, regardless of whether they were subject to this rule, avoided accessing health-promoting benefits for which they were eligible.[22]

The final 2022 rule restored the understanding that supplemental public health benefits, like Medicaid and nutritional assistance programs, are not part of the public charge inadmissibility determination.[21] However, the previous policy was seen to have a chilling effect on public program participation. In the months following the passage of the 2020 policy, health care centers reported that immigrant families declined to enroll themselves, their children, or both in Medicaid, along with other programs like the Special Supplemental Nutrition Program for Women, Infants, and Children.[19] A study from the Kaiser Family Foundation reported that pregnant women were delaying care or seeking prenatal care less frequently on the basis of their fear of enrollment.[20] Overall, these policy changes led to widespread misinformation and fear regarding seeking health care among many immigrant populations, including undocumented pregnant women, even if they were not subject to the rulings.

Federally qualified health centers are the backbone for preventive care among minoritized communities, including those who are undocumented. Federally qualified health centers qualify for funding under the Public Health Service Act and enhanced reimbursement from Medicare and Medicaid. They must offer a sliding fee scale and provide comprehensive services, importantly serving all community members, regardless of citizenship or documentation status. They must also be governed by a board with a majority of members who receive care at the federally qualified health center.[19,23]

AJPH October 2024, Vol. 114, No. 10

STATE PREGNANCY COVERAGE

According to federal requirements, CHIP, which is jointly funded by both the state and federal government, is administered by the individual state. Generally, CHIP provides coverage to eligible low-income uninsured children and pregnant women whose income is too high for Medicaid eligibility. States have broad flexibility in terms of the scope of services that are covered. Under federal regulations as of 2009,[24] states can provide pregnancy-related care through the CHIP state plan to low-income children from conception to birth. This program was called the "unborn child" option by Congress, though others have objected to the use of this term.[25] Advocates describe the use of the term unborn child as an attempt to integrate fetal personhood into policy in the context of the ongoing antiabortion movement, thereby narrowing eligibility for services specifically for the unborn child and indicating that the people carrying the pregnancies are not worthy of coverage themselves.[26] We will use the term "CHIP pregnancy care" to refer to this policy. This program allows states the option to provide prenatal, childbirth, and postpartum care to pregnant people regardless of immigration status.[25] Given that it is implemented through CHIP, the specificities of the CHIP pregnancy care option vary by state in regard to the income requirements and extent of prenatal and postpartum coverage.

Recently, some states have expanded their Medicaid programs to include coverage for undocumented immigrants with state funds, not federal funds. Some states have also expanded Medicaid or CHIP to "lawfully present" children and pregnant noncitizens.[15] People who are considered lawfully present may include those with qualified status, including asylees and refugees, persons from specific geographies or lawful permanent residents holding a green card, and others. States also have the option to remove a waiting period for all pregnant people if they are lawfully present rather than only those who are qualified. Eligibility criteria for coverage is complex and opaque. States vary in their coverage of what pregnancy services are included. Furthermore, there is proposed legislation in Congress that would repeal the arbitrary 5-year waiting period before accessing health care coverage and other public benefits created by the Personal Responsibility and Work Opportunity Reconciliation Act.[27] Figure 1 shows a timeline of relevant federal and state policies for health care coverage for undocumented immigrants.

Because there is no centralized resource that allows for easy access to information regarding health care coverage for undocumented immigrants, we searched each state Medicaid website, many of which were not user-friendly and described health care coverage with policy jargon. Furthermore, when this information could not be identified on state Medicaid websites, researchers reviewed secondary policy websites, such as the Kaiser Family Foundation website, which led to conflicting or outdated information. Despite the myriad challenges in corroborating and confirming some information, we report what was found to be most accurate at the time of data collection. A detailed list of websites and resources reviewed can be found in Table A (available as a supplement to the online version of this article at https://ajph.org).

PREGNANCY COVERAGE LANDSCAPE

We analyzed pregnancy coverage mechanisms by estimated total population and proportion of undocumented people in each state using data from the Pew Research Center. We present the landscape of policy mechanisms that provide health care coverage for pregnant people who are undocumented, including both state and jointly funded state and federal mechanisms, and the relative magnitude of the population affected by these policies.

Each state has distinct pregnancy care services that can be covered by different funding mechanisms. For example, many states use Emergency Medicaid funding to cover inpatient labor and delivery and apply CHIP to fund prenatal and postpartum services. Our research found that only 18 states and Washington, DC provided prenatal, labor and delivery, and postpartum coverage for undocumented individuals, although the cost to patients, specific services covered, and length of coverage within these pregnancy phases varied. In addition, 9 states provided limited coverage of some prenatal care services, labor and delivery services through Emergency Medicaid, and no postpartum care. The 23 remaining states had severely restricted coverage, offering only labor and delivery coverage through Emergency Medicaid. Figure 2 summarizes the state-based scope of pregnancy care coverage for undocumented people.

All states provided coverage for labor and delivery regardless of documentation status under Emergency Medicaid, though the scope of services covered is determined by each state. Twenty-seven states and the District of Columbia

Permanently Resided in the US Under Color of Law	Emergency Medical Treatment and Labor Act	Personal Responsibility and Work Opportunity Reconciliation Act	The Children's Health Insurance Program Reauthorization Act	Affordable Care Act	Expansion of the Scope of Public Charge	Restoration of the Lifting Immigrant Families Through Benefits Act
Pre-1996	1986	1996	2009	2010	2019	2024
• Interpreted eligibility category for individuals permanently residing in the US	• Required all hospitals with emergency departments to provide a medical screening examination • Hospitals are required to provide stabilizing treatments for individuals with emergency medical conditions	• Created a time requirement of at least 5 years for lawfully residing immigrants to fulfill before being eligible for coverage • Defined 2 categories for public benefit eligibility: qualified vs nonqualified immigrants. Qualified immigrants include asylees and refugees while nonqualified immigrants include undocumented individuals	• Allowed states the option to cover the fetus as a "targeted low-income child" and thus allowed for CHIP to cover pregnancy care	• Excluded undocumented people from state exchanges • Eligibility for Emergency Medicaid • In 2012, the Supreme Court made expansion voluntary for states	• Supplemental health benefits like Medicaid and SNAP are not part of public charge inadmissibility determination	• A proposed bill that would repeal the 5-year waiting period

FIGURE 1— Overview of Federal and State Policies Relevant to Health Care Coverage for Undocumented Immigrants: United States, 1990s–2020s

Note. CHIP = Children's Health Insurance Program; SNAP = Supplemental Nutrition Assistance Program.

provided additional coverage for prenatal care, postpartum care, or both, while 23 states did not. Twenty states opted in to the CHIP pregnancy care option, though with considerable variation. Some states, such as Louisiana and Nebraska, only provided coverage for pregnancy-related care, while other states, such as Connecticut, covered most medical needs as long as the individual qualified for the CHIP pregnancy care option. Limited information is available on the state websites regarding the details of this plan and how it is administered in each state. Of the information that could be found regarding this option, 12 states explicitly mention postpartum coverage, with only 7 states providing postpartum coverage for a full 12 months after birth. Details outlining the states that utilize the CHIP pregnancy care option and their respective postpartum coverage can be found in Table 1. An overview of the federal and state policies is available in Figure A (available as a supplement to the online version of this article at https://ajph.org).

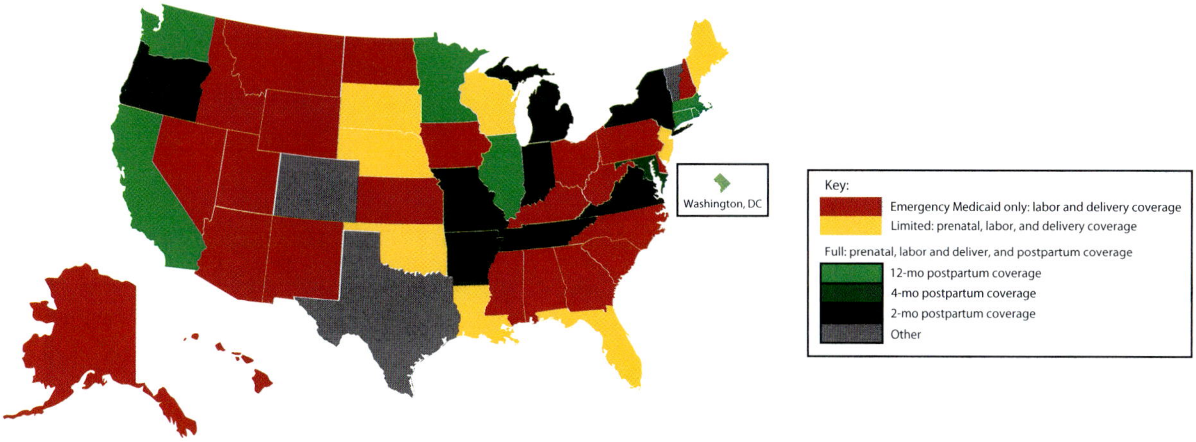

FIGURE 2— Map of State-Based Pregnancy Care Coverage for Undocumented Individuals: United States, 2023

TABLE 1— State-Based Pregnancy Care Coverage for Undocumented People: United States, 2023

State[a]	Unauthorized Immigrant Percentage of Population,[28] %	Uptake of the CHIP Pregnancy Care Option[24]	CHIP Pregnancy Care Option FPL Requirement,[24] %	Postpartum Coverage Through CHIP Pregnancy Care Option[b]	Inclusion in State Medicaid Program	State Medicaid FPL Requirement, %
Arkansas	1.9	Yes	214	60 d	No	. . .
California[c]	5.6	Yes	322	12 mo	Yes	213[d]
Connecticut	3.5	Yes	263	12 mo	No	. . .
Illinois[e]	3.2	Yes	213	12 mo	Yes	213
Louisiana	1.5	Yes	214	None	No	. . .
Maine	0.4	Yes	213	None	Yes	214
Maryland	4.5	No	. . .	. . .	Yes	250
Massachusetts	3.8	Yes	205	12 mo	Yes	200
Michigan	1.0	Yes	200	None	No	. . .
Minnesota	1.7	Yes	283	12 mo	No	. . .
Missouri	1.0	Yes	305	60 d	No	. . .
Nebraska	3.1	Yes	202	None	No	. . .
New York	3.6	No	. . .	. . .	Yes	223
Oklahoma	2.2	Yes	210	None	No	. . .
Oregon	2.6	Yes	190	None	Yes	185
Rhode Island	2.8	Yes	258	12 mo	Yes	258
South Dakota	0.7	Yes	138	None	No	. . .
Tennessee	2.0	Yes	255	60 d	No	. . .
Texas	5.7	Yes	207	2 postpartum care visits	No	. . .
Virginia	3.4	Yes	205	60 d	No	. . .
Washington	3.3	Yes	198	12 mo	Yes	193
Wisconsin	1.3	Yes	306	None	No	. . .

Note. CHIP = Children's Health Insurance Program; FPL = federal poverty level (according to the US Department of Health and Human Services).
[a]States that did not participate in the programs listed in the table are AL, AK, AZ, CO, DC, DE, FL, GA, HI, IA, ID, IN, KS, KY, MS, MT, NC, ND, NE, NH, NJ, NM, OH, PA, SC, UT, VT, WV, and WY.
[b]Several states extended coverage to 12 months under the CHIP pregnancy care option to align with Medicaid postpartum coverage extension from 60 days to 12 months established by the American Rescue Plan of 2021.
[c]Medi-Cal (Medicaid of CA) provides coverage for all young adults aged 19–26 years regardless of immigration status and adults aged ≥ 50 years.
[d]To meet eligibility requirements for Medi-Cal, applicants must have income meeting 213% FPL. Income that is meeting 214%–322% FPL qualifies applicants for the Medi-Cal Access Program, which provides low-cost comprehensive health care throughout pregnancy through 1 y postpartum to middle-income families.
[e]Illinois has a Medicaid/CHIP joint-funded program called Moms and Babies that covers health care for women while they are pregnant and up to 12 months after delivery. It is a full Medicaid benefit package including outpatient health care, inpatient hospital care, and prescription drugs.

A state-based mechanism to provide coverage for pregnant undocumented immigrants is using state funds to cover undocumented immigrants in Medicaid. See Box 1 for details about the programs. Five states and Washington, DC, have created other independent mechanisms to provide pregnancy-related services to undocumented immigrants. For example, in 2021, OmniSalud was created to provide a secure, online marketplace for undocumented persons living in Colorado to compare and purchase insurance plans without sharing their data with federal agencies. OmniSalud does not require information about immigration status by any user, and information provided to the online platform cannot be used for immigration enforcement. As a requirement of OmniSalud, all companies that sell health insurance in Colorado must provide an affordable plan for everyone, regardless of immigration or pregnancy status.

Washington, DC, has a similar program, Cover All D.C., which allows people who are undocumented to

BOX 1— Other State Programs of Pregnancy Care Coverage for Undocumented Individuals: United States

State	Programs	Description
Colorado	OmniSalud	• Established in 2021 • Facilitates undocumented residents in comparing and enrolling in affordable health insurance plans online • Insurers are mandated to offer Colorado Options Plans with a requirement to reduce premiums on these plans by 15% by 2025
District of Columbia	DC Healthcare Alliance Program Cover All DC	• Locally funded, for DC residents aged ≥ 21 y not eligible for Medicaid • Allows for the purchase of full-cost private health insurance without a qualifying immigration status
Indiana	Indiana Health Coverage Plans (Emergency Medicaid extension)	• Covers prenatal and postpartum services up to 60 d • Emergency Medicaid covers childbirth
Michigan	Maternity Outpatient Medical Services program (Emergency Medicaid extension)	• Provides immediate coverage for prenatal care and 2 mo postpartum • Family planning services and supplies covered using state general funds
New Jersey	New Jersey Supplemental Prenatal and Contraceptive Program	• Run by New Jersey Medicaid and provides prenatal and family planning services only to people who are undocumented • Does not cover hospital visits or labor and delivery
Vermont	Immigrant Health Insurance Plan	• State-funded health care program for pregnant individuals and children aged < 19 y who have an immigration status for which Medicaid is not available • Covers hospital, medical, and dental services and prescription drugs

purchase full-cost private health insurance. Washington, DC, also has a district-funded program, Healthcare Alliance, that provides medical care for DC residents who are not eligible for Medicaid. In 2021, Vermont created a new state-funded health care program to provide care for pregnant people who do not meet Medicaid requirements because of immigration status, called Immigrant Health Insurance Plan. This program covers hospital, medical, and dental services, as well as prescription drugs. While programs may allow undocumented immigrants to buy health care plans, this does not equate with meaningful access. Many of these plans can be very expensive, especially if they are not offered at a subsidized rate.

The Pew Research Center found that the 5 states with highest proportions of undocumented individuals were Nevada (7.1%), Texas (5.7%), California (5.6%), New Jersey (5.2%), and Maryland (4.5%).[28] Despite having the largest proportion of undocumented individuals, Nevada provides no pregnancy care coverage for this population aside from childbirth services through Emergency Medicaid only (Table 1). California, on the other hand, provides the most extensive pregnancy coverage for the undocumented population, while the other states provide variable coverage (Table 1).

LACK OF TRANSPARENCY AND ACCESSIBILITY OF STATE POLICIES

Lack of transparency of information about pregnancy care coverage for undocumented individuals was a major barrier. Websites were not up to date (e.g., had last been updated more than 5 years ago), or information was vague and incomplete. At times, there was contradictory information found on different web pages. Six follow-up phone calls to Medicaid offices were made. Only 1 office was able to provide accurate information within a period of less than 10 minutes of waiting. Out of the 5 other offices, 4 offices were unable to confirm the information because of automated messages or did not lead to a human contact within approximately 10 minutes of waiting. The remaining office did not know the information off hand, but pointed to the Medicaid website.

Language access for individuals who speak languages other than English was limited. While 31 state Medicaid websites integrated Google Translate functionality into the website itself, the quality of this translation mechanism for highly specialized policy jargon often poses challenges for accuracy and comprehension. Some websites only included information in English (n = 15), while only a few included information in both English and Spanish (n = 5). Given that 2 major barriers for immigrants in seeking care are lack of knowledge of the complex health care system and language barriers,[29] increasing accessibility to this information is critical. Our findings should be contextualized in the limitations of the approach we used in reviewing state Medicaid websites, which may have missed other relevant policies and programs for undocumented immigrants.

POLICY IMPLICATIONS

Understanding the labyrinth of programs and policies that allow access to pregnancy care coverage for undocumented individuals presents a challenge for clinicians, resource specialists, and pregnant people themselves. Overall, fragmented state- and federal-level mechanisms provide pregnancy care to undocumented individuals, such as CHIP and Medicaid on the state level and Emergency Medicaid on the federal level. As a result, the eligibility requirements and coverage for pregnancy care vary widely from state to state. The overall complexity and lack of transparency of these policies makes navigating these systems—for patients, for advocates and community organizations, for clinicians, and even for policymakers—extremely difficult. Given these findings, one important improvement would be for all states and federal agencies to adopt plain-language explanations in all public materials, enhance transparency and clarity of coverage policies, and provide multilingual access to information.

Reducing fragmentation across state policies and programs to expand coverage for full-spectrum pregnancy care, including miscarriage, prenatal, labor and delivery, and postpartum services, for all populations regardless of immigration status, is critical to enhance access and outcomes. Studies of Oregon's expansion of Medicaid found that increasing prenatal care coverage for undocumented immigrants led to an increase in infants receiving recommended preventive health services, a decrease in the probability of extreme low birth weight infants, and a decrease in infant mortality.[30] Increasingly restrictive legislation around access to reproductive health care and stigmatizing anti-immigrant rhetoric produce particular vulnerability for the pregnant undocumented population, especially in states like Florida that have begun to require hospitals accepting Medicaid to ask about a patient's immigration status.[31] Recent literature shows that immigrants living in states with public insurance restrictions are less likely to receive postpartum care.[32] It is essential that health policy efforts focus on increasing access to care for everyone, regardless of immigration status.

Eroding access to abortion care adds further complexity to the landscape of care for pregnant people who are undocumented who may experience heightened fears of seeking reproductive health care. We did not find any studies that analyzed the impact of abortion policy and coverage for abortion care specifically for pregnant people who are undocumented. The lack of studies on this topic is likely attributable to the challenges in collecting sensitive information about immigration status amid an increasingly restrictive landscape of abortion access.

Research on health outcomes among undocumented immigrants is limited because of challenges in identifying the marginalized population. Common proxies are absence of a social security number on a birth certificate[33] or enrollment in Emergency Medicaid at the time of delivery.[30,34] Studies that compare state policies often use utilization of health care as a primary outcome.[30,34] One study found that coverage of prenatal care for undocumented pregnant people was associated with increased prenatal care screening (anemia, blood typing) and influenza vaccinations.[35] Another study found expansion of Emergency Medicaid to cover prenatal care for undocumented immigrants in Oregon was associated with better detection of pregnancy complications, including diagnosis of diabetes, hypertensive diseases, and poor fetal growth.[34]

Another important policy option is expansion of postpartum care coverage through 12 months postpartum for undocumented immigrants. Given that one half of pregnancy-related deaths occur after birth,[36] health care coverage during the postpartum period is a critical opportunity for reducing overall pregnancy-related mortality and morbidity in the United States. Although there are a variety of different solutions that can be implemented to increase pregnancy care, California's Medi-Cal policy seems to be a promising approach, but it is still in need of studies to evaluate its long-term outcomes. Instead of using a patchwork of programs and funding sources for different stages of pregnancy, California uses Medicaid to cover all prenatal, childbirth, and postpartum services. Through Medi-Cal, California has extended Medicaid to all individuals, regardless of immigration status, through age 26, with plans to extend this program to individuals of all ages in 2024.

Nonprofits and advocacy organizations may aim to fill some of the current policy gaps and help individuals and families understand their eligibility for services. For example, the Nurse Family Partnership is a free program for low-income parents that connects nurses with first-time parents in the prenatal period.[37] Another key group of organizations include medical–legal partnerships, integrating lawyers into the health care setting to address legal concerns that perpetuate health inequities, such as access barriers to the health care system.[38]

PUBLIC HEALTH IMPLICATIONS

Human responses to climate change, increasing political instability, severe impoverishment, continued economic impacts of COVID-19, the asylum system backlog, and deteriorating economic conditions have led to an influx of migrants to the United States over the past few years.[39] Ensuring all individuals have access to health care coverage is a critical priority for public health with important economic benefits, especially for reproductive-aged individuals who make up a large proportion of the workforce.

Pregnancy care coverage for people who are undocumented remains a complex labyrinth of federal and state policies, which leads to variable, fragmented, and often inadequate access for undocumented pregnant individuals, which has important implications for maternal–newborn outcomes. In recent years, more states have moved toward enacting inclusive policies. While 20 states have applied the CHIP pregnancy care option for prenatal coverage regardless of documentation status, fewer states have expanded Medicaid or state programs to be inclusive of all pregnant people. More-inclusive policies are needed for this marginalized population at the crossroads of a complicated web of immigration policy and a maternal health crisis. Advocacy efforts around equitable maternal health care should include all regardless of immigration status. Increased clarity and accessibility of policies is needed on state and other public websites. Information should be updated for accuracy to ensure accountability, and resources should be made in accordance with national cultural and linguistic standards. AJPH

ABOUT THE AUTHORS

Amanda DiMeo is with Ariadne Labs at Brigham and Women's Hospital and Harvard T. H. Chan School of Public Health, Boston, MA. Rasheca Logendran is with Harvard Medical School, Boston. Benjamin D. Sommers is with Harvard Medical School and Harvard T. H. Chan School of Public Health. Alexandra Beecroft and Yessamin Pazos Herencia are with Brigham Young University, Provo, UT. Maria Bazan, Jeffrey Sprankle, and Rose L. Molina are with the Department of Obstetrics and Gynecology, Beth Israel Deaconess Medical Center, Boston. Carrie Wade is with Countway Library, Harvard Medical School. Margaret M. Sullivan is with François-Xavier Bagnoud Center for Health and Human Rights, Harvard University, Boston.

CORRESPONDENCE

Correspondence should be sent to Rose L. Molina, MD, MPH, Department of Obstetrics and Gynecology, Beth Israel Deaconess Medical Center, 330 Brookline Ave, Boston, MA 02215 (e-mail: rmolina@bidmc.harvard.edu). Reprints can be ordered at https://www.ajph.org by clicking the "Reprints" link.

PUBLICATION INFORMATION

Full Citation: DiMeo A, Logendran R, Sommers BD, et al. Navigating the labyrinth of pregnancy-related coverage for undocumented immigrants: an assessment of current state and federal policies. *Am J Public Health*. 2024;114(10):1051–1060.

Acceptance Date: June 2, 2024.

DOI: https://doi.org/10.2105/AJPH.2024.307750

ORCID iDs:

Amanda DiMeo https://orcid.org/0000-0001-7827-2258

Alexandra Beecroft https://orcid.org/0000-0001-8966-3705

Maria Bazan https://orcid.org/0000-0002-9818-7699

Jeffrey Sprankle https://orcid.org/0009-0003-4429-1831

Margaret M. Sullivan https://orcid.org/0000-0003-2669-8139

Rose L. Molina https://orcid.org/0000-0001-7977-7960

CONTRIBUTORS

A. DiMeo, C. Wade, M. M. Sullivan, and R. L. Molina conceptualized the work. A. DiMeo, R. Logendran, A. Beecroft, Y. P. Herencia, M. Bazan, C. Wade, and J. Sprankle contributed to data collection. A. DiMeo, R. Logendran, B. D. Sommers, J. Sprankle, M. M. Sullivan, and R. L. Molina contributed to data analysis and interpretation. A. DiMeo, R. Logendran, and R. L. Molina drafted the article. All authors contributed to critical revision of the article and final approval of the version to be published.

ACKNOWLEDGMENTS

This project was supported by grant K12HS026370 from the Agency for Healthcare Research and Quality.

Note. The content is solely the responsibility of the authors and does not necessarily represent the official views of the Agency for Healthcare Research and Quality.

CONFLICTS OF INTEREST

The authors have no potential or actual conflicts of interest to disclose.

HUMAN PARTICIPANT PROTECTION

This study does not constitute human participant research.

REFERENCES

1. Al-Kire R, Pasek M, Tsang J-A, Leman J, Rowatt W. Protecting America's borders: Christian nationalism, threat, and attitudes toward immigrants in the United States. *Group Process Intergroup Relat.* 2022;25(2):354–378. https://doi.org/10.1177/1368430220978291
2. Craft-Blacksheare M, Kahn P. Midwives' and other perinatal health workers' perceptions of the Black maternal mortality crisis in the United States. *J Midwifery Womens Health.* 2023;68(1):62–70. https://doi.org/10.1111/jmwh.13433
3. Martinez O, Wu E, Sandfort T, et al. Evaluating the impact of immigration policies on health status among undocumented immigrants: a systematic review. *J Immigr Minor Health.* 2015;17(3):947–970. https://doi.org/10.1007/s10903-013-9968-4
4. Conway KS, Kutinova A. Maternal health: does prenatal care make a difference? *Health Econ.* 2006;15(5):461–488. https://doi.org/10.1002/hec.1097
5. Larrea-Schiavon S, Vázquez-Quesada LM, Bartlett LR, et al. Interventions to improve the reproductive health of undocumented female migrants and refugees in protracted situations: a systematic review. *Glob Health Sci Pract.* 2022;10(6):1–15. https://doi.org/10.9745/GHSP-D-21-00418
6. Molina RL, Beecroft A, Pazos Herencia Y, et al. Pregnancy care utilization, experiences, and outcomes among undocumented immigrants in the United States: a scoping review. *Womens Health Issues.* 2024:S1049-3867(24):6–9. https://doi.org/10.1016/j.whi.2024.02.001
7. Phillippi JC. Women's perceptions of access to prenatal care in the United States: a literature review. *J Midwifery Womens Health.* 2009;54(3):219–225. https://doi.org/10.1016/j.jmwh.2009.01.002
8. Budiman A. *Key Findings About US Immigrants.* Pew Research Center. August 20, 2020. Available at: https://www.pewresearch.org/short-reads/

2020/08/20/key-findings-about-u-s-immigrants. Accessed August 2, 2023.

9. Boundless. Deferred Action for Childhood Arrivals (DACA). Explained. Available at: https://www.boundless.com/immigration-resources/what-is-daca. Accessed April 18, 2024.
10. *Fact Sheet: The Use of Parole Under Immigration Law*. Washington, DC: American Immigration Council; 2024.
11. National Immigration Forum. *Immigration Primer*. December 16, 2019. Available at: https://immigrationforum.org/article/immigration-primer/#current-system. Accessed September 7, 2023.
12. Health care for immigrants: ACOG committee statement no. 4. *Obstet Gynecol*. 2023;141(2): e427–e433. https://doi.org/10.1097/AOG.0000000000005061
13. Kaiser Family Foundation. *Health Coverage and Care of Immigrants*. December 20, 2022. Available at: https://www.kff.org/racial-equity-and-health-policy/fact-sheet/health-coverage-and-care-of-immigrants. Accessed August 2, 2023.
14. Broder T. *Overview of Immigrant Eligibility for Federal Programs*. National Immigration Law Center. March 2023. Available at: https://www.nilc.org/issues/economic-support/overview-immeligfed programs. Accessed September 8, 2023.
15. Healthcare.gov. Coverage for lawfully present immigrants. Available at: https://www.healthcare.gov/immigrants/lawfully-present-immigrants. Accessed August 11, 2023.
16. MyMedicare.com. Emergency Medicaid. 2018. Available at: https://mymedicare.com/medicaid/emergency-medicaid. Accessed September 13, 2023.
17. Park JK, Reyes-Becerra C, Makhlouf MD. State flexibility in Emergency Medicaid to care for uninsured noncitizens. *JAMA Health Forum*. 2023;4(7): e231997. https://doi.org/10.1001/jamahealthforum.2023.1997
18. National Immigrant Law Center. Immigrants and the Affordable Care Act (ACA). January 2014. Available at: https://www.nilc.org/issues/health-care/immigrantshcr. Accessed September 8, 2023.
19. Daval CJR. Immigration law, public health, and the future of public charge policymaking. *J Law Med Ethics*. 2022;50(2):336–338. https://doi.org/10.1017/jme.2022.60
20. Pillai D. *2022 Changes to the Public Charge Inadmissibility Rule and the Implications for Health Care*. KFF. May 5, 2022. Available at: https://www.kff.org/racial-equity-and-health-policy/issue-brief/2022-changes-to-the-public-charge-inadmissibility-rule-and-the-implications-for-health-care. Accessed April 18, 2024.
21. US Citizen and Immigration Services. Clarifying the 2022 Public Charge Final Rule. Available at: https://www.uscis.gov/sites/default/files/document/flyers/PublicChargeFinalRule2022_Infographic_V4_508.pdf. Accessed October 21, 2023.
22. Haq C, Hostetter I, Zavala L, Mayorga J. Immigrant health and changes to the Public-Charge Rule: family physicians' response. *Ann Fam Med*. 2020;18(5):458–460. https://doi.org/10.1370/afm.2572
23. Centers for Medicare and Medicaid Services. *Federally Qualified Health Center*. September 2019. Available at: https://www.hhs.gov/guidance/sites/default/files/hhs-guidance-documents/FQHC-Text-Only-Factsheet.pdf. Accessed April 22, 2024.
24. KFF. Medicaid and CHIP income eligibility limits for pregnant women as a percent of the federal poverty level. January 1, 2023. Available at: https://www.kff.org/health-reform/state-indicator/medicaid-and-chip-income-eligibility-limits-for-pregnant-women-as-a-percent-of-the-federal-poverty-level. Accessed September 8, 2023.
25. Manatt Health. *Supporting Health Equity and Affordable Health Coverage for Immigrant Populations: CHIP Coverage Option for Pregnant Immigrants and Their Children. State Health & Value Strategies: Driving Innovation Across States*. January 1, 2022. Available at: https://www.shvs.org/wp-content/uploads/2022/01/Supporting-Health-Equity-and-Affordable-Health-Coverage-for-Immigrant-Populations_CHIP-Coverage-Option-for-Pregnant-Immigrants-and-their-Children.pdf. Accessed August 1, 2023.
26. National Women's Law Center. CHIP must be reauthorized and it must also be improved to better cover pregnant women. December 14, 2017. Available at: https://nwlc.org/chip-must-be-reauthorized-and-it-must-also-be-improved-to-better-cover-pregnant-women. Accessed April 18, 2024.
27. Jayapal H. Cárdenas introduce bicameral legislation to expand public benefits to immigrants. Pramila Jayapal Congresswoman for WA-07. June 15, 2023. Available at: https://jayapal.house.gov/2023/06/15/jayapal-hirono-cardenas-introduce-bicameral-legislation-to-expand-public-benefits-to-immigrants. Accessed September 23, 2023.
28. Pew Research Center. US unauthorized immigrant population estimates by state, 2016. Pew Research Center. May 2, 2019. Available at: https://www.pewresearch.org/hispanic/interactives/u-s-unauthorized-immigrants-by-state. Accessed December 3, 2023.
29. Hacker K, Anies M, Folb BL, Zallman L. Barriers to health care for undocumented immigrants: a literature review. *Risk Manag Healthc Policy*. 2015; 8:175–183. https://doi.org/10.2147/RMHP.S70173
30. Swartz JJ, Hainmueller J, Lawrence D, Rodriguez MI. Expanding prenatal care to unauthorized immigrant women and the effects on infant health. *Obstet Gynecol*. 2017;130(5):938–945. https://doi.org/10.1097/AOG.0000000000002275
31. Chang D. Doctors hesitate to ask about patients' immigration status despite new Florida law. *KFF Health News*. August 17, 2023. Available at: https://kffhealthnews.org/news/article/doctors-patient-immigration-status-new-florida-law. Accessed October 21, 2023.
32. Steenland MW, Fabi RE, Bellerose M, Desir A, White MS, Wherry LR. State public insurance coverage policies and postpartum care among immigrants. *JAMA*. 2023;330(3):238–246. https://doi.org/10.1001/jama.2023.10249
33. Atkins DN, Held ML, Lindley LC. The impact of expanded health insurance coverage for unauthorized pregnant women on prenatal care utilization. *Public Health Nurs*. 2018;35(6):459–465. https://doi.org/10.1111/phn.12524
34. Swartz JJ, Hainmueller J, Lawrence D, Rodriguez MI. Oregon's expansion of prenatal care improved utilization among immigrant women. *Matern Child Health J*. 2019;23(2):173–182. https://doi.org/10.1007/s10995-018-2611-1
35. Rodriguez MI, Kaufman M, Lindner S, Caughey AB, DeFede AL, McConnell KJ. Association of expanded prenatal care coverage for immigrant women with postpartum contraception and short interpregnancy interval births. *JAMA Netw Open*. 2021;4(8):e2118912. https://doi.org/10.1001/jamanetworkopen.2021.18912
36. Kassebaum NJ, Bertozzi-Villa A, Coggeshall MS, et al. Global, regional, and national levels and causes of maternal mortality during 1990–2013: a systematic analysis for the Global Burden of Disease Study 2013. *Lancet*. 2014;384(9947): 980–1004. https://doi.org/10.1016/S0140-6736(14)60696-6
37. US Department of Health and Human Services. Implementing Nurse-Family Partnership (NFP). Home visiting evidence of effectiveness. 2019. Available at: https://homvee.acf.hhs.gov/implementation/Nurse-Family%20Partnership%20(NFP)%C2%AE/Model%20Overview#Intendedpopulation-M. Accessed April 18, 2024.
38. National Center for Medical Legal Partnership. Available at: https://medical-legalpartnership.org. Accessed April 18, 2024.
39. Gramlich J, Scheller A. What's happening at the US-Mexico border in 7 charts. Pew Research Center. November 9, 2021. Available at: https://www.pewresearch.org/short-reads/2021/11/09/whats-happening-at-the-u-s-mexico-border-in-7-charts. Accessed July 3, 2024.

Regulation of Added Substances in the Food Supply by the Food and Drug Administration Human Foods Program

Jennifer L. Pomeranz, JD, MPH, Emily M. Broad Leib, JD, and Dariush Mozaffarian, MD, DrPH

See also Aaron, p. 968.

The US food supply is increasingly associated with diet-related diseases, toxicity, cancer, and other health harms. These public health concerns are partly attributable to a loophole in federal law.

The Food and Drug Administration (FDA) evaluates the premarket safety of ingredients regulated as food additives but allows the food industry to self-regulate and determine which substances to classify as generally recognized as safe (GRAS) based on undisclosed data and conclusions that the FDA never sees. Furthermore, the FDA lacks a formal approach for reviewing food additives and GRAS substances already found in the food supply. Substances in the food supply thus include innocuous ingredients (e.g., black pepper), those that are harmful at high levels (e.g., salt), those that are of questionable safety (e.g., potassium bromate), and those that are unknown to the FDA and the public.

A recent court decision codified these gaps in the FDA's current approach, leaving states to try to fill the regulatory void. The FDA and Congress should consider several policy options to ensure that the FDA is meeting its mission to ensure a safe food supply. (*Am J Public Health*. 2024;114(10):1061–1070. https://doi.org/10.2105/AJPH.2024.307755)

AJPH October 2024, Vol. 114, No. 10

The Food and Drug Administration's (FDA's) mission includes protecting the "public health by ensuring that foods are safe, wholesome, sanitary, and properly labeled."[1] Yet concerns have been raised that, because of weak statutory requirements, the FDA's interpretation of its authorities, and lack of sufficient funding, the FDA's oversight for ingredients in our food supply is inadequate to ensure a safe and wholesome food supply.[2–4]

The Federal Food Drug and Cosmetics Act (FDCA) distinguishes between—but does not clearly define—substances that are considered food additives and those that are deemed generally recognized as safe (GRAS). Both categories include complex chemical substances, but their regulatory frameworks are quite different. Food additives are subject to FDA premarket review because they are presumed to be unsafe. Consequently, foods containing food additives are considered adulterated unless the use of the substance complies with an FDA regulation prescribing the conditions of safe use.[5] By contrast, GRAS substances are presumed to be safe and thus exempt from such requirements. This exemption allows the food industry to define a wide array of new substances as GRAS and introduce them into the food supply without FDA or public knowledge of their existence, use, or safety.

A stark example of the FDA's regulatory gap was seen in October 2023, when California banned 4 substances from being used as ingredients in food sold or manufactured in the state.[6] These substances are banned in Europe because of their association with an increased risk of cancer and other health, behavioral, developmental, and reproductive harms.[6] A month later, the FDA proposed revoking the approved food additive status for 1 of the 4 substances banned in California: brominated vegetable oil (BVO).[7] BVO was considered GRAS decades ago.[7] In 1970, the FDA determined that BVO was no longer GRAS and designated it as an approved food additive.[7] After this reclassification, BVO remained in food products such as Gatorade and Mountain Dew, while science mounted questioning its safety. It was not until California banned BVO that the FDA announced it was taking action, leaving questions on how proactive the FDA is over ingredients already in the food supply.

Indeed, a 2021 court case, *Center for Food Safety v Becerra* (*Center for Food Safety*), highlighted that GRAS substances are not necessarily safe and that ingredients already in the food supply are not regularly reexamined for safety.[8] Although the FDA has clear authority to take postmarket action, the FDCA does not provide the FDA with a clear or well-resourced pathway to systematically review food additives or GRAS substances already in the food supply. As a result, foods contain ingredients that may be harmful in high doses (e.g., salt), are of questionable safety (e.g., nonnutritive sweeteners), or are unknown to the FDA or the public.

Concerns about ingredients in the US food supply have been increasing in recent years.[9] In 2022, at the FDA's request, the Reagan–Udall Foundation released a report noting the need for the FDA to adapt to a changing food supply, including increasing its oversight of the chemicals in food.[9] In response, the FDA announced a restructuring of its Human Foods Program to improve and coordinate its prevention and response activities. As part of these new efforts, in May 2023, the FDA announced that it was "embarking on a more modernized, systematic reassessment" of chemicals in the food supply "with a focus on postmarket review."[10] The proposed activities are crucial. However, the announcement raises questions about how the FDA will accomplish such an evaluation and, perhaps more critically, how ingredients make their way into the food supply in the first place and whether the FDA is aware of all of the ingredients that should be subject to this postmarket review.

We set forth the history of the GRAS notification and food additive approval processes and examine the decision and implications of *Center for Food Safety*, which solidified the FDA's anemic GRAS oversight. (Color additives are treated under a different framework, and we do not address them.) We conclude with recommendations for future action for the FDA to achieve its duty of ensuring a safe food supply.

FOOD ADDITIVES AND GRAS SUBSTANCES

Congress passed the Food Additives Amendment of 1958 to establish a rigorous statutory scheme for the FDA to review and approve food additives before they go to market.[11] An entity seeking to introduce a food additive into the food supply petitions the FDA requesting that the FDA promulgate a regulation prescribing the conditions under which the substance may safely be used.[2,11] The FDA evaluates the petition in light of scientific data to determine whether the data demonstrate that the food additive is safe—using the standard of "a reasonable certainty of no harm"—for the proposed conditions of use.[12] If the FDA believes it is safe, it publishes a draft regulation in the Federal Register for public notice and comment.[2,12] Consequently, for food additives, the FDA must go through a full regulatory process that requires a transparent demonstration of safety before approval.

By contrast, the Food Additives Amendment of 1958 carved out GRAS substances as those that are "generally recognized, among experts qualified by scientific training and experience to evaluate its safety, as having been adequately shown through scientific procedures" to be safe under the conditions of its intended use or, for a substance used in food before 1958, through experience based on common use in food (e.g., salt, pepper).[11] The separate designation for GRAS was designed to permit substances commonly used in food to remain in the food supply without the necessity of companies supplying evidence to prove safety and the FDA using its finite resources to review such data.[2] GRAS substances are thus explicitly exempted from food additive regulations and therefore the FDA's current premarket review process.

However, for the decade or so after passage of the Food Additives Amendment, the FDA exercised rigorous oversight over GRAS substances and published and updated a list of all existing and new substances considered GRAS in the Code of Federal Regulations.[13] But in 1972, the FDA began using a voluntary GRAS affirmation process in which manufacturers had the option to voluntarily submit a GRAS affirmation petition with data for FDA review.[2,13] When submitted, the FDA would publish a notice and request for comments and then issue its GRAS determination on the substance.[2] During this period, concerns arose about the safety of cyclamate salts, which were in the food supply. President Richard Nixon directed the FDA to review the safety of GRAS substances already in the food supply.[2] The FDA worked with an independent scientific organization to conduct a safety review of 422 substances from 1972 to 1982, but then the agency did not adopt the recommendations of the committee.[2]

In 1997 the FDA proposed a rule to replace the GRAS voluntary affirmation process with a voluntary notification process "whereby any person may notify the FDA of a determination that a particular use of a substance is GRAS."[14] Although the rule was not formally finalized until 2016, the FDA has operated under this proposed rule since 1997 (Table 1 provides a timeline of relevant activities).

Under the GRAS notification rule, manufacturers have the choice of either engaging in "self-GRAS" or submitting a notification. Through self-GRAS, a company is supposed to determine through their own internal research that an ingredient is GRAS, and then they can market the food with the ingredient without any notification to—or oversight by—the FDA.[15] Alternatively, companies can go through the more onerous process of submitting a GRAS notification to the FDA describing the substance, the applicable conditions of use, and the basis for the GRAS determination (i.e., common use in food or scientific procedures) before using the ingredient. The company then waits for the FDA to issue either a "no question letter" stating that it does not question the company's GRAS decision—allowing the company to go to market with this letter—or an "insufficient basis" letter—meaning the FDA finds insufficient information to substantiate the GRAS claim, suggesting the company can submit additional data.[16] If a company submits a GRAS notification but then chooses to withdraw it, the FDA issues a "cease to evaluate" letter, and the company can still go to market with the substance.[2,3]

Thus, in practice, a strong impetus exists for the food industry to self-GRAS so it can manufacture and market food products with new substances without ever notifying the FDA of either its determination or the research underlying its determination that the substance is safe.[2,3,16] Moreover, if the food industry actually notifies the FDA that it considers a new substance to be GRAS, the FDA does not need to engage in its own research to confirm the industry's conclusions or the ingredient's safety.[16]

Another result of the self-GRAS allowance is that a company may self-GRAS an ingredient that otherwise should be considered a food additive subject to the FDA's premarket oversight. Therefore, numerous ingredients that should be appropriately regulated as food additives are likely in the food supply through the self-GRAS mechanism. Indeed, research published by Neltner et al. found that between 1990 and 2010, an estimated 1000 manufacturer ingredient-safety decisions were never reported to the FDA or the public.[17] An industry panel of experts (known as a "GRAS panel") determined an additional 2702 ingredients to be GRAS.[15] Since this review was completed back in 2011, there are likely numerous more ingredients in the food supply that have never been reviewed by the FDA and that are of unknown safety to the FDA and the public.

CENTER FOR FOOD SAFETY V BECERRA

After the FDA finalized its GRAS rule in 2016, nonprofit organizations sued the FDA, arguing that the rule violates the FDCA and that the agency abdicated its responsibility to ensure a safe food supply and unlawfully delegated its duties to the food industry through the self-GRAS mechanism.[8] In 2021, a federal district court upheld the FDA's final rule in *Center for Food Safety*, finding that the FDA did not unlawfully delegate its authority over food safety to private parties and that the rule does not violate the FDCA.[8]

According to the court, because the FDCA is "silent" on the question of whether GRAS notifications must be mandatory, the FDA's allowance for voluntary notification was a reasonable interpretation of the statute.[8] The court thus deferred to the FDA's interpretation of its authority under what is called the *Chevron* doctrine, which is when a court provides deference to an agency's interpretation of its own authority under an ambiguous statute.[8] The court reasoned that because the FDCA sets forth a rigorous scheme for food additive approvals—and GRAS substances were specifically exempt from that scheme—it was within the FDA's authority to adopt a voluntary notification system for GRAS substances.[8]

In terms of the self-GRAS determinations themselves, the court explained that self-GRAS conclusions must be based on "the same quantity and quality of scientific evidence as is required to obtain approval of a food additive," which is "based upon the application of generally available and accepted scientific data, information, or methods" or "common knowledge throughout the scientific community."[8] However, it found that this requirement does not translate into a need for self-GRAS determinations to be based on published studies, nor are companies required to publicly disclose the basis for their self-GRAS decisions.[8] The court highlighted that the FDA retains the postmarket power to disagree with manufacturers' self-GRAS determinations and bring enforcement actions.[8]

Yet, as the plaintiffs noted, the FDA's ability to bring postmarket enforcement is complicated by the voluntary GRAS notification process, which allows industry to add new substances to food without the FDA's knowledge. The FDA is thus hindered from using its

TABLE 1— Timeline of Key Actions Related to the US Food and Drug Administration's Generally Recognized as Safe and Food Additive Substances Regulations

Date	Action
1958	Congress passes the Food Additives Amendment of 1958, establishing the current framework for food substances that are GRAS or food additives
1961	FDA amends its regulations to include a list of food substances that are GRAS under certain conditions of use
1969	FDA removes cyclamate salts from its GRAS list as a result of safety questions
1969	President Nixon directs the FDA to make a critical evaluation of the safety of GRAS food substances
1970	FDA starts its critical review of the GRAS process and finds it to be resource intensive
1972	FDA conducts rulemaking to establish the affirmation process to affirm the GRAS status of substances that are subject to GRAS review
1977	FDA approves caffeine as a GRAS substance when used in cola-type beverages at 0.02%
1978	CSPI submits a citizen petition to the FDA requesting it to revoke the GRAS status of salt
1982	FDA holds "GRAS Safety Review of Sodium Chloride" and declines to regulate salt using its GRAS/food additive authority but announces its policy of encouraging food manufacturers to voluntarily reduce sodium in processed foods and notes that it is proposing a sodium-labeling regulation
1984	FDA proposes and finalizes labeling regulations to define terms such as "sodium free," "low sodium," and "reduced sodium," among other acts (effective July 1, 1986)
1990	Congress passes NLEA, which requires the disclosure of the nutrition facts label and ingredient list on packaged food
1993	FDA promulgates regulations to carry out the NLEA
1996	FDA promulgates a regulation affirming high fructose corn syrup is GRAS
1997	FDA proposes a rule to replace the GRAS affirmation process with a GRAS notification process and starts functioning under this proposed rule
2003	FDA promulgates a final rule requiring trans fatty acids be declared in the nutrition facts label of foods (effective January 1, 2006)
2004	CSPI submits a citizen petition to the FDA to revoke the GRAS status of PHOs and declare PHOs as food additives
2005	The IOM suggests limiting consumption of artificial trans fat to as low as possible
2005	CSPI submits a citizen petition to the FDA requesting it revoke the GRAS status of salt
2007	FDA holds a public hearing on CSPI's 2005 petition requesting it to revoke the GRAS status of salt
2009	Fred A. Kummerow, trans fat researcher, submits a citizen petition to the FDA requesting the FDA ban partially hydrogenated fat from the food supply
2010	The IOM issues a report on strategies to reduce sodium in the food supply, which includes a recommendation that the FDA use its GRAS regulatory authority to mandate limits on the amount of sodium allowed in food
2010	The US Government Accountability Office releases a report criticizing the FDA's 1997 proposed GRAS rule
2013	FDA makes a preliminary determination that the trans fats generated from PHOs are no longer GRAS
2013	CSPI submits a citizen petition to the FDA to ensure the safe use of "added sugars" using the FDA's authority over GRAS substances
2014	FDA promulgates a proposed rule to revise the nutrition facts label to include an "added sugar" disclosure among other updates
2015	FDA promulgates its final determination that PHOs are no longer GRAS
2016	FDA promulgates final rule updating the nutrition facts label to include "added sugar" among other updates (compliance set for 2018 for large manufacturers and 2019 for small manufacturers)
2016	FDA finalizes its 1997 GRAS notification rule
2017	Nonprofit consumer and environmental protection organizations file a lawsuit challenging the FDA's final GRAS notification rule
2018	FDA denied a petition by Grocery Manufacturers Association to allow PHOs as a food additive
2021	The US District Court for the Southern District of New York upholds the FDA's voluntary GRAS notification rule in *Center for Food Safety v Becerra*
2021	FDA establishes "Voluntary Sodium Reduction Goals," which provide voluntary sodium reduction targets
May 2022	US Senator Markey introduces the bill Ensuring Safe and Toxic-Free Foods Act of 2022 to address deficiencies in the FDA's GRAS notification procedure; bill fails to pass
July 2022	FDA Commissioner Robert Califf requests that the Reagan-Udall Foundation convene an independent expert panel to conduct a comprehensive evaluation of the FDA Human Foods Program to strengthen the FDA's food regulatory role
September 2022	The White House holds the Conference on Hunger, Nutrition, and Health
December 2022	The Reagan-Udall Foundation issues its report *Operational Evaluation of the FDA's Human Foods Program*

Continued

TABLE 1— Continued

Date	Action
December 2022	FDA issues guidance document "Best Practices for Convening a GRAS Panel"
January 2023	FDA announces the proposed restructuring of its Human Foods Program
October 2023	California bans 4 substances permitted to be in food by the FDA (red dye no. 3, potassium bromate, brominated vegetable oil, and propylparaben) from being used as an ingredient in food sold or manufactured in California
November 2023	FDA announces its proposal to revoke the approved food additive status of brominated vegetable oil
November 2023	US senators Edward J. Markey (D, MA) and Cory Booker (D, NJ) announce the introduction of the bill Ensuring Safe and Toxic-Free Foods Act of 2023
March 2024	FDA announcement that it would conduct postmarket review of 21 chemicals in the food supply

Note. CSPI = Center for Science in the Public Interest; FDA = US Food and Drug Administration; GRAS = generally recognized as safe; IOM = Institute of Medicine; NLEA = Nutrition Labeling and Education Act of 1990; PHO = partially hydrogenated vegetable oil.

postmarket authority for substances that are unknown to it. Finally, the court agreed that the plaintiffs' "legitimate concerns" about potential industry conflicts of interest "may be valid," but the FDCA was also silent on this issue, so the FDA was not required to address potential conflicts of interest for self-GRAS reviews.[8]

The plaintiffs also argued that the FDA's GRAS rule contravenes the FDCA's Delaney Clause. The Delaney Clause, incorporated into the FDCA by the Food Additives Amendment of 1958, explicitly requires the FDA to ban food additives that are found to cause or induce cancer in humans or animals.[18] The FDA successfully argued that "the Delaney Clause governs food additives, not GRAS" substances.[8] Although the court agreed that GRAS substances linked to cancer are exempt from the FDA's premarket review, the court noted that "inherent in the GRAS Rule are criteria that would likely prevent a carcinogenic substance from being deemed GRAS," because it would not be generally recognized as safe.[8] However, without required premarket notification, this may be difficult for the FDA to ensure in practice.

In assessing the reasonableness of the FDA's interpretation of the statute, the court noted approvingly that the number of GRAS notifications the FDA receives since amending its rule in 1997 had increased.[8] The court cited FDA data showing that under the previous voluntary affirmation process, the FDA received approximately 8 GRAS affirmation petitions per year between 1987 and 1996 but approximately 34 per year between 1997 and 2015.[8] However, these numbers are complicated by an obvious fact: the denominator of new substances added to the food supply each year is unknown. Moreover, as Neltner et al. found, only a small percentage of all GRAS substance determinations actually ever cross the FDA's desk.[17] Given the advances in food-processing technologies, it seems plausible that the increase in filings is explained by a growing number of new substances being developed each year.[8]

Lastly, the court agreed with the FDA that it could choose, as it did, to not require GRAS substance notification because a mandatory system would consume the FDA's resources.[8] Indeed, a more robust system would require Congress to dedicate additional resources to the FDA—something Congress has historically failed to do.[9] In conclusion, the court did not find that the FDA's GRAS rule supports the safety of the food supply but that the rule did not violate the FDCA despite the safety concerns raised by the plaintiffs.

IMPLICATIONS

Even before the FDA finalized its GRAS rule, it was aware of gaps in its oversight highlighted by the *Center for Food Safety* plaintiffs. In 2010, the US Government Accountability Office (GAO) released a report determining that the FDA's oversight process does not "ensure the safety" of new GRAS substances or those based on previous GRAS determinations.[19] The report recommended that the FDA strengthen its GRAS oversight, including by developing strategies to require companies to provide the FDA with basic information about GRAS substances and to minimize the potential for conflicts of interest in companies' self-GRAS determinations. The GAO also recommended that the FDA create a more systematic mechanism to review and reconsider existing GRAS determinations.[19] The FDA issued guidance documents clarifying its thinking on several issues in this report[20]; however, in 2016 the FDA chose to finalize its GRAS notification rule without modifying it in accordance with GAO recommendations. Thus, the problems the GAO identified remain.[3]

As a result of the FDA's GRAS rule, and the supportive ruling in *Center for Food Safety*, the food industry is free to self-determine the GRAS status of a substance and add that substance to food products without notifying the FDA or the public. Although some food companies may choose to undertake the voluntary public notification process to obtain the "no question" letter from the FDA, a company that seeks to maintain confidentiality over its proprietary information (or does not wish to bring attention to a new substance it has added) will choose to self-GRAS.

The FDA has reminded companies that choose to self-GRAS that they must still have the data to support their safety decisions or they will be noncompliant. Even with such data, very real concerns about conflict of interest remain. Neltner et al. found that of the 451 GRAS notifications voluntarily submitted to the FDA between 1997 and 2012, 100% of them were decided by people with a conflict of interest, including employees of—or consulting firms selected by—the manufacturers themselves or by a GRAS panel with conflicts of interest.[21] A subsequent 2023 analysis of these GRAS panels found that food industry GRAS panels are made up of experts whose income is derived from GRAS panel participation.[22] The authors identified 7 people (all with financial conflicts of interest) who essentially determine the safety of GRAS ingredients in our food supply by serving on the majority of self-GRAS determination panels.[22]

The court in *Center for Food Safety* focused on the FDA's postmarket authority as a safeguard to self-GRAS. However, the FDA has revoked the GRAS status of substances very few times, likely in part because of the lack of a resourced and robust systematic process for the FDA to conduct a postmarket review of GRAS substances or food additives. For example, the FDA's inventory of postmarket determinations that the use of a substance is not GRAS includes only 14 substances for which GRAS status has been revoked.[23] Yet, this database is incomplete, as it excludes 4 examples of GRAS revocations mentioned in the FDA's 2015 Federal Register entry when it revoked the GRAS status of partially hydrogenated vegetable oils (PHOs).[24]

The FDA's treatment of PHOs exemplifies its ability to exercise postmarket authority over GRAS ingredients. Scientific literature on the health harms of industrially produced trans fat from PHOs began accumulating in the 1950s.[25] In the early 1990s, a seminal editorial identified a significant association between trans fat consumption and heart disease among more than 100 000 US women, and growing experimental evidence documented harmful effects of trans fat on blood cholesterol concentrations.[25] In 2005, the Institute of Medicine (IOM; now the National Academies of Sciences, Engineering, and Medicine) issued a report identifying the health harms of PHOs and recommending reduced consumption. Citizens' petitions were filed with the FDA in 2004 and 2009. Despite this strong evidence that there was no longer a consensus among qualified experts that PHOs were generally recognized as safe, the FDA did not alter the GRAS designation but merely required the disclosure of trans fat on the nutrition facts label, effective 2006.[26]

It was not until 2013 that the FDA proposed revoking the GRAS status of PHOs, a rule that was not finalized until 2015 and did not go into effect until 2018.[24] This example highlights the extensive weight of science and time required for the FDA to remove a previous GRAS designation from an industrially produced food ingredient, illustrating the barriers the FDA faces in its ability to exercise postmarket authority for a known substance even when there is clear information questioning its safety.

POSTMARKET REVIEW OF CHEMICALS IN FOOD

In March 2024, the FDA announced that it identified 21 chemicals in the food supply for which it would conduct postmarket review.[27] However, only a few of these chemicals are food ingredients. Moreover, this is only a small fraction of the thousands of food additives, GRAS-affirmed ingredients, and—especially concerning—self-GRAS ingredients now in the US food supply.

Notably, the FDA has not proposed to reevaluate or conduct postmarket review of common GRAS-designated substances that may be safe at low levels but unsafe when added at high levels. This is true even when the current GRAS approval is level specific. For example, in 1977, the FDA approved caffeine as a GRAS substance when used in cola-type beverages at 0.02%.[28] Currently, caffeine is added to energy drinks at levels far exceeding this GRAS tolerance level, with resulting hospitalizations and even deaths among children and adults.[28] Yet, the FDA has not acted on caffeine in energy drinks even though the FDA regulates the use of GRAS substances, meaning the FDA can set limits on the amount of caffeine in energy drinks.

Similarly, given the documented health harms of excess added salt and sugar in the food supply,[29] there is a public health need for the FDA to conduct a postmarket review of the health implications of high levels of added salt and sugar. The Center for Science in the Public Interest unsuccessfully petitioned the FDA to revoke salt's GRAS status in 1978 and again in 2005.[30] In 2010, the IOM issued a report on strategies to reduce sodium in the US food supply that included a recommendation that the FDA use its food regulatory authority to mandate limits.[31] Ralston Aoki et al. suggested compelling strategies for the FDA to implement the IOM's sodium recommendations by classifying and regulating sodium as either GRAS or a food additive with safe harbor provisions or specific regulations for use.[32]

Instead of exercising its postmarket regulatory authority, the FDA has focused on labeling and voluntary targets for sodium.[32,33] The FDA's proposed voluntary sodium reduction goals provide carefully determined levels across 163 categories of commercially processed packaged and prepared foods, each based on amounts already present in multiple products in each category.[34] The FDA could use these evidence-based levels as the basis for a determination that foods that exceed these limits are no longer considered GRAS. In addition, evidence exists that current levels of salt added to certain products far exceed the amount reasonably acceptable under conditions of "good manufacturing practice."[35] Good manufacturing practices require that the "quantity of the substance added to food does not exceed the amount reasonably required to accomplish its intended physical, nutritive, or other technical effect in food."[35] This violation of good manufacturing practice has been empirically demonstrated by widely varying sodium contents of otherwise very similar food items.[34]

FUTURE DIRECTIONS

The FDA recognizes its authority to conduct postmarket review and reclassification of GRAS substances found to "produce not just cancer but any disease or disability"[24(p34654)] to regulate them as food additives. Yet, the sheer number of GRAS substances and food additives to be reviewed, combined with the lack of knowledge about the existence of self-GRAS ingredients, insufficient resources, and documented time delays for well-supported action, renders reliance on postmarket authority an ineffective and unreliable method for ensuring a safe food supply. The FDA is only starting to use its postmarket powers to review a tiny number of ingredients in the food supply, even though evidence of harm has been present for decades.

Our analysis indicates that a new framework is needed to assess the safety of GRAS substances and food additives. This could include (1) a new, mandatory premarket GRAS notification or public affirmation process aligned with continued use of the mandatory food additive premarket review process; (2) user fees for the FDA to be able to engage in robust premarket review of GRAS substances and food additives; (3) a new framework for regular, robust, and transparent postmarket FDA review of both GRAS substances and food additives currently in the food supply; and (4) additional resources allocated by Congress. Table 2 sets forth recommendations for action by Congress and the FDA to help achieve these goals.

In the background of these recommendations was the expectation that in June 2024, the US Supreme Court would overturn the *Chevron* doctrine—which it did. The *Chevron* doctrine provided judicial deference to agencies' interpretation of their own authorities. This may result in huge swaths of regulatory actions subject to judicial review without the benefit of such deference, rendering courts the final arbiter of whether Congress granted an agency the authority in question. Based on the issues we have identified, the FDA could still take the position of requiring premarket review of all GRAS substances—a position it mentioned it would consider during its 2016 rulemaking based on implicit authority it acknowledged possessing.[36,37] However, the court's finding in *Center for Food Safety* that the FDCA is "silent" on the FDA's premarket GRAS authorities and the FDA's position that it lacks express statutory authority to require companies to submit GRAS notices leaves questions on how courts would interpret a reverse in the FDA's position absent congressional action indicating that Congress disagrees with the FDA's position or the court's decision in *Center for Food Safety*.

Congressional action would shield the FDA from lawsuits by food industry entities claiming the FDA does not have authority for mandatory GRAS review. The growing evidence for the harms of ultraprocessed foods[38]—a category defined in particular by the presence of industrial compounds added for functional purposes—may provide additional impetus for both Congress and the FDA to act. Congress could revise the Food Additives Amendment of 1958 to require the FDA use a methodologically sound premarket approval or required notification process with transparent data based on publicly available research for GRAS substances. Separately, Congress should provide meaningful new resources to the FDA for both pre- and postmarket review efforts, coupled with a user fee program created by Congress, as it did for tobacco, or negotiated

TABLE 2— Recommendations to Strengthen the FDA's GRAS and Food Additive Processes to Protect the Food Supply

Recommendations	Suggested Actions[a]	Alternative Actions[b]
Appropriations	Congress should allocate sufficient appropriations to the FDA's Human Foods Program, especially to oversee the safety of ingredients in the US food supply.	Congress should increase appropriations specifically to support the FDA's current (and additional more robust) premarket authorities and postmarket review of substances in the food supply.
User fees	Congress should establish a user fee program for the FDA to complete premarket review of food additives. Congress should establish a user fee program for the FDA to complete premarket review of GRAS substances if or when authorities are changed to require mandatory premarket review for GRAS substances.	FDA should negotiate a user fee program to complete premarket review of food additives and—if authorities are changed to require mandatory premarket review for GRAS substances—GRAS substances. Industry will oppose the FDA-negotiated user fees unless they benefit industry, in this case by ensuring premarket review is more efficient and timely.
Premarket review food additives	FDA should maintain premarket review of food additives.	
Premarket review of GRAS substances	Congress should amend the Food Additives Amendment of 1958 to require a mandatory premarket GRAS review process whereby data are submitted to the FDA for review before a company can market the ingredient. This is consistent with the method proposed in the bill Ensuring Safe and Toxic-Free Foods Act of 2023.[39]	FDA should promulgate regulations requiring premarket review (through notification or affirmation) for GRAS substances. If the FDA does not do full premarket review, it should at least promulgate regulations to review substances premarket to determine whether they can go through GRAS designation or must go through food additive review.
Distinguishing food additives from GRAS substances	Congress should amend the Food Additives Amendment of 1958 to better define GRAS substances and more clearly distinguish between GRAS and food additives so that substances that should rightly be food additives are required to go through the approval process.	FDA should promulgate regulations to clarify the distinction between GRAS substances and food additives.
Conflict-free GRAS determinations	FDA should require all GRAS determinations and panels to be free from conflicts of interest and follow best practices for convening GRAS panels. This includes prohibiting people with industry-related conflicts of interest from serving as experts on GRAS review panels,[39] ensuring GRAS panel members have appropriate and balanced expertise,[40] requiring public data and information to form the basis of GRAS review, and limiting the data provided to a GRAS panel to public information (e.g., not allowing trade secret information).[39]	Congress should mandate that GRAS panels are conflict-free.
Robust and systematic postmarket review	FDA should create a robust and systematic postmarket review process to reevaluate substances previously determined to be GRAS and approved food additives, with scheduled rereview time frames (building substantially on the process it announced in March 2024). FDA should undertake these systematic reviews on a regular basis.	Congress should require the FDA to create a robust procedure to systematically and regularly review the safety of approved food additives, substances previously determined to be GRAS by industry, and substances that went through a previous FDA GRAS affirmation or notification process.
Prohibit harmful substances from receiving or maintaining a GRAS designation	FDA should act to prohibit substances that show evidence of carcinogenic, reproductive, developmental, or metabolic toxicity from receiving GRAS designation or maintaining GRAS designation if postmarket evidence of this arises.[39]	Congress could authorize the FDA to fine or otherwise penalize food manufacturers that self-GRAS and market a substance without sufficient premarket evidence to ensure absence of such harms.
Transparency	Congress should require the food industry to identify all GRAS substances they have determined are safe through the self-GRAS process. FDA should disclose a list of all known GRAS substances in the food supply on its Web site. FDA should also post a clear list or database of all substances for which GRAS status has been revoked or limited.	
Reevaluating GRAS substances associated with health harm at high levels of consumption	FDA should develop and implement a framework to reevaluate the GRAS status of current levels and uses of added caffeine, sodium, and sugar, which are associated with health harms at high levels. FDA should consider imposing limits as part of the good manufacturing practices required for use of those substances.	

Note. FDA = US Food and Drug Administration; GRAS = generally recognized as safe.
[a]Recommended actions are those that have the most evidence or for which the actor (Congress or the FDA) has the most authority to act on that issue.
[b]Alternative actions are those that should be implemented if the recommended action is not implemented.

by the FDA with food companies, as it did for drug regulation (Table 2).

In November 2023, Senators Edward J. Markey (D, MA) and Cory Booker (D, NJ) introduced the Ensuring Safe and Toxic-Free Foods Act, which would address some of the gaps left in the wake of the FDA's current interpretation of its regulatory authority over GRAS substances.[39] Key points in this bill include requiring FDA premarket review of GRAS substances, reducing conflicts of interest in GRAS panels,[40] improving the FDA's postmarket review to reevaluate substances already in the food supply, and prohibiting carcinogenic substances and substances with evidence of reproductive or developmental toxicity from receiving GRAS designation.[39]

Our analysis demonstrates the very real challenges of the FDA's current framework for evaluating and regulating substances added to food products. Several policy pathways are available for Congress and the FDA to rectify these challenges and provide resources to the FDA to protect public health in the United States with a robust framework to ensure the safety of our food supply. AJPH

ABOUT THE AUTHORS

Jennifer L. Pomeranz is with the Department of Public Health Policy and Management, School of Global Public Health, New York University, New York, NY. Emily M. Broad Leib is with the Center for Health Law and Policy Innovation, Harvard Law School, Cambridge, MA. Dariush Mozaffarian is with the Friedman School of Nutrition Science and Policy, Tufts University, Boston, MA and the Tufts School of Medicine and Division of Cardiology, Tufts Medical Center, Boston, MA.

CORRESPONDENCE

Correspondence should be sent to Jennifer L. Pomeranz, Department of Public Health Policy and Management, School of Global Public Health, New York University, 708 Broadway, 7th Floor, New York, NY 10003 (e-mail: jlp284@nyu.edu). Reprints can be ordered at https://www.ajph.org by clicking the "Reprints" link.

PUBLICATION INFORMATION

Full Citation: Pomeranz JL, Broad Leib EM, Mozaffarian D. Regulation of added substances in the food supply by the Food and Drug Administration Human Foods Program. *Am J Public Health.* 2024;114(10): 1061–1070.

Acceptance Date: June 9, 2024.

DOI: https://doi.org/10.2105/AJPH.2024.307755

CONTRIBUTORS

J. L. Pomeranz and E. M. Broad Leib conducted the legal analysis. All authors conceptualized the work and contributed to the writing.

ACKNOWLEDGMENTS

This research was supported by National Institutes of Health (NIH; project 2R01HL115189-06A1 Cost-Effectiveness of Health System and State-Level Strategies to Improve Diet and Reduce Cardiometabolic Diseases; principal investigator: D. Mozaffarian).

The authors wish to thank Michael Jacobson and Jerold Mande for their thoughts on previous drafts of this work and Noelle Musolino and Jessica Pe for their research assistance.

CONFLICTS OF INTEREST

The authors have no potential or actual conflicts of interest to disclose.

HUMAN PARTICIPANT PROTECTION

No protocol approval was necessary because no human participants were involved in this study.

REFERENCES

1. US Food and Drug Administration. Food and Drugs: Mission. 21 USC § 393(b).
2. Beyranevand LJ. Generally recognized as safe? Analyzing flaws in the FDA's approach to GRAS additives (November 13, 2013). *Vermont Law Review.* 2013;37(4). Vermont Law School Research Paper No. 33-13. Available at: https://ssrn.com/abstract=2353837. Accessed July 16, 2024.
3. Soroudi RR. Government repudiation of Americans' safety: a call for reformulation of the FDA's GRAS notification program. *Food Drug Law J.* 2020;75(1):39–64.
4. Aaron DG. The fall of the FDA review. *Yale J. Health Pol'y L. & Ethics.* 2023;22(95). University of Utah College of Law Research Paper No. 545. Available at: https://ssrn.com/abstract=4413047. Accessed July 16, 2024.
5. Food and Drugs: Food Additives. 21 US Code § 348 (1958).
6. Medintz S. Four dangerous food additives banned in California. *Consumer Reports.* October 7, 2023. Available at: https://www.consumerreports.org/health/food-additives/four-dangerous-food-additives-banned-in-california-a9426571060. Accessed July 16, 2024.
7. US Food and Drug Administration. FDA proposes to ban food additive, continues assessments of additional chemicals. November 2, 2023. Available at: https://www.fda.gov/news-events/press-announcements/fda-proposes-ban-food-additive-continues-assessments-additional-chemicals. Accessed July 16, 2024.
8. *Center for Food Safety v Becerra*, 565 F. Supp. 3d 519 (SDNY, 2021).
9. Henney J, Diez-Gonzalez F, Jones J, Kowalcyk B, Kumanyika S, Taylor J. Operational evaluation of the FDA Human Foods Program: a report of the Human Foods Independent Expert Panel Reagan–Udall Foundation for the FDA. 2022. Available at: https://reaganudall.org/operational-evaluation-fdas-human-foods-programs. Accessed July 16, 2024.
10. US Food and Drug Administration. How the FDA's new approach to reviewing chemicals added to food will strengthen food safety. May 26, 2023. Available at: https://www.fda.gov/news-events/fda-voices/how-fdas-new-approach-reviewing-chemicals-added-food-will-strengthen-food-safety. Accessed July 16, 2024.
11. Food Additives Amendment. PL 85-929, 72 Stat. (September 6, 1958). Available at: https://www.govinfo.gov/content/pkg/STATUTE-72/pdf/STATUTE-72-Pg1784.pdf. Accessed July 16, 2024.
12. US Food and Drug Administration. Understanding how the FDA regulates food additives and GRAS ingredients. July 6, 2023. Available at: https://www.fda.gov/food/food-additives-and-gras-ingredients-information-consumers/understanding-how-fda-regulates-food-additives-and-gras-ingredients. Accessed July 16, 2024.
13. US Food and Drug Administration. FDA's approach to the GRAS provision: a history of processes. January 4, 2018. Available at: https://www.fda.gov/food/generally-recognized-safe-gras/fdas-approach-gras-provision-history-processes. Accessed July 16, 2024.
14. Department of Health and Human Services. Substances generally recognized as safe. *Fed Regist.* 1997;62(74):18938–18964. Available at: https://www.govinfo.gov/content/pkg/FR-1997-04-17/pdf/97-9706.pdf. Accessed July 16, 2024.
15. Jockel S, Wolf B. Food ingredient GRAS conclusions: what you should know. Available at: https://www.foodmanufacturing.com/ingredients/article/21271894/food-ingredient-gras-conclusions-what-you-should-know. Accessed July 16, 2024.
16. US Food and Drug Administration. How US FDA's GRAS notification program works. February 9, 2018. Available at: https://www.fda.gov/food/generally-recognized-safe-gras/how-us-fdas-gras-notification-program-works. Accessed July 16, 2024.
17. Neltner TG, Kulkarni NR, Alger HM, et al. Navigating the US Food Additive Regulatory Program. *Compr Rev Food Sci Food Saf.* 2011;10(6):342–368. https://doi.org/10.1111/j.1541-4337.2011.00166.x
18. US Government Accountability Office. Regulation of cancer-causing food additives—time for a change. December 11, 1981. Available at: https://www.gao.gov/products/hrd-82-3#. Accessed July 16, 2024.
19. US Government Accountability Office. Food safety: FDA should strengthen its oversight of food ingredients determined to be generally recognized as safe (GRAS). March 5, 2010. Available at: https://www.gao.gov/assets/gao-10-246.pdf. Accessed July 16, 2024.
20. US Government Accountability Office. Food safety: FDA should strengthen its oversight of food ingredients determined to be generally recognized as safe (GRAS). Recommendations for executive action. Available at: https://www.gao.gov/products/gao-10-246. Accessed July 16, 2024.
21. Neltner TG, Alger HM, O'Reilly JT, Krimsky S, Bero LA, Maffini MV. Conflicts of interest in approvals

of additives to food determined to be generally recognized as safe: out of balance. *JAMA Intern Med.* 2013;173(22):2032–2036. https://doi.org/10.1001/jamainternmed.2013.10559

22. Matouskova K, Neltner TG, Maffini MV. Out of balance: conflicts of interest persist in food chemicals determined to be generally recognized as safe. *Environ Health.* 2023;22(1):59. https://doi.org/10.1186/s12940-023-01004-8
23. US Food and Drug Administration. Post-market determinations that the use of a substance is not GRAS. Available at: https://www.cfsanappsexternal.fda.gov/scripts/fdcc/?set=Postmarket. Accessed April 28, 2024.
24. US Food and Drug Administration. Final determination regarding partially hydrogenated oils. *Fed Regist.* 2015;80(116):34650–34670. Available at: https://www.govinfo.gov/content/pkg/FR-2015-06-17/pdf/2015-14883.pdf. Accessed July 16, 2024.
25. Willett WC, Stampfer MJ, Manson JE, et al. Intake of trans fatty acids and risk of coronary heart disease among women. *Lancet.* 1993;341(8845):581–585. https://doi.org/10.1016/0140-6736(93)90350-P
26. US Food and Drug Administration. Proposed rules. *Fed Regist.* 2003;68(133):41434–41506. Available at: https://www.govinfo.gov/content/pkg/FR-2003-07-11/pdf/03-17525.pdf. Accessed July 29, 2024.
27. US Food and Drug Administration. List of select chemicals in the food supply under the FDA review. March 4, 2024. Available at: https://www.fda.gov/food/food-chemical-safety/list-select-chemicals-food-supply-under-fda-review. Accessed July 16, 2024.
28. Pomeranz JL, Munsell CR, Harris JL. Energy drinks: an emerging public health hazard for youth. *J Public Health Policy.* 2013;34(2):254–271. https://doi.org/10.1057/jphp.2013.6
29. Micha R, Peñalvo JL, Cudhea F, Imamura F, Rehm CD, Mozaffarian D. Association between dietary factors and mortality from heart disease, stroke, and type 2 diabetes in the United States. *JAMA.* 2017;317(9):912–924. https://doi.org/10.1001/jama.2017.0947
30. Center for Science in the Public Interest. Petition to revoke the GRAS status of salt. Filed November 8, 2005. Available at: https://www.cspinet.org/sites/default/files/media/documents/resource/fda_salt_petition.pdf. Accessed July 16, 2024.
31. Henney JE, Taylor CL, Boon CS, eds; Institute of Medicine, Committee on Strategies to Reduce Sodium Intake. *Strategies to Reduce Sodium Intake in the United States.* Washington, DC: National Academies Press; 2010. https://doi.org/10.17226/12818.
32. Ralston Aoki J, Dawkins SA, Bishop SK. Implementing the IOM's recommendations for reducing sodium in the US food supply: considerations and approaches. *Food Drug Law J.* 2014;69(1):53–85.
33. US Food and Drug Administration. Salt and sodium; petition to revise the regulatory status of salt and establish food labeling requirements regarding salt and sodium; public hearing; request for comments. *Fed Regist.* 2007;72(204):59973–59979. Available at: https://www.govinfo.gov/content/pkg/FR-2007-10-23/pdf/07-5216.pdf. Accessed July 16, 2024.
34. US Food and Drug Administration. Voluntary sodium reduction goals: target mean and upper bound concentrations for sodium in commercially processed, packaged, and prepared foods. October 2021. Available at: https://www.fda.gov/media/98264/download. Accessed July 16, 2024.
35. Substances added directly to human food affirmed as generally recognized as safe (GRAS). 21 CFR § 184.1 (2023).
36. Faustman C, Aaron D, Negowetti N, Broad Leib E. Ten years post-GAO assessment, the FDA remains uninformed of potentially harmful GRAS substances in foods. *Crit Rev Food Sci Nutr.* 2020;61(8):1260–1268. https://doi.org/10.1080/10408398.2020.1756217
37. US Food and Drug Administration. Substances generally recognized as safe. *Fed. Reg.* 2016;81(159):54960–55055. Available at: https://www.govinfo.gov/content/pkg/FR-2016-08-17/pdf/2016-19164.pdf. Accessed July 29, 2024.
38. Lane MM, Gamage E, Du S, et al. Ultra-processed food exposure and adverse health outcomes: umbrella review of epidemiological meta-analyses. *BMJ.* 2024;384:e077310. https://doi.org/10.1136/bmj-2023-077310
39. Ensuring Safe and Toxic-Free Foods Act of 2023. Available at: https://www.markey.senate.gov/imo/media/doc/ensuring_safe_and_toxic-free_foods_act_one-pager_-_112123pdf.pdf. Accessed July 16, 2024.
40. US Food and Drug Administration. FDA issues final guidance on best practices for convening a GRAS panel. December 20, 2022. Available at: https://www.fda.gov/food/cfsan-constituent-updates/fda-issues-final-guidance-best-practices-convening-gras-panel. Accessed July 16, 2024.

Mortality Surveillance for the COVID-19 Pandemic: Review of the Centers for Disease Control and Prevention's Multiple System Strategy

Diba Khan, PhD, MS, Meeyoung Park, MPH, Peter Grillo, BS, Lauren Rossen, PhD, MS, B. Casey Lyons, MPH, Sarah David, MPH, Matthew D. Ritchey, PT, DPT, MPH, Farida B. Ahmad, MPH, A. D. McNaghten, PhD, MS, Adi V. Gundlapalli, MD, PhD, and Amitabh B. Suthar, PharmD, MPH

See also Lee, p. 963.

Mortality surveillance systems can have limitations, including reporting delays, incomplete reporting, missing data, and insufficient detail on important risk or sociodemographic factors that can impact the accuracy of estimates of current trends, disease severity, and related disparities across subpopulations.

The Centers for Disease Control and Prevention used multiple data systems during the COVID-19 emergency response—line-level case–death surveillance, aggregate death surveillance, and the National Vital Statistics System—to collectively provide more comprehensive and timely information on COVID-19–associated mortality necessary for informed decisions.

This article will review in detail the line-level, aggregate, and National Vital Statistics System surveillance systems and the purpose and use of each. This retrospective review of the hybrid surveillance systems strategy may serve as an example for adaptive informational approaches needed over the course of future public health emergencies. (*Am J Public Health*. 2024;114(10):1071–1080. https://doi.org/10.2105/AJPH.2024.307743)

AJPH October 2024, Vol. 114, No. 10

In December 2019, officials in Wuhan, China, reported the first cases of a novel virus of unknown etiology associated with pneumonia. China's World Health Organization Country Office received the first notification of an outbreak on December 31, 2019.[1,2] The National Center for Immunization and Respiratory Diseases at the Centers for Disease Control and Prevention (CDC) activated a center-level response to the 2019 novel coronavirus outbreak on January 5, 2020, to monitor the progression of the outbreak overseas. Following the first laboratory-confirmed case in Washington State,[3] CDC scaled to an agency-wide response by activating the Emergency Operations Center on January 20, 2020[1]; the World Health Organization (WHO) declared the 2019 novel coronavirus outbreak a Public Health Emergency of International Concern on January 30, 2020.[4] In the United States, state, tribal, local, and territorial (STLT) jurisdictions mandated reporting requirements based on the Council of State and Territorial Epidemiologists' (CSTE's) interim case definitions[5,6] and began publicly reporting the number of people with severe acute respiratory syndrome coronavirus-2 (SARS-CoV-2) infection.[7]

On February 29, 2020, the first confirmed COVID-19 death in the United States was reported in Washington State.[8] COVID-19 was the third leading cause of death in the United States by the end of 2020, with 350 831 deaths.[9] By January 20, 2024, the United States reached 1 172 229 COVID-19–associated deaths and continues to record more than 1000 deaths per week as of January 20, 2024.

COVID-19 MORTALITY SURVEILLANCE SYSTEMS

During the COVID-19 emergency response, CDC used 3 data sources to provide COVID-19 mortality data for decision-making and resource allocation. "Line-level" data, comprising individual case records, are used to conduct epidemiological analyses on COVID-19 cases and deaths and characterize demographic trends for COVID-19 severity. Aggregate Case and Death Surveillance (ACS) provided situational awareness based on provisional, cumulative case, and death counts to monitor recent trends in severity and geographic spread of COVID-19. The National Vital Statistics System (NVSS) provides the most comprehensive information on overall and cause-specific mortality in the United States, including for COVID-19. We describe the 3 surveillance systems used by CDC for tracking COVID-19 mortality—line-level, ACS, and NVSS—and the purpose and use of each. CDC used data from multiple surveillance systems to assess accurate, complete, and timely information on COVID-19–associated deaths to develop evidence-based guidance for safeguarding the nation's health, and lessons learned from this experience can help to prepare for future public health emergencies.

Line-Level Death Surveillance

COVID-19 is a nationally notifiable disease, for which case notification by STLT jurisdictions to CDC for national surveillance is recommended but voluntary in nature (https://bit.ly/3XNafwg).[6] The case report form has more than 200 data elements to capture information such as patient demographics, including age, race, and ethnicity; signs and symptoms of illness; underlying health conditions; hospitalization status; laboratory results; vaccination history; possible routes of exposure; death status; and date of death.[10]

CSTE published their first interim case definition for COVID-19–associated deaths on April 5, 2020, which states a death certificate must "list COVID-19 disease or SARS-CoV-2 as a cause of death or a significant condition contributing to death" for classification as a death attributable to COVID-19.[6] Because of the evolving nature of the COVID-19 pandemic, CSTE issued a revised definition in January 2022 and additional guidance in November 2022[11] to address concerns such as the increasing levels of transmissibility, prevalence of at-home rapid over-the-counter SARS-CoV-2 tests (generally not reported to STLT public health departments), and the reduction of universal case investigation and contact tracing.[12] The current case definition for a COVID-19–associated death is "A person whose death certificate lists COVID-19 disease or SARS-CoV-2 or an equivalent term as an underlying cause of death or a significant condition contributing to death."[12(p13)]

Brief system design overview and implementation. STLT jurisdictions mandate hospitals, health care providers, laboratories, and various other institutions to report case data for reportable conditions, such as COVID-19. Mandated reporters may indicate whether the patient is deceased as part of their case report to public health departments. Public health departments may also establish whether the patient is deceased during case investigation[13] or through routine cross-referencing with death registries.

Jurisdictions voluntarily send COVID-19 case reports to CDC via standardized electronic messaging to the Nationally Notifiable Disease Surveillance System or directly upload comma-separated values (CSV) files[10,14] into CDC's data management and analytic platform built for COVID-19, Department of Health and Human Services (HHS) Protect (Figure 1). Before transmission to CDC, STLTs remove personally identifiable information, such as name and home address, to de-identify COVID-19 line-level case data. At CDC, COVID-19 case data from both sources are ingested into the US Department of Health and Human Services (HHS) platform HHS Protect, combined, and cleaned to produce a single line-level data set (Figure 1). On October 20, 2022, CDC transitioned from daily to weekly reporting of COVID-19 data to reduce reporting burden on jurisdictions.

A jurisdiction may iteratively update a case record as it gathers additional information; because of the potential lag between when a case is identified, reported, and subsequently dies, death status is often updated after the initial COVID-19 notification has been submitted. Each production of the combined COVID-19 line-level data set overwrites the previously submitted data to capture these updates. Because of the large number of data elements collected on COVID-19 case reports and changes in case status (e.g., hospitalization or death) that can occur over time, a COVID-19 record may take weeks to finalize. Some jurisdictions initially submit individual case reports with minimal data, providing additional data as they become available, while other jurisdictions share the case record only when it is considered complete.

Purpose and use. Line-level data provide detailed information about each COVID-19 case and can be used to answer emerging clinical, epidemiological, and scientific questions about COVID-19 severity for specific populations. Analysis of COVID-19 death information captured

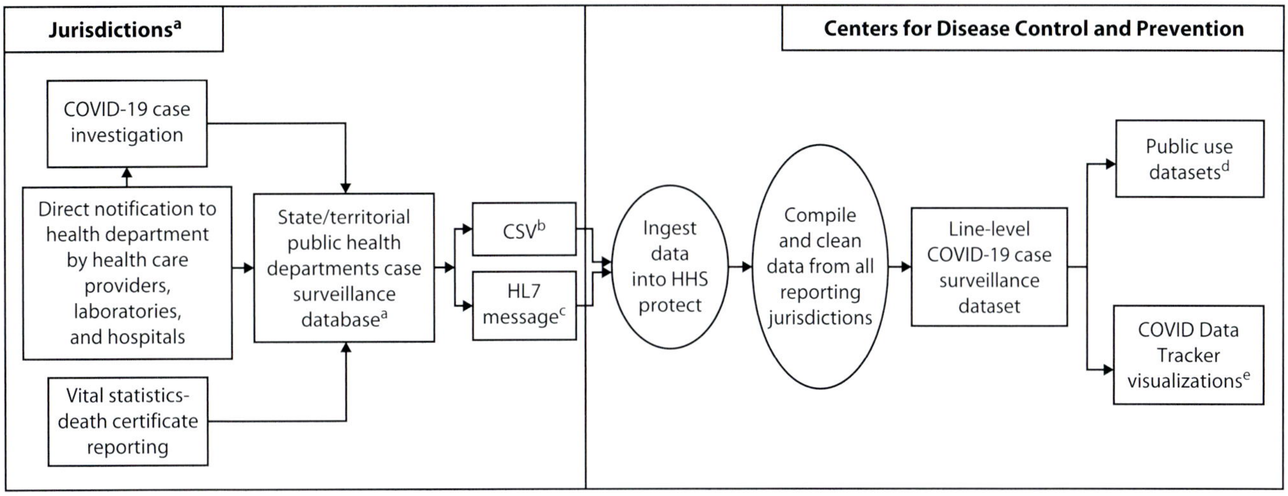

FIGURE 1— COVID-19 Mortality Data Collection, Transmission, and Collation for Line-Level Reporting: United States, January 1, 2020–Present

Note. CSV = comma separated value; HHS = Department of Health and Human Services; HL7 = Health Level 7.
[a]Reporting public health department may include local, state, or territorial jurisdictions. New York City reported as its own jurisdiction, separate from New York State. Death status and death date are 2 of many variables collected about each individual COVID-19 case.
[b]To report to the Centers for Disease Control and Prevention (CDC), jurisdictions may format deidentified case records into comma-separated value and upload to HHS Protect via a secured Web site.
[c]Alternatively, jurisdictions may utilize deidentified Health Level 7 messages to submit case information to the Nationally Notifiable Disease Surveillance System, a database maintained at CDC. Records are ingested from this database to HHS Protect.
[d]Death status is available with suppression in certain public-use data sets available on https://data.cdc.gov.
[e]Death data from line-level case surveillance is used in visualizations by demographic groups on COVID Data Tracker.

in the line-level data can help determine sociodemographic mortality trends, identify vulnerable populations, and target interventions. CDC publishes 3 COVID-19 line-level case surveillance data sets for public use and research with various levels of privacy protection.[15–17] Because of decreased reporting by jurisdictions as a result of at-home testing and reporting fatigue, among other factors, CDC discontinued use of line-level data as a leading indicator for COVID-19 monitoring at the end of the COVID-19 national public health emergency (PHE) on May 11, 2023.[18] CDC's COVID Data Tracker included dynamic data visualizations using line-level data to track trends in COVID-19 cases and deaths by age, race, ethnicity, and sex until November 2023, when the case visualizations were discontinued and the death visualizations were transitioned to using NVSS data.[19,20]

Aggregate Case and Death Surveillance

Given the time needed to collect and transmit individual case details from the line-level data and immediate operational need for situational awareness, CDC established the ACS for tracking cumulative COVID-19 case and death data in January 2020.[21] Initially, CDC worked with jurisdictions to systematically collect daily cumulative COVID-19 case and death totals at the state level using an Epi-Info Web entry form.[22]

From March to August 2020, CDC used open-source data from USAFacts, a third-party aggregator of COVID-19 data, for enumeration of cases and deaths at the county level, after additional data cleaning by CDC and HHS staff. Starting in August 2020, CDC expanded the ACS to electronically gather cumulative COVID-19 case and death counts from official jurisdictional and county-level online sources to monitor the current transmission of COVID-19 (via cases) and severity (via deaths).

CDC collected ACS data daily until October 2022, and on a weekly basis thereafter until the end of the COVID-19 PHE.[18] ACS data were based on preliminary COVID-19 case reports, often before case investigations were considered complete, and were subjected to changes including the deletion of cases if duplicate records were identified or if the case definition was not met; for these reasons, it was not uncommon for the number of overall deaths in a jurisdiction or county to change from week to week as records were updated.

Brief system design and implementation. Before October 2022, aggregate COVID-19 case and death data were simultaneously collected at the county as well as at the state level. To streamline the data collection process and to align county- and state-level totals, CDC began using the sum of the county-level counts to reflect the state-level totals. CDC collected county-level aggregate COVID-19 death data for more than 3200 counties by automated processes, including Web-scraping (a process by which Web-based publicly available information on COVID-19 cases and deaths were extracted from the jurisdictions' official Web pages, dashboards, and official press releases, which were further validated by the jurisdictions[21]), direct data transfer through application programming interfaces, and comma-separated value file transmissions using a standard template (Figure 2). CDC recorded aggregate COVID-19 deaths by the date (in order of preference) they were reported to the health department, notified by the health department to CDC, or reported publicly, but the actual date of death likely occurred before the date of report, with lag times varying by jurisdiction.

CDC used a variety of data quality and anomaly detection techniques to indicate potential issues, such as inconsistent reporting or trends that deviated significantly from the historic patterns. If data anomalies were identified, CDC data analysts coordinated directly with the corresponding STLT health departments to verify and correct issues. CDC routinely conducted historical data reconciliation for many jurisdictions to assign or redistribute COVID-19 cases and deaths to their correct dates of reporting. The reconciliation process also accounted for data cleaning or retroactively applied case definitions by jurisdictions and kept the COVID-19 timeseries data aligned with jurisdictional corrections to the county-level information for improved data quality and more accurate trends.

The final county-level and state-level time series data sets of COVID-19 deaths were disseminated as official public use data sets on https://data.cdc.gov and visualizations on COVID Data Tracker. After the PHE, the aggregate COVID-19 case and death data sets have been archived on https://data.cdc.gov.[23,24]

Purpose and use. The aggregate county- and state-level COVID-19 death data[23,24] were used for near-real-time spatial–temporal surveillance and forecasting the severity of the pandemic.[25] National ensemble forecasting estimates used ACS data to predict trends in reported COVID-19 deaths and enabled CDC to anticipate potential near-term mortality outcomes for risk mitigation.[25] Because the ACS provided the most up-to-date accounting of jurisdictions' mortality burden across the 3 systems, CDC used ACS throughout the COVID-19 response as the official current count of COVID-19 deaths at the national level published on CDC's

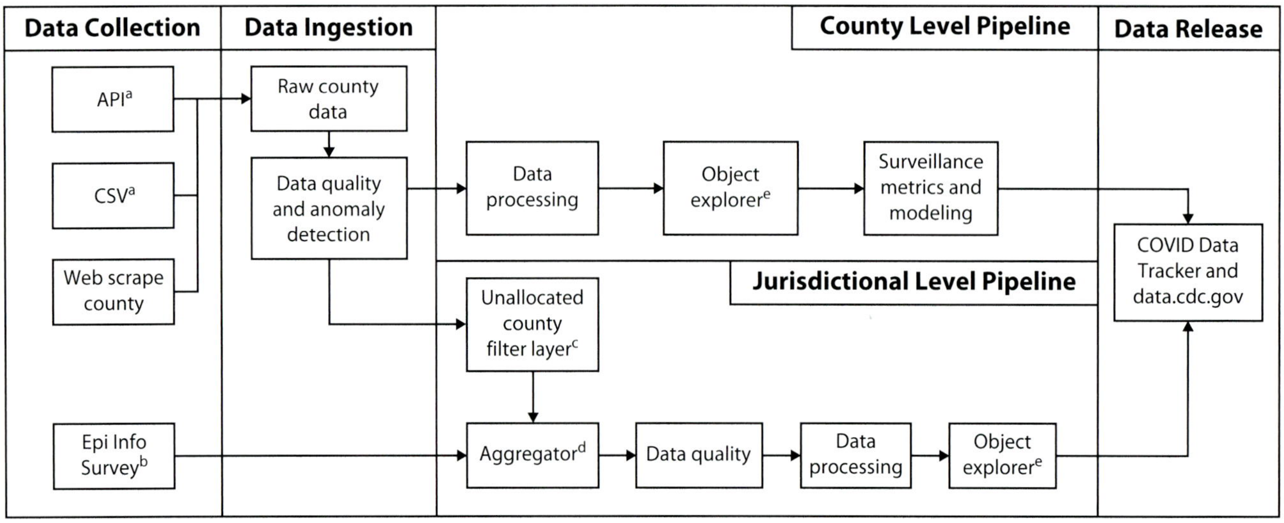

FIGURE 2— Aggregate COVID-19 Mortality Data Collection: United States, January 22, 2020–May 10, 2023

Note. API = application programming interfaces; CSV = comma separated values.
[a]API and CSV data transmissions allow for full time series data corrections by jurisdictions.
[b]Epi Info Survey allows for states to make weekly corrections to state totals. In addition, it feeds District of Columbia data to the county pipeline.
[c]Filter layer node handles variabilities in how states use unallocated counties. Each jurisdiction has an unallocated county that is designed to record cases and deaths without county assignments or account for differences between state- and county-level reporting.
[d]Aggregator node aggregates county cases and deaths to the state level.
[e]Object explorer allows for Centers for Disease Control and Prevention, on behalf of a jurisdiction, to make weekly corrections to COVID-19 cases and death totals.

COVID Data Tracker until the end of the PHE.[18]

National Vital Statistics System

NVSS aggregates and disseminates the nation's mortality statistics using death certificate data submitted by the 50 states, New York City, the District of Columbia, and the 5 US territories. Provisional NVSS mortality data are based on nonfinal death certificates processed as of a given analysis date. Because of the many steps needed to complete, verify, process, code, and disseminate death certificate data, NVSS data can be subject to a reporting lag. As of January 2024, NVSS mortality data were approximately 98% complete within 4 weeks.[26]

Brief system design overview and implementation. The NVSS provides the most comprehensive information for all deaths occurring in the United States.[27] Though each jurisdiction is responsible for the registration of vital events, including deaths, standard forms and model procedures for the uniform registration of events help ensure consistent collection of death certificate data, with several different steps. First, demographic information on the death certificate is completed by funeral directors (Figure 3). Cause-of-death information is completed by a physician (typically for natural causes of death including deaths occurring in a medical setting) or by a coroner or medical examiner (for injury-related deaths and deaths occurring outside of a medical setting). The underlying cause of death represents "the disease or injury which initiated the train of morbid events leading directly to death."[28(p1)] Death certificate data are then submitted to the state vital registration offices,[28] who in turn submit the death records to National Center for Health Statistics (NCHS) through the Vital Statistics Cooperative Program.[29] Cause-of-death information is then assigned *International Classification of Diseases, 10th Revision* (*ICD-10*; Geneva, Switzerland: World Health Organization; 1992) codes through a combination of automated coding algorithms, which process data within minutes, or manual coding of records by trained nosologists.[27] Approximately 80% to 90% of deaths are electronically processed and coded using the automated software, while the remaining 10% to 20% require manual coding by a trained nosologist.

Once death certificate data have been coded and processed, NCHS tabulates COVID-19–associated deaths and deaths from other causes, providing mortality statistics by demographic and geographic variables. Based on published guidance for certifiers,[28] the COVID-19 death counts may consist of either laboratory-confirmed COVID-19 deaths or clinically confirmed COVID-19 deaths.[29] The COVID-19 death counts also include death records where

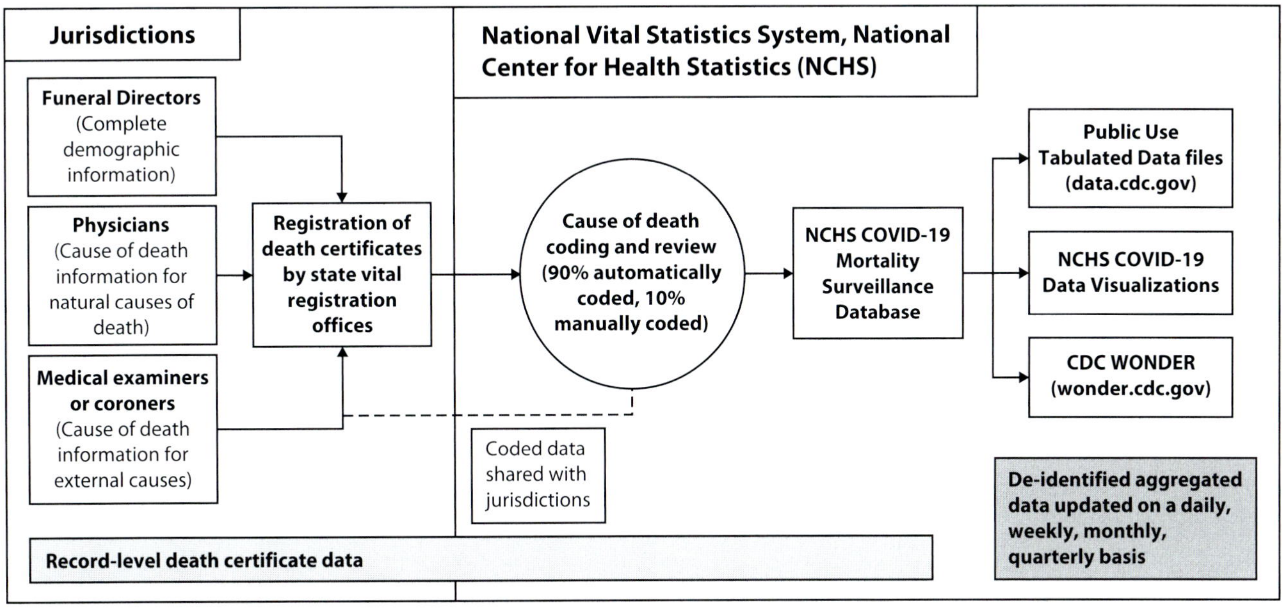

FIGURE 3— US National Vital Statistics Data Collection

Note. CDC WONDER = The Centers for Disease Control and Prevention Wide-ranging Online Data for Epidemiologic Research.

COVID-19 is listed as a "presumed" or "probable" cause, based on a reasonable degree of certainty on the part of the certifier that COVID-19 was a cause of death. Counts of deaths where COVID-19 is the underlying cause and counts where COVID-19 is either the underlying or a contributing cause are provided in many provisional mortality data files. From 2020 through 2022, COVID-19 was listed as the underlying cause of death in around 80% to 90% of deaths and dropped to 65% in 2023, where COVID-19 appears on the death certificate as an underlying cause of death.[29–31]

The NCHS provided preliminary guidance in March and full guidance in April 2020 to assist officials with certifying COVID-19–associated deaths and to ensure consistent collection of COVID-19 information on death certificates, facilitating accurate *ICD-10* coding and ascertainment of COVID-19 deaths from death certificate data.[28] NCHS expanded this guidance in February 2023 to include certification of deaths involving long COVID or postacute sequelae of COVID-19.[28]

Purpose and use. NVSS has historically collected, coded, and processed data for all causes of death in a consistent manner over time and across jurisdictions.[27] Because of the rich set of sociodemographic variables available on death certificates and the consistent manner of data collection, coding, and dissemination, NVSS mortality data are widely used to compare mortality across geographies, genders, races/ethnicities, and age groups.[30,32,33]

In April 2020, NVSS began releasing provisional COVID-19 death counts with daily and, later, weekly updates.[31,32] Provisional COVID-19 mortality data from NVSS are now available on a monthly basis on CDC Wide-ranging Online Data for Epidemiologic Research (WONDER),[33] allowing data users to query the database by many of the variables available on the death certificate (e.g., age, sex, race/ethnicity, geography of residence, urban–rural classification, cause of death, time period, place of death, and autopsy status). Final mortality data for a given calendar year are published annually, typically 10 to 11 months after the end of the data year. CDC uses final NVSS data as the official annual count of COVID-19 deaths for that year.

After the PHE, NVSS is used as the primary data source for monitoring COVID-19 deaths.[18] The percentage of COVID-19 deaths is used as a timely disease severity indicator for surveillance of COVID-19 on the COVID Data Tracker[19,20] because this metric remains relatively stable and therefore is unaffected by incomplete reporting in recent weeks, given that NVSS data on COVID-19 deaths and deaths from all causes have similar timeliness.

CDC used all-cause mortality data to estimate excess deaths associated with COVID-19,[34] including unreported COVID-19 deaths and deaths from other causes linked to secondary effects of the COVID-19 pandemic, such as reduced access to health care. The analysis of excess deaths provided a clearer picture of the total mortality burden of the COVID-19 pandemic. Excess death analyses have also offered valuable insights about the degree to which COVID-19 deaths may have been undercounted and how this has varied over time and place. CDC also published weekly death counts from the most prevalent COVID-19 comorbidities (respiratory diseases, circulatory diseases, malignant neoplasms, Alzheimer's disease, dementia, and other causes that may have been affected by the COVID-19 pandemic).[34] NVSS is the only system able to track trends in mortality from non–COVID-19 causes of death, allowing for the evaluation of the impact of the pandemic on other causes of death and on overall life expectancy.

COMPARISON OF THE 3 MORTALITY SURVEILLANCE SYSTEMS

The 3 CDC COVID-19 mortality surveillance systems vary in terms of representation (i.e., number of reporting jurisdictions), timeliness, variables in data systems, and completeness of COVID-19 death counts; a summary of comparisons based on these criteria, as established by CDC's Updated Guidelines for Evaluating Public Health Surveillance Systems,[35] is outlined in Table A (available as a supplement to the online version of this article at https://ajph.org).

Timeliness of COVID-19 death data has varied throughout the pandemic. Early in the pandemic, the ACS provided the fastest estimation of COVID-19 mortality among the 3 systems at the national, state, and county levels, followed by line-level surveillance and NVSS death data (Table A). Because of the advancements in vital registration systems over the course of the COVID-19 pandemic, timeliness for the NVSS and ACS systems became more similar, and NVSS COVID-19 death counts at times exceeded that of line-level and ACS systems (Figure 4, panel a). In 1 retrospective study, NVSS COVID-19 death trends were identified to be strongly correlated with ACS (correlation coefficient = 0.79) and also timelier than ACS during April 1, 2022, to March 22, 2023.[36] NVSS counts may

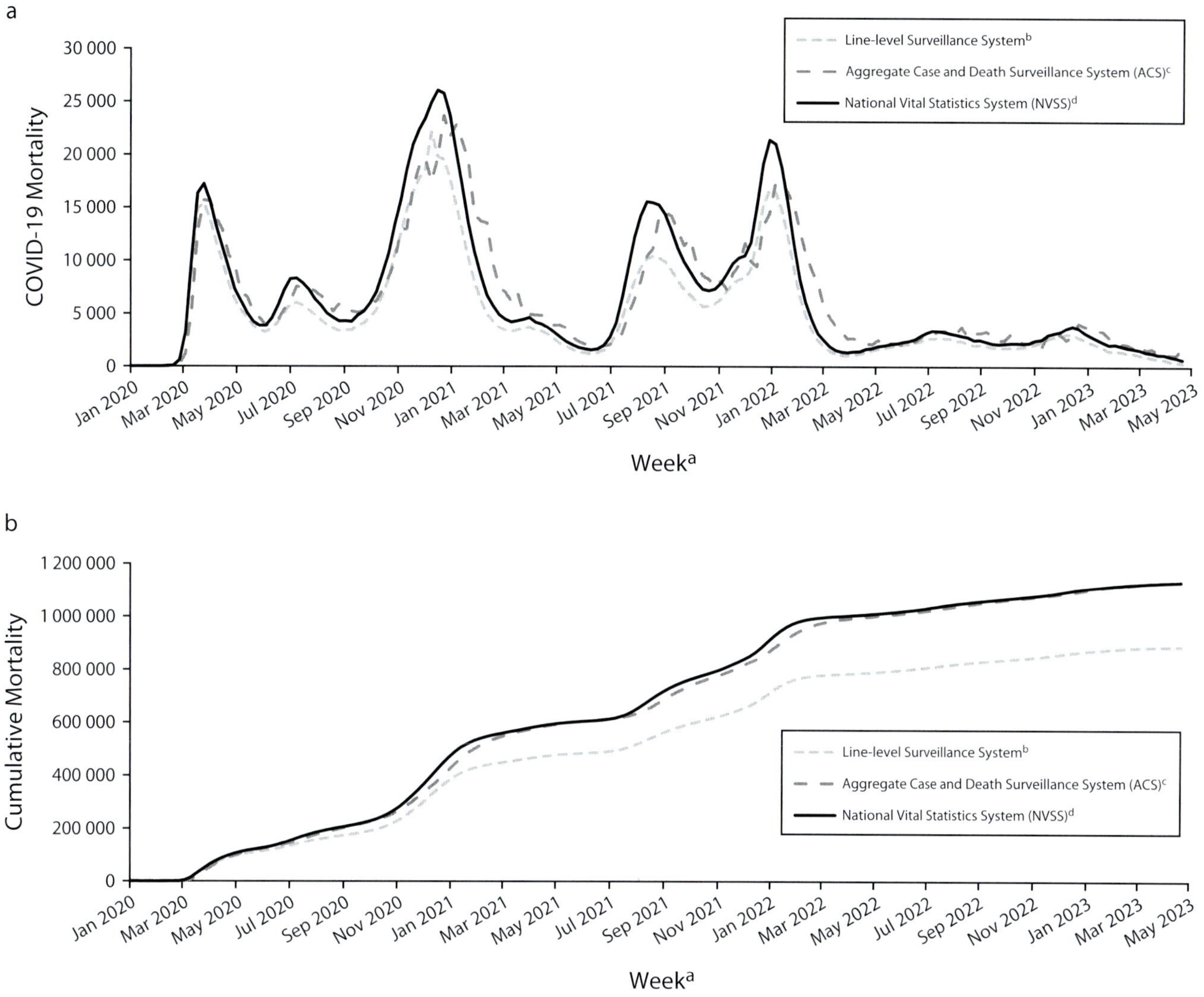

FIGURE 4— Line-Level, Aggregate Case and Death Counts and National Vital Statistics System National COVID-19 Deaths, (a) Weekly, (b) Cumulative: United States, January 20, 2020–May 13, 2023

Note. Data accessed on June 1, 2023. Line-level and National Vital Statistics System (NVSS) are organized by *Morbidity and Mortality Weekly Report* weeks and are presented up to week ending date May 13, 2023. (These visualizations include all COVID-19 deaths data from NVSS and line-level recorded as of June 1, 2023. ACS COVID-19 death data are reported as of May 10, 2023 [end of Public Health Emergency]. The reporting lag for NVSS and line-level is not as evident because sufficient time elapsed [by June 1] for data to be fully processed.) Due to data update cadences, ACS defined a week as the previous Wednesday to the current Thursday, and data are presented up to May 11, 2023.

[a]ACS data based on date reported to the Centers for Disease Control and Prevention (CDC); line-level, and NVSS are based on the date the death occurred.

[b]n = 888 357. Death date was unknown for 8.6% of deaths from the line-level surveillance system. As of March 15, 2022, the CDC changed its method for cleaning line-level death information to remove an outdated piece of cleaning code to better reflect the data jurisdictions' share and to improve alignment with other data sources. This removal resulted in a decrease of 72 277 deaths in the data set, as well as 270 health care worker deaths. Decreases were observed in 18 jurisdictions' data.

[c]n = 1 133 807. A total of 2 807 historical deaths were reported to ACS as of May 11, 2023. Historical deaths are not reflected in new weekly death counts.

[d]n = 1 132 394.

differ from ACS and line-level counts because (1) COVID-19 cases may not have been reported or case reports may have been delayed in ACS and line-level surveillance data, (2) some COVID-19 case reports may have closed without updating the death status in line-level surveillance data, (3) NVSS collects a comprehensive record of all causes of death and could be subject to delay, and (4) NVSS data are based on COVID-19 being documented as an underlying or contributing cause of death on the death certificate and coded according to *ICD-10* coding rules. ACS and line-level surveillance data use CSTE case definitions to classify COVID-19 deaths, and, thus, death counts may not align with those captured via NVSS, even where reporting lags are not a reason for discrepancy.

All 3 surveillance systems experienced increased delays in reporting during heightened volumes of deaths.[37] The existing variation in terms of timeliness, consistent submission of initial case reports, and subsequent death status updates by the different STLTs have made the line-level data difficult to use for assessing current overall mortality trends. NVSS experienced additional delays in earlier waves of the pandemic, as periodic increases in deaths led to backlogs as COVID-19 deaths needed manual coding and review. ACS data were therefore deemed most suitable for routine public reporting during the PHE. While manual coding typically takes an average of 7 days, backlogs increased the wait time to as high as 29 days following a major surge in COVID-19 deaths. Subsequent improvements to NVSS coding systems have increased the proportion of records automatically coded such that 90% of all death records (including COVID-19) are now auto-coded.

The sensitivity in terms of number of COVID-19 death records captured varied across the 3 mortality surveillance systems, with NVSS being the gold standard. As of May 13, 2023, CDC recorded the most COVID-19 deaths from ACS (n = 1 133 807), followed by NVSS (n = 1 132 394), then the line-level system (n = 888 357; Figure 4, panel b). During the initial period of the COVID-19 response, cumulative COVID-19 death counts from provisional NVSS data consistently lagged behind cumulative death counts from ACS because of the time associated with reporting, coding, and processing death certificate data (which can take 1 to 8 weeks to be complete). With advancements in vital registration systems, as more COVID-19 new and updated death certificates are received and processed by NCHS, the discrepancy between the total COVID-19 death counts in the 3 systems has been reduced, though some differences may remain. Moreover, ACS presented death counts by date of report, rather than by event date (i.e., the date the death occurred). This made the impact of reporting delays more apparent, and the death trends in ACS to be more pronounced, because backfilled death counts were assigned to recent report dates rather than the dates when the deaths occurred. This reporting artifact is not present in line-level and NVSS data, which use date of death.

In terms of completeness, data from the NVSS provide the most accurate and complete information on the demographics of COVID-19 mortality[38,39] (Table A). By contrast, race and ethnicity data in the line-level data source are subject to higher levels of incompleteness[38] (approximately 36% of the data set) as are other details such as symptoms and comorbid conditions, and the ACS could only be stratified by case classification status and geographic level.[21] The ACS allowed publication of COVID-19 case and death data at more granular geographies (e.g., county-level) and time intervals (e.g., daily) because of how the data were reported and summarized. In addition, NVSS has data-suppression restrictions for displaying data for smaller geographies and time intervals because of agreements with reporting jurisdictions. Similarly, line-level data require suppression at more granular geographic levels and time intervals.

CHALLENGES AND STRENGTHS

The balance between accuracy and timeliness presents a unique challenge when providing meaningful COVID-19–associated mortality estimates based on provisional death data, which are by definition incomplete and continually updated over time. The need for real-time data on COVID-19–associated mortality necessitates the reliance on incomplete, provisional data, as decision-makers and public health officials cannot wait weeks or months for complete, final data to be available. However, this also presents challenges in terms of evolving numbers over time and potential differences between provisional and final estimates.

The use of multiple COVID-19 mortality surveillance systems also presented some challenges related to the communication of the total burden of COVID-19 mortality, given that the 3 sources did not perfectly align in their estimates. Each data source was used for specific purposes during the PHE based on its strengths and limitations (Table B, available as a supplement to the online version of this article at https://ajph.org). ACS was timely enough to provide top-line, near-real-time counts for daily visualizations on COVID Data Tracker from its inception to until the end of the PHE, while line-level data provided basic information on demographic trends. However, line-level data suffered from a large degree of missing data on key variables such as race/ethnicity, which hindered the ability to accurately assess and address the inequitable impact of the pandemic. NVSS data, because of its standardization and more complete information on demographic variables such as race/ethnicity, was preferred for in-depth analysis and monitoring the disproportionate impact of the pandemic across various subpopulations throughout the PHE, eventually replacing line-level data on COVID Data Tracker as well.[20]

CONCLUSIONS

Mortality data continue to play a key role in monitoring the impact and trajectory of the COVID-19 pandemic. The complementary nature of the 3 surveillance systems established by CDC for monitoring COVID-19 mortality enabled unique inferences to be obtained from each surveillance system to accurately assess COVID-19–associated mortality and may serve as an example in preparing for future public health emergencies. In the beginning and middle phases of the COVID-19 PHE, combining information from the 3 surveillance systems provided a more complete and near-real-time picture of COVID-19 mortality. Multiple data streams informed CDC recommendations, helped in dissemination of critical information to the public, and established new data collection methods in preparation for future responses. With the launch of the Data Modernization Initiative in 2020, CDC has been continually working to further streamline and integrate the data collection processes and modernize the public health surveillance infrastructure to prepare for future threats. Considerable improvements have been made in the speed of death certificate reporting and coding as part of Data Modernization Initiative–related work, and continued progress will ensure that the information derived from death certificates is as timely as possible to track trends in mortality.[29] As the timeliness of deaths reported through NVSS continues to improve, the need for supplemental aggregate and line-level systems has decreased. With recent advances and investments in NVSS over the course of the PHE, NVSS is now used as a primary mortality surveillance tool to assess disease severity and provides the most complete picture of COVID-19–associated mortality.

CDC continues to examine data collection procedures for producing accurate and reliable data and is working to apply lessons learned from the COVID-19 pandemic for responding to future public health emergencies. AJPH

ABOUT THE AUTHORS

Diba Khan, Peter Grillo, and Sarah David are with the National Center for Immunization and Respiratory Diseases, Coronavirus and Other Respiratory Viruses Division (CORVID), Centers for Disease Control and Prevention (CDC), Atlanta, GA. Meeyoung Park is with Situational Awareness Team, Division of Emergency Operations, Office of Readiness and Response, CDC, Atlanta. Lauren Rossen and Farida B. Ahmad are with National Center for Health Statistics, CDC, Hyattsville, MD. B. Casey Lyons is with Epidemiology and Surveillance Branch, Division of Overdose Prevention, National Center for Injury Prevention and Control, CDC, Atlanta. Mathew D. Ritchey and Adi V. Gundlapalli are with the Office of Public Health Data, Surveillance, and Technology, CDC, Atlanta. A. D. McNaghten is with the Division of HIV Prevention, CDC, Atlanta. Amitabh B. Suthar is with the Clinical Surveillance and Epidemiology Team, Division of Global HIV and TB, Global Health Center, CDC, Atlanta.

Note. The findings and conclusions in this article are those of the authors and do not necessarily represent the official position of the Centers for Disease Control and Prevention.

CORRESPONDENCE

Correspondence should be sent to Diba Khan, PhD, MS, Biostatistics, Economic and Modeling (BEaM) Unit, Coronavirus and Other Respiratory Viruses Division, National Center for Immunization and Respiratory Diseases, Centers for Disease Control and Prevention, 1600 Clifton Rd NE, Atlanta, GA 30329 (e-mail: ild1@cdc.gov). Reprints can be ordered at https://www.ajph.org by clicking the "Reprints" link.

PUBLICATION INFORMATION

Full Citation: Khan D, Park M, Grillo P, et al. Mortality surveillance for the COVID-19 pandemic: review of the Centers for Disease Control and Prevention's multiple system strategy. *Am J Public Health*. 2024;114(10):1071–1080.

Acceptance Date: May 24, 2024.

DOI: https://doi.org/10.2105/AJPH.2024.307743

ORCID iD:

Diba Khan https://orcid.org/0000-0001-7314-8709

CONTRIBUTORS

All authors contributed to the initial conceptualization and design of the article, provided detailed content related to the drafting of the article, and have reviewed and approved the submitted article and agreed to be accountable for its contents.

ACKNOWLEDGMENTS

The authors acknowledge CORVID staff for their constructive criticism, support, and encouragement during the writing of this article.

CONFLICTS OF INTEREST

The authors report that they have no conflicts of interest.

HUMAN PARTICIPANT PROTECTION

The activities captured in this essay are a descriptive narrative of the CDC COVID-19 mortality surveillance systems. Thus, this body of work does not meet the definition of research as defined by the Revised Common Rule 45 CFR 46 and is therefore not subject to review by an institutional review board. However, the contents have undergone review and approval by the Office of the Associate Director for Epidemiologic Science at CORVID, CDC.

REFERENCES

1. Centers for Disease Control and Prevention. *CDC Museum COVID-19 Timeline*. Available at: https://www.cdc.gov/museum/timeline/covid19.html. Accessed February 13, 2023.
2. World Health Organization. *COVID-19 – China*. Available at: https://www.who.int/emergencies/disease-outbreak-news/item/2020-DON233. Accessed February 13, 2023.
3. Holshue ML, DeBolt C, Lindquist S, et al. First case of 2019 novel coronavirus in the United States. *N Engl J Med*. 2020;382(10):929–936. https://doi.org/10.1056/NEJMoa2001191
4. World Health Organization. *Statement on the Second Meeting of the International Health Regulations (2005) Emergency Committee Regarding the Outbreak of Novel Coronavirus (2019-nCoV)*. Available at: https://www.who.int/news-room/detail/30-01-2020-statement-on-the-second-meeting-of-the-international-health-regulations-(2005)-emergency-committee-regarding-the-outbreak-of-novel-coronavirus-(2019-ncov). Accessed February 13, 2023.
5. World Health Organization. Global surveillance for human infection with novel coronavirus (2019-nCoV)—interim guidance. January 31, 2020. Available at: https://apps.who.int/iris/bitstream/handle/10665/330857/WHO-2019-nCoV-SurveillanceGuidance-2020.3-eng.pdf?sequence=1%26isAllowed=y. Accessed February 13, 2023.

6. Council of State and Territorial Epidemiologists. Standardized surveillance case definition and national notification for 2019 novel coronavirus disease (COVID-19). Available at: https://cdn.ymaws.com/www.cste.org/resource/resmgr/ps/positionstatement2020/Interim-20-ID-01_COVID-19_NO.pdf. Accessed February 13, 2023.
7. Patel A, Jernigan DB. Initial public health response and interim clinical guidance for the 2019 novel coronavirus outbreak—United States, December 31, 2019–February 4, 2020 [erratum in *MMWR Morb Mortal Wkly Rep*. 2020;69(6):173]. *MMWR Morb Mortal Wkly Rep*. 2020;69(5):140–146. https://doi.org/10.15585/mmwr.mm6905e1
8. Centers for Disease Control and Prevention. Washington State report first COVID-19 death. February 29, 2020. Available at: https://archive.cdc.gov/#/details?url=https://www.cdc.gov/media/releases/2020/s0229-COVID-19-first-death.html. Accessed June 22, 2024.
9. Murphy S, Kochanek K, Xu J, Arias E. Mortality in the United States, 2020. *NCHS Data Brief*. 2021;(427):1–8. https://doi.org/10.15620/cdc:112079
10. Centers for Disease Control and Prevention. *Information for Health Departments on Reporting Cases of COVID-19*. May 25, 2022. Available at: https://www.cdc.gov/coronavirus/2019-ncov/php/reporting-pui.html. Accessed February 23, 2023.
11. Council of State and Territorial Epidemiologists. *CSTE Revised COVID-19-Associated Death Classification Guidance for Public Health Surveillance Programs (Version 2)*. 2022. Available at: https://preparedness.cste.org/wp-content/uploads/2022/12/CSTE-Revised-Classification-of-COVID-19-associated-Deaths.Final_.11.22.22.pdf. Accessed April 18, 2023.
12. Council of State and Territorial Epidemiologists. *Update to the Standardized Surveillance Case Definition and National Notification for SARS-CoV-2 Infection (the Virus That Causes COVID-19)*. Available at: https://cdn.ymaws.com/www.cste.org/resource/resmgr/ps/ps2022/22-ID-01_COVID19.pdf. Accessed February 13, 2023.
13. Council of State and Territorial Epidemiologists. Public health agencies transitioning away from universal case investigation and contact tracing for individual cases of COVID-19. January 24, 2022. Available at: https://cdn.ymaws.com/www.cste.org/resource/resmgr/covid-19/4e509e47-08ec-4e93-a7be-f301.pdf. Accessed June 28, 2024.
14. Gold JAW, DeCuir J, Coyle JP, et al. COVID-19 case surveillance: trends in person-level case data completeness, United States, April 5–September 30, 2020. *Public Health Rep*. 2021;136(4):466–474. https://doi.org/10.1177/00333549211006973
15. Centers for Disease Control and Prevention. *COVID-19 Case Surveillance Restricted Access Detailed Data*. January 1, 2020–February 3, 2023. Available at: https://data.cdc.gov/Case-Surveillance/COVID-19-Case-Surveillance-Restricted-Access-Detai/mbd7-r32t. Accessed June 28, 2024.
16. Centers for Disease Control and Prevention. *COVID-19 Case Surveillance Public Use Data With Geography*. January 1, 2020–February 3, 2023. Available at: https://data.cdc.gov/Case-Surveillance/COVID-19-Case-Surveillance-Public-Use-Data-with-Ge/n8mc-b4w4. Accessed June 28, 2024.
17. Surveillance Review Response Group. *COVID-19 Case Surveillance Public Use Data*. January 1, 2020–February 3, 2023. Available at: https://data.cdc.gov/Case-Surveillance/COVID-19-Case-Surveillance-Public-Use-Data/vbim-akqf. Accessed June 28, 2024.
18. Silk BJ, Scobie H, Duck W, et al. COVID-19 surveillance after expiration of the public health emergency declaration—United States, May 11, 2023. *MMWR Morb Mortal Wkly Rep*. 2023;72(19):523–528. https://doi.org/10.15585/mmwr.mm7219e1
19. National Center for Health Statistics. *Provisional COVID-19 Death Counts, Rates, and Percent of Total Deaths, by Jurisdiction of Residence*. February 1, 2024. Available at: https://data.cdc.gov/NCHS/Provisional-COVID-19-death-counts-rates-and-percen/mpx5-t7tu/about_data. Accessed February 6, 2024.
20. Centers for Disease Control and Prevention. COVID-19 monthly death rates per 100,000 population by age group, race and ethnicity, and sex. January 16, 2024. Available at: https://covid.cdc.gov/covid-data-tracker/#demographicsovertime. Accessed February 6, 2024.
21. Khan D, Park MP, Burkholder J, et al. Tracking COVID-19 in the United States with surveillance of aggregate cases and deaths. *Public Health Rep*. 2023;138(3):428–437. https://doi.org/10.1177/00333549231163531
22. Centers for Disease Control and Prevention. Epi Info™ for Web and Cloud. Available at: https://www.cdc.gov/epiinfo/cloud.html. Accessed September 16, 2021.
23. Centers for Disease Control and Prevention. Weekly United States COVID-19 cases and deaths by county - ARCHIVED. June 22, 2023. Available at: https://data.cdc.gov/dataset/Weekly-United-States-COVID-19-Cases-and-Deaths-by-/yviw-z6j5. Accessed June 28, 2024.
24. Centers for Disease Control and Prevention. Weekly United States COVID-19 cases and deaths by state - ARCHIVED. June 1, 2023. Available at: https://data.cdc.gov/Case-Surveillance/Weekly-United-States-COVID-19-Cases-and-Deaths-by-/pwn4-m3yp. Accessed June 28, 2024.
25. National Center for Immunization and Respiratory Diseases. *COVID-19 Forecasts: Deaths* - ARCHIVED. Centers for Disease Control and Prevention. Available at: https://archive.cdc.gov/#/details?url=https://www.cdc.gov/coronavirus/2019-ncov/science/forecasting/forecasting-us.html. Accessed February 13, 2023.
26. National Center for Health Statistics. *Deaths by Week and State - Provisional Death Counts for COVID-19*. Centers for Disease Control and Prevention. July 11, 2023. Available at: https://www.cdc.gov/nchs/nvss/vsrr/COVID19/index.htm. Accessed July 11, 2023.
27. National Center for Health Statistics. *About the National Vital Statistics System*. Available at: https://www.cdc.gov/nchs/nvss/about_nvss.htm. Accessed February 13, 2023.
28. National Center for Health Statistics. *Guidance for Certifying Deaths Due to Coronavirus Disease 2019 (COVID-19). Vital Statistics Reporting Guidance*. Vol. 3. April 2020. Available at: https://www.cdc.gov/nchs/data/nvss/vsrg/vsrg03-508.pdf. Accessed February 13, 2023.
29. Ahmad FB, Anderson RN, Knight K, Rossen LM, Sutton PD. Advancements in the National Vital Statistics System to meet the real-time data needs of a pandemic. *Am J Public Health*. 2021;111(12):2133–2140. https://doi.org/10.2105/AJPH.2021.306519
30. National Center for Health Statistics. *COVID-19 Death Data and Resources*. September 14, 2021. Available at: https://www.cdc.gov/nchs/nvss/covid-19.htm. Accessed February 13, 2023.
31. National Center for Health Statistics. *Technical Notes - Provisional Death Counts for Coronavirus Disease (COVID-19)* - ARCHIVED. Available at: https://www.cdc.gov/nchs/nvss/vsrr/covid19/tech_notes.htm. Accessed February 13, 2023.
32. National Center for Health Statistics. *Provisional COVID-19 Deaths by Week, Sex, and Age* - ARCHIVED. Available at: https://data.cdc.gov/NCHS/Provisional-COVID-19-Deaths-by-Week-Sex-and-Age/vsak-wrfu. Accessed February 13, 2023.
33. National Center for Health Statistics. *Mortality Data on CDC WONDER*. Available at: https://wonder.cdc.gov/mcd.html. Accessed March 3, 2023.
34. National Center for Health Statistics. *Excess Deaths Associated With COVID-19* - ARCHIVED. Centers for Disease Control and Prevention. Available at: https://www.cdc.gov/nchs/nvss/vsrr/covid19/excess_deaths.htm. Accessed February 13, 2023.
35. German RR, Lee LM, Horan JM, Milstein RL, Pertowski CA, Waller MN; Guidelines Working Group Centers for Disease Control and Prevention. Updated guidelines for evaluating public health surveillance systems. *MMWR Recomm Rep*. 2001;50(RR-13):1–35.
36. Scobie H, Panaggio M, Binder A, et al. Correlations and timeliness of COVID-19 surveillance data sources and indicators—United States, October 1, 2020–March 22, 2023. *MMWR Morb Mortal Wkly Rep*. 2023;72(19):529–535. https://doi.org/10.15585/mmwr.mm7219e2
37. Rosenbaum JE, Stillo M, Graves N, Rivera R. Timeliness of provisional United States mortality data releases during the COVID-19 pandemic: delays associated with electronic death registration system and weekly mortality. *J Public Health Policy*. 2021;42(4):536–549. https://doi.org/10.1057/s41271-021-00309-7
38. Zhang G, Rose CE, Zhang Y, et al. Multiple imputation of missing race and ethnicity in CDC COVID-19 case-level surveillance data. *Int J Stat Med Res*. 2022;11:1–11. https://doi.org/10.6000/1929-6029.2022.11.01
39. Arias E, Heron M, Hakes J. The validity of race and Hispanic-origin reporting on death certificates in the United States: an update. *Vital Health Stat 2*. 2016;(172):1–21.

Trends in Drug Overdose Deaths by Intent and Drug Categories, United States, 1999–2022

Anallely Nguyen, MPH, Jing Wang, MD, MPH, Kristin M. Holland, PhD, MPH, Daniel C. Ehlman, ScD, MPH, Laura E. Welder, DrPH, MPH, Kimberly D. Miller, MPH, and Deborah M. Stone, ScD, MSW, MPH

See also Bohnert and Sen, p. 966.

Objectives. To examine trends in overdose deaths by intent and drug category to better understand the recent decrease in overdose suicides amid the overdose epidemic.

Methods. We examined trends in rates of overdose deaths by intent (unintentional, suicide, or undetermined) across 9 drug categories from 1999 to 2022 using US National Vital Statistics System mortality data.

Results. Unintentional overdoses involving synthetic opioids, polydrug toxicity involving synthetic opioids, psychostimulants, and cocaine increased exponentially with annual percentage changes ranging from 15.0% to 104.9% during 2010 to 2022. The death rates also increased for suicides involving these drugs, especially for psychostimulants (annual percentage change = 12.9% for 2010–2022; $P < .001$). However, these drugs accounted for relatively small percentages of overdose suicides. The leading drug categories among suicides were antidepressants, prescription opioids, and benzodiazepines, though these deaths have decreased or leveled off in recent years.

Conclusions. Different drugs commonly involved in suicides and unintentional overdoses may contribute to their divergent trends.

Public Health Implications. Amid the overdose epidemic, safe storage of medications remains a crucial strategy to prevent overdose suicides. The large increases in suicides involving psychostimulants warrant monitoring. (*Am J Public Health*. 2024;114(10):1081–1085. https://doi.org/10.2105/AJPH.2024.307745)

AJPH October 2024, Vol. 114, No. 10

The rates of unintentional drug overdose deaths increased 7.5-fold from 2001 to 2022.[1] Meanwhile, the rates for overdose suicides have been decreasing since the mid-2010s.[2] Given that unintentional overdose and suicide share many risk factors,[3] more concordant trends between the 2 outcomes may be anticipated. One plausible explanation for the discrepant trends may be the misclassification of suicides. This misclassification differs across demographic groups and jurisdictions because of factors including the frequent absence of suicide notes and psychiatric histories,[4] diverse practice and training between medical examiners and coroners, variations in scene investigation, presence and completeness of toxicology testing, legal concerns, stigma associated with suicide as a manner of death, and limited resources.[5]

In light of these challenges, it remains of significant public health interest to understand the burden of suicides during the overdose epidemic for prevention efforts.[6] Thus, we analyzed the trends in overdose deaths stratified by intent across drug categories, aiming to reveal where discrepant patterns exist and provide insights into the recent decrease in overdose suicides.

METHODS

Drug overdose deaths were identified from National Vital Statistics System multiple cause of death data for 1999 to 2022 (2022 data were provisional).[1] We determined the intent for overdose deaths by using the *International Classification of*

Disease, 10th Revision (*ICD-10*; Geneva, Switzerland: World Health Organization; 2004) as X40–X44 (unintentional), X60–X64 (suicide), and Y10–Y14 (undetermined). We excluded homicides. We used *ICD-10* codes to identify the involved drug categories (synthetic opioids excluding methadone, heroin, prescription opioids [i.e., natural or semisynthetic opioids or methadone], psychostimulants with abuse potential, cocaine, benzodiazepines, and antidepressants; Figure A, available as a supplement to the online version of this article at https://ajph.org). Given the recently increasing co-involvement of synthetic opioids with other drugs,[7] we defined a "polydrug toxicity involving synthetic opioids" category as co-listing synthetic opioids with any of the aforementioned drugs. Drug categories selected were identified as fueling the 3 waves of overdose epidemic or being frequently co-involved with synthetic opioids.[7,8] Lastly, other overdose deaths not included explicitly in listed drug categories were classified as involving "miscellaneous" drugs (e.g., sedative-hypnotic drugs, antipsychotics, and neuroleptics). All defined drug categories, except for miscellaneous drugs, were not mutually exclusive, and cases involving multiple drug categories were counted in each.

Detailed methods for the calculation of age-adjusted rates are provided in Table A (available as a supplement to the online version of this article at https://ajph.org). We assessed trends in age-adjusted rates for drug overdose deaths by intent and drug categories using Joinpoint regression software (version 4.9.1.0; National Cancer Institute, Bethesda, MD). We considered a 2-sided $P < .05$ statistically significant. We restricted trend analyses involving psychostimulants to 2010 to 2022 because of small counts before 2010. The results for undetermined overdoses are presented (Table B, available as a supplement to the online version of this article at https://ajph.org) but not described. As a sensitivity analysis to partially justify underreporting of suicide intent, we examined the suicide trends with undetermined overdoses included.

RESULTS

Drug overdose deaths, excluding homicides, increased from 16 809 in 1999 to 106 850 in 2022. Compared with unintentional overdoses, suicides had more older adults (> 65 years), females, and non-Hispanic Whites (Table C, available as a supplement to the online version of this article at https://ajph.org). Synthetic opioids, polydrug toxicity involving synthetic opioids, psychostimulants, and cocaine were predominant categories of unintentional overdoses, accounting for 71.2%, 47.6%, 33.2%, and 26.7% of cases, respectively, in 2022 (Figure B, available as a supplement to the online version of this article at https://ajph.org). However, these 4 drug categories were uncommon among overdose suicides, each accounting for less than 15% in both 1999 and 2022. Of note, polydrug toxicity involving synthetic opioids was generally rare (< 3%) in 1999 but exponentially increased to 47.6% for unintentional overdoses and to 9.6% for suicides in 2022. In contrast, antidepressants, prescription opioids, benzodiazepines, and miscellaneous drugs were the top drug categories involved in suicides, accounting for 30.6%, 21.0%, 19.6%, and 36.9%, respectively, in 2022.

Overall, unintentional overdose death rates increased 12.2% annually from 1999 to 2006, stabilized through 2013, and resumed a 12.1% annual increase from 2013 to 2022 (Table B; Figure C, available as supplements to the online version of this article at https://ajph.org). Overdose suicide rates increased 3.7% annually from 1999 to 2008, stabilized through 2014, and then decreased 4.3% annually thereafter until leveling off in 2020 to 2022. In sensitivity analyses, when undetermined overdoses were included in suicides, the trend still showed a decrease from 2003 to 2022.

Death rates for unintentional overdoses involving synthetic opioids, polydrug toxicity involving synthetic opioids, psychostimulants, and cocaine steeply increased in recent years (annual percentage changes [APCs] ranged from 15.0% [for cocaine in 2017–2022] to 104.9% [for polydrug toxicity involving synthetic opioids in 2013–2016]; Figure 1; Table B). Rates of unintentional overdose for all other drug categories increased until the late 2000s, then either increased at a slower pace (prescription opioids, antidepressants, and benzodiazepines) or decreased (miscellaneous drugs).

Among overdose suicides, the rates increased for those involving synthetic opioids (1999–2022: APC = 3.5%) and polydrug toxicity involving synthetic opioids (1999–2022: APC = 6.7%; Figure 1; Table B). The rates also increased notably for suicides involving psychostimulants (2010–2022: APC = 12.9%) and cocaine (2013–2022: APC = 9.1%). Conversely, rates decreased in recent years for suicides involving benzodiazepines (2017–2022: APC = −5.2%), prescription opioids (2016–2022: APC = −7.5%), and miscellaneous drugs (2012–2020: APC = −7.3%) and leveled off for suicides involving antidepressants from 2015 to 2022.

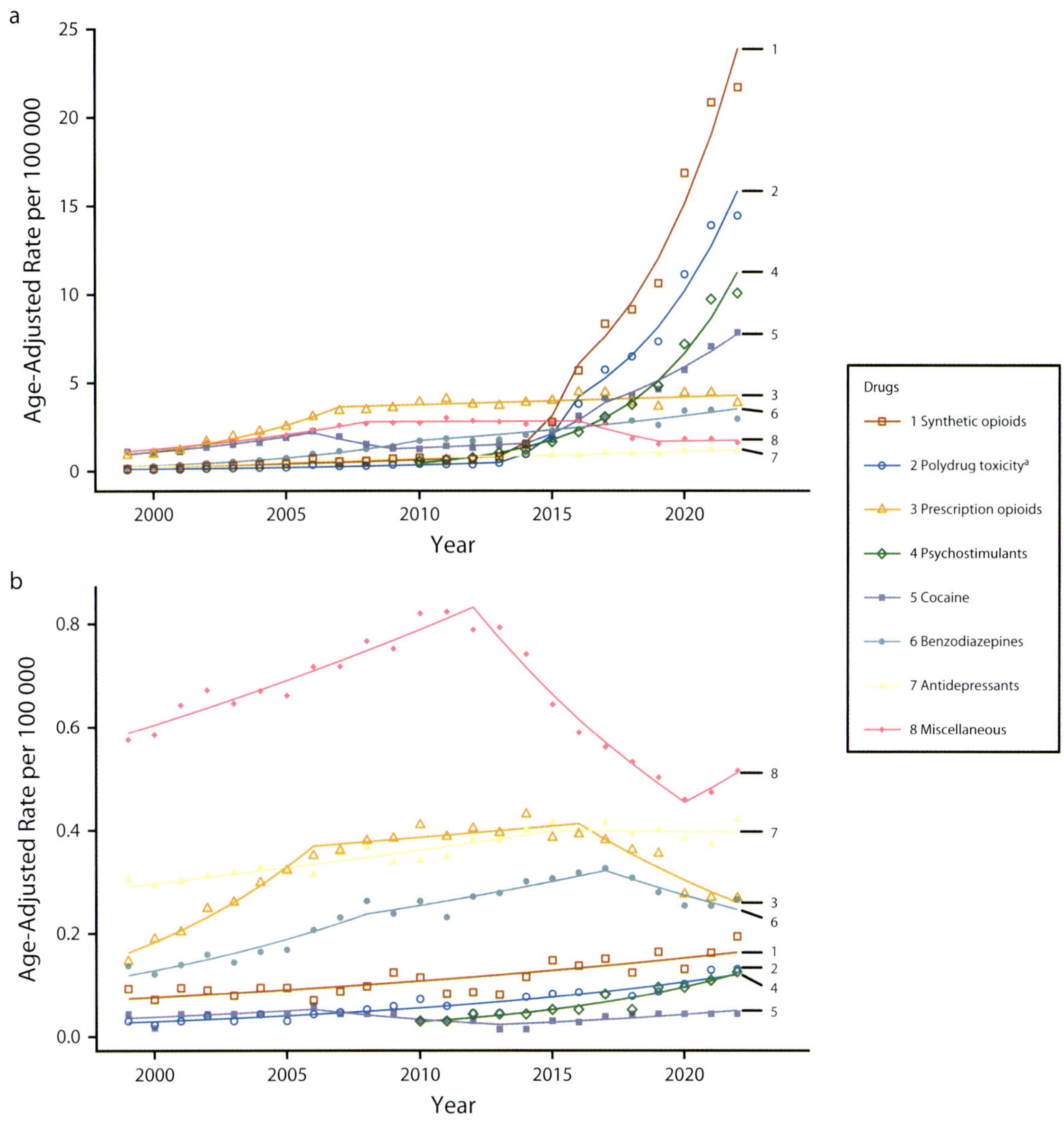

FIGURE 1— Trends in the Age-Adjusted Rates (per 100 000 Persons) for Drug Overdose Deaths by Drug Categories and by (a) Unintentional and (b) Suicide: United States, 1999–2022

Note. The dots indicate observed rates, and the lines indicate modeled rates from Joinpoint regression software (version 4.9.1.0; National Cancer Institute, Bethesda, MD). Scales are different by chart. Because of small counts, the trends were not examined for suicides involving heroin or undetermined overdoses involving polydrug toxicity involving synthetic opioids, and the trends for overdoses involving psychostimulants were only assessed for 2010 to 2022. All drug categories, except for miscellaneous drugs, were not mutually exclusive. Each drug category indicated the involvement of the specified drug; however, other drugs could also have been involved.

Source. National Vital Statistics System mortality data queried via CDC WONDER (https://wonder.cdc.gov). The 2022 data were provisional as of July 13, 2023, when the data were downloaded. As a sensitivity analysis, we analyzed the data up to 2021 and found minimum changes in the trends.

[a]Polydrug toxicity refers to polydrug toxicity involving synthetic opioids.

DISCUSSION

Between 1999 and 2022, increasing trends were observed for suicides involving synthetic opioids, polydrug toxicity involving synthetic opioids, psychostimulants, and cocaine, although to a lesser extent compared with the corresponding trends for unintentional overdose deaths. However, because these drugs were not commonly involved in suicides, these increases did not noticeably affect the trend for overall overdose suicides. Conversely, upward trends for overdoses involving benzodiazepines, antidepressants, prescription opioids, and miscellaneous drugs have slowed for unintentional overdoses and leveled off or decreased for suicides in recent years. Because these drugs had been commonly involved in suicides, their decreases may have driven the reduction in overall overdose suicide rates.

Historically, approximately 10% to 30% of overdose suicides have been estimated to be misclassified as unintentional or undetermined deaths.[5] With recent rapid increases in overdose deaths involving synthetic opioids, limited resources for investigating deaths may exacerbate underreporting of suicides. As a sensitivity analysis, we included undetermined overdoses in suicides and still found a decreasing trend in recent years. Yet, true overdose suicide trends remain uncertain without accounting for suicides hidden in unintentional overdoses, calling for effective strategies including continued training and standardization of death investigation in addressing the misclassification issue.[5]

The current phase of the opioid epidemic primarily involves synthetic opioids, particularly illicitly manufactured fentanyl.[8] However, our findings showed that this drug category was not documented as commonly used in suicides. While this pattern may partly stem from underreporting, individuals might opt to use prescription medications they already possess for suicide. Therefore, the recent steep rise in unintentional overdose deaths fueled by illicit opioids may not be equally seen in overdose suicides.

The noticeable increase in suicides involving psychostimulants or cocaine, albeit at low rates, suggest an emerging pattern that requires continued monitoring. Particularly, methamphetamine use has been on the rise, with approximately 2.5 million Americans reporting use in 2021.[9]

Our study limitations include the increased listing of specific drugs for overdose deaths as toxicology testing improved over time,[10] We did not classify drugs in mutually exclusive categories, yet assessing the overall involvement of a drug is an essential step.

PUBLIC HEALTH IMPLICATIONS

Different drug involvements for suicides and unintentional overdoses underscore the safe storage of prescription medications as a critical downstream strategy for suicide prevention. A comprehensive public health approach to addressing upstream shared risk factors for suicide and substance use may include ensuring access to mental health services, strengthening economic supports, and teaching coping and problem-solving skills.[11] AJPH

ABOUT THE AUTHORS

Anallely Nguyen, Jing Wang, Daniel C. Ehlman, and Deborah M. Stone are with the Division of Injury Prevention, National Center for Injury Prevention and Control, Centers for Disease Control and Prevention (CDC), Atlanta, GA. Kristin M. Holland is with the Division of Violence Prevention, National Center for Injury Prevention and Control, CDC. Laura E. Welder and Kimberly D. Miller are with the Division of Overdose Prevention, National Center for Injury Prevention and Control, CDC.

Note. The findings and conclusions in this report are those of the authors and do not necessarily represent the official position of the CDC.

CORRESPONDENCE

Correspondence should be sent to Jing Wang, MD, MPH, Division of Injury Prevention, National Center for Injury Prevention and Control, Centers for Disease Control and Prevention, 4770 Buford Hwy NE, S106-9, Atlanta, GA 30341-3724 (e-mail: zrr4@cdc.gov). Reprints can be ordered at https://www.ajph.org by clicking the "Reprints" link.

PUBLICATION INFORMATION

Full Citation: Nguyen A, Wang J, Holland KM, et al. Trends in drug overdose deaths by intent and drug categories, United States, 1999–2022. *Am J Public Health*. 2024;114(10):1081–1085.

Acceptance Date: May 24, 2024.

DOI: https://doi.org/10.2105/AJPH.2024.307745

CONTRIBUTORS

D. M. Stone, J. Wang, and K. M. Holland contributed to the concept and design. A. Nguyen, J. Wang, D. C. Ehlman, and K. Miller contributed to the acquisition, analysis, or interpretation of data. A. Nguyen, J. Wang, and D. M. Stone drafted the article. J. Wang, K. M. Holland, D. C. Ehlman, L. E. Welder, K. Miller, and D. M. Stone critically revised the article for important intellectual content. A. Nguyen, J. Wang, and K. Miller performed the statistical analysis. D. M. Stone provided supervision.

CONFLICTS OF INTEREST

The authors have no known competing financial interests or personal relationships that could have appeared to influence the work reported in this brief.

HUMAN PARTICIPANT PROTECTION

This study used de-identified publicly available data and was exempt from an institutional review board review.

REFERENCES

1. Centers for Disease Control and Prevention, National Center for Health Statistics. National Vital Statistics System, provisional mortality on CDC WONDER online database. Available at: https://wonder.cdc.gov. Accessed June 13, 2023.
2. Han B, Compton WM, Einstein EB, et al. Intentional drug overdose deaths in the United States. *Am J Psychiatry*. 2022;179(2):163–165. https://doi.org/10.1176/appi.ajp.2021.21060604
3. Bohnert ASB, Ilgen MA. Understanding links among opioid use, overdose, and suicide. *N Engl J Med*. 2019;380(1):71–79. https://doi.org/10.1056/NEJMra1802148
4. Rockett IRH, Caine ED, Connery HS, et al. Discerning suicide in drug intoxication deaths: paucity and primacy of suicide notes and psychiatric history. *PLoS One*. 2018;13(1):e0190200. https://doi.org/10.1371/journal.pone.0190200
5. Stone DM, Holland KM, Bartholow B, et al. Deciphering suicide and other manners of death associated with drug intoxication: a Centers for Disease Control and Prevention consultation meeting summary. *Am J Public Health*. 2017;107(8):1233–1239. https://doi.org/10.2105/AJPH.2017.303863

6. Oquendo MA, Volkow ND. Suicide: a silent contributor to opioid-overdose deaths. *N Engl J Med*. 2018;378(17):1567–1569. https://doi.org/10.1056/NEJMp1801417
7. Jones CM, Einstein EB, Compton WM. Changes in synthetic opioid involvement in drug overdose deaths in the United States, 2010–2016. *JAMA*. 2018;319(17):1819–1821. https://doi.org/10.1001/jama.2018.2844
8. Ciccarone D. The triple wave epidemic: supply and demand drivers of the US opioid overdose crisis. *Int J Drug Policy*. 2019;71:183–188. https://doi.org/10.1016/j.drugpo.2019.01.010
9. Substance Abuse and Mental Health Services Administration. *Key Substance Use and Mental Health Indicators in the United States: Results From the 2021 National Survey on Drug Use and Health* (HHS Publication No. PEP22-07-01-005, NSDUH Series H-57). Center for Behavioral Health Statistics and Quality. 2022. Available at: https://www.samhsa.gov/data/report/2021-nsduh-annual-national-report. Accessed July 13, 2023.
10. Hedegaard HMA, Warner M. Drug overdose deaths in the United States, 1999–2019. *NCHS Data Brief, no* 394. Hyattsville, MD: National Center for Health Statistics; 2020.
11. *Suicide Prevention Resource for Action. A Compilation of the Best Available Evidence.* Atlanta, GA: National Center for Injury Prevention and Control, Centers for Disease Control and Prevention; 2022.

The War on Drugs, Racialized Capitalism, and Health Care Utilization Among White People Who Use Drugs in 22 Rural Appalachian Counties

Hannah L. F. Cooper, ScD, Melvin "Douglas" Livingston, PhD, Natalie D. Crawford, PhD, Judith Feinberg, MD, Chandra L. Ford, PhD, Vivian Go, PhD, Umed Ibragimov, PhD, Tasfia Jahangir, MPH, Anna Mullany, PhD, William C. Miller, PhD, Snigdha Peddireddy, MPH, Leslie Salas-Hernandez, PhD, Gordon Smith, PhD, April M. Young, PhD, William Zule, PhD, and Ali Sewell, PhD

AJPH October 2024, Vol. 114, No. 10

Objectives. To analyze War on Drugs encounters and their relationships to health care utilization among White people who use drugs (PWUD) in 22 Appalachian rural counties in Kentucky, West Virginia, Ohio, and North Carolina.

Methods. We recruited White PWUD using chain referral sampling in 2018 to 2020. Surveys asked about criminal–legal encounters, unmet health care needs, and other covariates. We used generalized estimating equations to regress unmet need on criminal–legal encounters in multivariable models.

Results. In this sample (n = 957), rates of stop and search, arrest, incarceration, and community supervision were high (44.0%, 26.8%, 36.3%, and 31.1%, respectively), as was unmet need (68.5%). Criminal–legal encounters were unrelated to unmet need (stops: adjusted prevalence ratio [APR] = 1.13; 95% confidence interval [CI] = 0.97, 1.32; arrest: APR = 0.95; 95% CI = 0.78, 1.15; incarceration: APR = 1.01; 95% CI = 0.89, 1.14; community supervision: APR = 0.99; 95% CI = 0.90, 1.09).

Conclusions. Contrasting with findings from predominantly Black urban areas, criminal–legal encounters and unmet need were unrelated among White Appalachian PWUD. Research should explore whether and under what conditions White supremacy's benefits might buffer adverse impacts of the War on Drugs in Appalachia. (*Am J Public Health*. 2024;114(10):1086–1096. https://doi.org/10.2105/AJPH.2024.307744)

The United States is experiencing a shift in a potent driver of racialized capitalism: the domestic War on Drugs is expanding from predominantly Black urban neighborhoods into rural areas,[1] including majority White Appalachian counties.[2] This expansion is striking: President Richard Nixon launched the War on Drugs as a form of anti-Black structural discrimination designed to bolster racialized capitalism in the wake of midcentury mobilizations for racial and economic justice.[3,4] Subsequently, relentless drug-related stops and frisks, mass incarceration, and community supervision have become essential strategies to perpetuate this system in urban, impoverished, predominantly Black neighborhoods.[3,4] Guided by racial justice lenses, decades of public health studies analyzing the consequences of this war in US cities have consistently found adverse health and health care impacts.[5–7] Black, Indigenous, and Latine/x people and other People of Color (BILPOC) who use drugs are targeted and suffer acutely.[3,4,8–11] Their utilization of essential health care services is particularly damaged.[3]

We followed the expanding War on Drugs into 22 rural, impoverished Appalachian counties in 4 states (Kentucky, West Virginia, Ohio, and North Carolina) to learn whether its effects on White people who use drugs (PWUD) in these counties parallel its effects among PWUD in the predominantly Black urban neighborhoods where it started. Rural Appalachia bears high rates of drug-related harms, including overdoses, hepatitis C virus (HCV) infection, and neonatal opioid withdrawal syndrome.[12–14] At issue here is whether the War on Drugs escalates these harms in these predominately White rural Appalachian areas.

We dedicate the remainder of this introductory section to considering the War on Drugs in Appalachia as part of the US racialized capitalist system and its ongoing construction of Whiteness. Current equity work tends to narrowly consider racialized capitalism as a determinant of BILPOC health alone. By melding racialized capitalism with critical Whiteness studies, we sought to support progress in research and interventions that comprehensively consider its role in shaping White health. Racialized capitalism establishes and reinforces the highly differentiated racialized and racializing landscapes required to maximize White profit, landscapes that are sharpened along intersecting hierarchies of labor–owner, rural–urban, gender, and other dimensions of social position.[15–18] Integrating this framework with critical Whiteness studies supports analyses of how Whiteness evolves to bolster, and benefit from, this system.[19–21]

LEGACIES OF CRIMINAL–LEGAL INITIATIVES

As in impoverished urban Black communities, criminal–legal terrorism targeting working-class White communities in rural Appalachia has been integral to the construction of race and class in the region for centuries.[22,23] The nature of this terrorism, however, has differed across these 2 communities because the racial groups and economic classes forged have differed.

Criminal–legal strategies have been deployed in rural Appalachian counties when White working-class people have challenged their position in racialized capitalism. The first such deployment was the Whiskey Rebellion (1794), in which White Appalachians rioted against Secretary of the Treasury Alexander Hamilton's whiskey tax. The region's barter economy threatened capitalism in the new republic: currency is a precondition for capital accumulation because it separates value from labor.[24] To bring Appalachia into capitalism's orbit, Hamilton demanded that Appalachians pay this tax in dollars.[24] When White Appalachians rioted, President George Washington deployed 12 000 troops to enforce the tax.

The Coal Wars (1890–1930) were the second deployment. These conflicts were waged sporadically when miners struck repeatedly to keep greater shares of the profits they generated.[25] Consequent deployments of law enforcement and armed forces sometimes precipitated brutal battles: in the 1921 Battle of Blair Mountain, for example, 3000 law enforcement officers joined with the National Guard to quash an uprising of 10 000 people, killing 100 Appalachians.

These Appalachian deployments sharply contrast with criminal–legal deployments against impoverished Black communities. A defining feature of race and class for impoverished Black people in the United States has been standing cycles of saturating state criminal–legal terrorism.[3,4,26] Deployed even without instigation, these deployments form an unbroken chain of state-sponsored structural violence to criminalize Black bodies and control segregated places where Black people live.[3,4,26] Deployments against Appalachian Whites, by contrast, have been rare, time-limited, and precise: troops and law enforcement withdrew when the Whiskey Rebellion and mining strikes ended.

Moreover, deployments against White Appalachians occurred in a broader context where Whiteness continued to yield benefits and may have buffered these deployments' harms. During the United States's early years, for example, Whiteness manifested as the power to expropriate land from Native nations and, for landowning men, to vote.[20,21] White Appalachians circa the time of the Whiskey Rebellion were actively seizing Native lands; White Appalachian men used this colonized land to secure enfranchisement. Appalachian Whites likewise maintained their racial position during the Coal Wars: although these conflicts unfolded in an era spanning Black Codes, lynchings, and ongoing violent expropriation of Indigenous land and Black labor,[3,4,26] White Appalachians could raise families where they chose, and White men could vote, earn wages, and travel freely.

SACRIFICE ZONES OF ORGANIZED ABANDONMENT

The present-day expansion of the War on Drugs into Appalachia hews to this pattern of deploying criminal–legal interventions targeting Whites to protect racialized capitalism, while still allowing them to benefit from White supremacy.

Over the past decades, rural Appalachian counties have evolved into "sacrifice zones of organized abandonment," characterized by (1) a descent from productive, essential engines of the US economy to its exhausted, peripheral remnants; (2) economic immiseration; and (3) environmental degradation.[16,18,27] For centuries, rural Appalachia was heralded as essential to US urbanization and industrialization: its salt mines preserved the food that sustained workers in emerging cities, and its timber and coal fueled US factories.[24,28,29]

Its resources, however, have been exhausted through centuries of extraction or rendered peripheral as factories migrated overseas. Resource extraction precipitated ecologic devastation in the form of routine "100-year floods" and contaminated land and water. Debt payments are primary ways residents of sacrifice zones participate in the 21st-century economy, and debt burdens are far higher in rural Appalachia than elsewhere in the United States.[30] Economic immiseration is also evident in the median regional household income, which is 69.2% that of the US average.

War on Drugs strategies are exquisitely suited to controlling residents of sacrifice zones and other restive regions, whether in the places they originated or elsewhere.[3] Drug-related policing, for example, must be highly proactive to detect street-level drug activity, because people possessing, purchasing, or selling illegalized substances are unlikely to report themselves to the police.[3] For example, police stops for drug-related offenses must involve highly invasive searches to locate the small quantities of drugs that are typically involved.[3] Consequent mass incarceration removes parents, friends, and neighbors from families and communities.[3] Proactive, invasive policing and mass incarceration, in turn, dismantle the individual, family, and community resources that could facilitate resident mobilization.[3]

Appalachian incarceration rates testify to the burgeoning War on Drugs in this sacrifice zone. To illustrate, in 12 predominantly White impoverished Appalachian Kentucky counties at the heart of the opioid epidemic, jail-based incarceration rates—calculated using incarcerated peoples' home addresses—surged 588% between 1980 (when coal mining started to flag) and 2006 and have remained relatively stable ever since.[2] Strikingly, these incarceration rates surpassed those in the 12 most populous urban counties in the United States in 2000 and by 2013 were 138% higher.[2]

Notably, although War on Drugs strategies may be more saturating and sustained than previous criminal–legal deployments targeting White Appalachians, they still follow historical patterns by unfolding alongside efforts to bolster White supremacy in the region. Even as the local War on Drugs raged, for example, President Donald Trump repeatedly promised to restore Appalachian centrality in the US economy by reviving mining and supported violence in the region to advance White supremacy.[31,32]

At issue here is whether the expansion of War on Drugs strategies into rural Appalachian sacrifice zones adversely affects health care engagement among White PWUD, as has been found previously among BILPOC urban PWUD. Engagement in health care is essential to PWUD's survival, given high rates of drug-related harms.[3] Appalachian rural PWUD confront multiple barriers to engaging in this essential care, including health care provider shortages, providers' antidrug stigma, and travel challenges.[33,34] We analyzed whether stops and searches, arrests, incarceration, and community supervision forms another barrier that escalates the unmet need for medical care among White PWUD in the region.

METHODS

We performed a cross-sectional analysis of data that we gathered through the Rural Opioid Initiative. The Rural Opioid Initiative is a federally funded multisite collaborative designed, in part, to describe the patterns and impacts of drug-related epidemics across 8 rural US communities. Public state universities with decades-long presences in the region were the lead universities at the sites; local community advisory boards guided the sites. Methods were harmonized across sites. We collected data from 2018 through March 2020.

Sample

Eligibility criteria were (1) using opioids or injecting any drug to "get high" in the past 30 days, (2) being aged 18 years or older, and (3) residing in a county participating in the Rural Opioid Initiative. We further restricted the analytic sample to participants recruited at any 1 of the initiatives' 4 Appalachian sites, as defined by the Appalachian Regional Commission (i.e., Kentucky, West Virginia, Ohio, and North Carolina); Appalachian sites spanned 22 counties. Participation rates (i.e., the percentage of eligible people who participated) for these 4 sites ranged from 93% to 100%. We further restricted the sample to non-Hispanic White PWUD (88% of the original Appalachian sample).

We recruited individuals using chain referral sampling. We recruited seeds through harm reduction programs, other community-based programs, and previous studies. Participants could recruit up to 3 peers (incentives varied across sites from $10 to $20 for each eligible individual recruited).

Data Collection

A harmonized survey was administered by trained local interviewers or audio computer-assisted self-interview. Participants completed surveys in 90 minutes or less (incentives varied across sites from $20 to $45).

Measures

We measured "unmet need for medical care" in the past 6 months using 12 indicators asking why a participant did not seek necessary care (Table 1); we coded participants endorsing any of the 12 items as experiencing an unmet need for health care.

The 4 focal exposures were past 6-month experiences of being (1) stopped and searched by law enforcement, (2) arrested, (3) incarcerated in a jail or prison, or (4) on probation, parole, supervised release, or another form of community supervision. Measures were binary.

Control covariates were informed by the Behavioral Model of Healthcare Utilization for Vulnerable Populations.[35] Domains included need (e.g., HCV diagnosis, recent substance use) and factors that predispose an individual to health care utilization (e.g., age, educational attainment, gender) or enable it (e.g., health insurance, distance to a syringe service program; Table 1).

Analyses

We applied Poisson models with log-link and robust SEs to estimate

TABLE 1— Characteristics of the 957 White Participants Who Used Drugs in the Rural Opioid Initiative's Appalachian Sample: Kentucky, West Virginia, Ohio, North Carolina, 2018–2020

Variable	No. (%) or Mean ±SD
Outcome	
Unmet need for medical care[a]	638 (68.5)
Unable to pay	256 (28.5)
Unsure where to get care	119 (13.2)
Lacked transportation	287 (31.4)
Inconvenient clinic hours	117 (13.1)
Treated poorly in the past	195 (21.1)
Did not want to be seen at clinic	167 (18.3)
Did not trust doctors	168 (18.5)
Did not care about taking care of self	187 (20.8)
Did not have childcare	76 (8.3)
Too drunk or high	252 (27.1)
Feared mistreatment	380 (41.1)
Treated myself or by another	282 (30.7)
Criminal–legal encounters[b]	
Stop and search	420 (44.0)
Arrest	255 (26.8)
Incarceration	347 (36.3)
Community supervision[b]	294 (31.1)
Predisposing covariates	
Age, y	37.2 ±0.5
Education	
<high school	251 (26.3)
High school or general equivalency diploma	438 (45.8)
Some college	191 (20.0)
Associate's degree or higher	76 (7.9)
Gender	
Male	524 (54.8)
Female	433 (45.2)
Experienced houselessness[a]	399 (41.9)
Employed full-time	170 (17.8)
Sold sex for money[a]	20 (2.1)
Sold drugs for money[a]	201 (21.0)
Has cell phone with active service	588 (61.8)
Frequency of Internet use[c]	
Never	103 (10.8)
Several times a month	117 (12.2)
Several times a week	74 (7.7)
About once a day	164 (17.2)
Several times a day	498 (52.1)
Enabling covariates	
Has health insurance	683 (72.9)

Continued

TABLE 1— Continued

Variable	No. (%) or Mean ±SD
Distance to SSP from residence	
Within walking distance	252 (32.5)
< 30-min drive	356 (45.9)
30–60-min drive	96 (12.4)
> 60-min drive	32 (4.1)
No SSP within reasonable distance	39 (5.0)
SUD treatment[a,d]	387 (40.5)
Needs covariates	
Positive HCV diagnosis	419 (44.0)
Prescription opioid misuse[c]	566 (59.5)
MOUD treatment misuse[c,d]	523 (55.0)
Illicit opioid use[d]	666 (70.8)
Stimulant use[d]	792 (82.8)
Injection drug use frequency[c]	
Never	192 (20.1)
Weekly or less	144 (15.1)
More than weekly	66 (6.9)
Daily	182 (19.0)
More than once daily	372 (38.9)
Study site	
Kentucky	330 (34.5)
North Carolina	242 (25.3)
Ohio	231 (24.1)
West Virginia	154 (16.1)

Note. HCV = hepatitis C virus; MOUD = medications for opioid use disorder; SSP = syringe service program; SUD = substance use disorder.
[a]Within past 6 months.
[b]Includes probation, parole, supervised release, or other forms of community supervision.
[c]Within past 30 days.
[d]Includes outpatient counseling, inpatient or residential treatment, oral buprenorphine or injections, methadone maintenance treatment, or naltrexone injections.

unadjusted and adjusted relationships between criminal–legal encounter variables and overall unmet need for care and to estimate relationships between criminal–legal encounter measures and each of the 12 items making up the unmet need variable. The latter step allowed us to learn whether associations varied according to the specific reason for unmet need. Seeds functioned as the clustering unit.

We used prevalence ratios (PRs) when overall unmet need was an outcome because of its high prevalence. Multivariable models controlled for study site as a fixed effect (i.e., Kentucky, Ohio, North Carolina, West Virginia) as well as other covariates (e.g., age, educational attainment, gender, HCV diagnosis, recent substance use, health insurance). We reran multivariable models excluding variables that might lie in the causal pathways (i.e., health insurance, housing status, injection frequency, HCV status, substance use disorder treatment, employment status). We estimated all models as generalized estimating equations assuming exchangeability by referral chain using PROC GENMOD in SAS version 9.4 (SAS Institute, Cary, NC). Variance inflation factor values testing multicolinearity across criminal–legal variables ranged from 1.13 to 2.95, which is below standard cutpoints, and so we entered all 4 variables as independent variables into multivariable models.

To account for missing data, we used multiple imputation by chained equations with 20 imputations in all unadjusted and adjusted models. All imputation models included the unmet need outcome, all criminal–legal exposures, and all modeled covariates. We used multiple imputation via chained equations to model variables on their natural scale and to avoid the assumption of joint normality.

We complemented data on individual PWUD with descriptive statistics about the 22 counties where participants lived. We drew variables from the American Community Survey, the Vera Institute of Justice, and the Federal Reserve.

RESULTS

According to administrative data on the 22 counties we studied, a median of 92.7% of residents were non-Hispanic White (25th percentile = 89.6%; 75th percentile = 95.7%; Table A, available as a supplement to the online version of this article at http://www.ajph.org). Aligned with sacrifice zones, the median poverty rate was 18.7% (25th percentile = 16.7%; 75th percentile = 22.7%), far exceeding the national poverty rate of 11.6%. The median debt to income ratio was 1.84 (25th percentile = 1.3; 75th percentile = 2.4), exceeding the national ratio of 1.45. Beginning approximately a decade before data collection, rates of jail- and prison-based incarceration in these 22 rural Appalachian counties surpassed rates in the 22 most populous urban counties (Figure 1).

Survey participants (n = 957; 291 clusters) who lived in these counties were aged 37 years on average (SD = 0.5; Table 1), and more than half were male (54.8%; n = 524). Participants were deeply impoverished: 41.9% were unhoused in the past 6 months.

The majority (68.5%) reported at least 1 instance of unmet need for health care (Table 1). The most commonly cited reason was fear of disrespectful treatment by providers (41.1%), followed by lack of transportation (31.4%) and being cared for by self or another layperson (30.7%). There were no differences in the overall measure of unmet need across predisposing characteristics (e.g., gender, educational attainment), but people who were unhoused had higher rates of unmet need (76.1% vs 61.9%; $P < .001$; Table 2. Two enabling characteristics mattered: people who lived within a 30-minute drive to a syringe service program reported the lowest prevalence of unmet need for care, as did insured participants. Multiple factors in the need category were positively associated with this outcome, including using stimulants, prescription opioids, and illicit opioids.

Almost half (44.0%) of the participants reported being stopped by police; 26.8% reported being arrested; 36.3% reporting being incarcerated in a jail or prison; and 31.1% reported some form of supervised release (Table 1). Men were more likely than were women to be arrested (29.6% vs 23.6%, respectively; $P = .03$), incarcerated (40.8% vs 30.8%, respectively; $P < .001$), or on community supervision (35.5% vs 25.7%, respectively; $P < .001$; Table B, available as a supplement to the online version of this article at http://www.ajph.org). The prevalence of all criminal–legal encounters except community supervision were higher among recently unhoused participants.

Unadjusted regression models showed statistically significant positive relationships between the overall measure of unmet need and being stopped

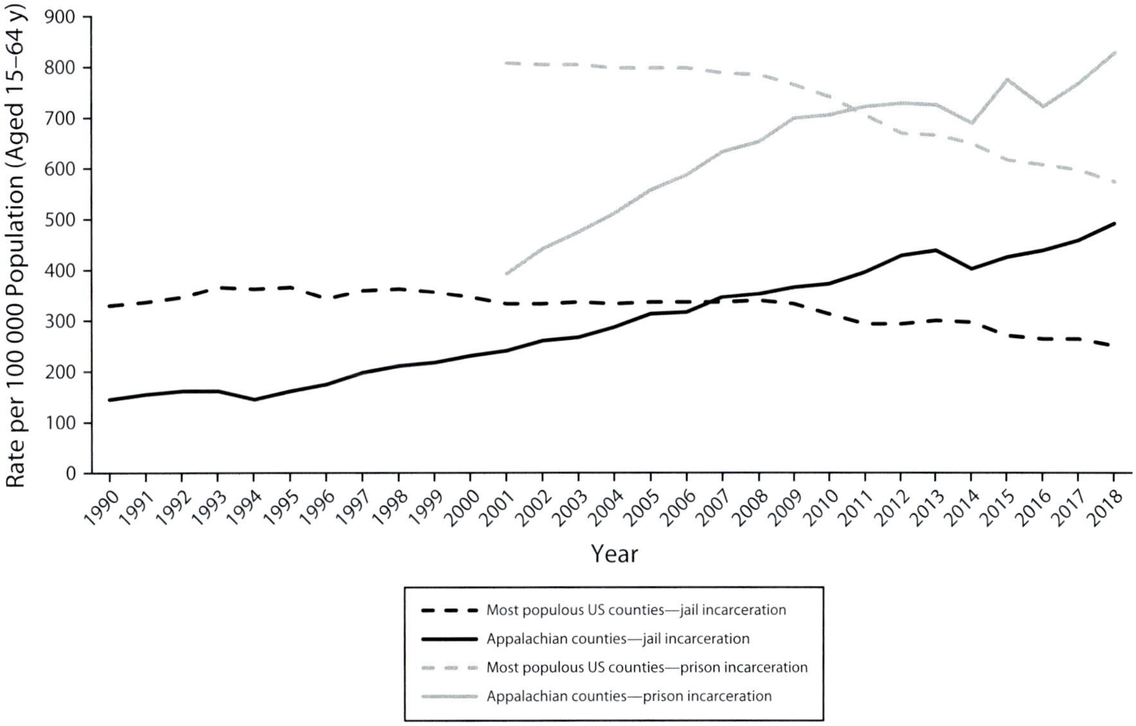

FIGURE 1— Jail and Prison Incarceration Trends for 22 Appalachian Counties and the 22 Most Populous US Counties per 100 000 Population (Aged 15–64 Years): Kentucky, West Virginia, Ohio, North Carolina, 1990–2018

Note. Prison population data reflect the number of people in state prisons who came from each county. For 28 county-years, prison data are regional and reported for all counties sharing a detention center. The prison population for an individual county is based on the target county's proportion of the total adult population across regional counties. Calculated for Kentucky (2017–2018) were Elliot and Morgan counties and for West Virginia (2015–2018) were Boone, Logan, McDowell, Mercer, Mingo, and Wyoming counties. Prison population data were available for all 22 of the most populous US counties starting in 2001. First year of Maricopa County, AZ, prison population data was reported in 2001.
Source. Mass incarceration data are from the Vera Institute of Justice. Incarceration Trends. Available at: https://trends.vera.org. Accessed January, 31, 2023.

TABLE 2— Frequency of Unmet Need for Medical Care by Predisposing, Enabling, and Needs Characteristics: Kentucky, West Virginia, Ohio, North Carolina, 2018–2020

Variable	% With Unmet Need for Care (95% CI)	P[a]
Predisposing		
Education		.22
<high school	63.7 (52.0, 75.4)	
High school or general equivalency diploma	68.2 (59.2, 77.2)	
Some college	71.0 (61.8, 80.2)	
Associate's degree or higher	72.1 (59.7, 84.4)	
Gender		.06
Male	64.6 (56.2, 73.0)	
Female	71.8 (60.9, 82.7)	
Experienced houselessness[b]		<.001
No	61.9 (52.1, 71.7)	
Yes	76.1 (67.5, 84.8)	
Employed full-time		.03
No	69.0 (60.0, 78.1)	
Yes	62.4 (52.2, 72.6)	
Sold sex for money[b]		.01
No	67.4 (58.4, 76.4)	
Yes	90.0 (77.1, 100.0)	
Sold drugs for money[b]		<.001
No	65.6 (56.5, 74.8)	
Yes	76.2 (66.8, 85.5)	
Has cell phone with active service		.01
No	72.6 (65.4, 79.8)	
Yes	64.9 (54.2, 75.6)	
Frequency of Internet use[c]		.04
Never	68.1 (59.1, 77.1)	
Several times a month	74.9 (65.6, 84.2)	
Several times a week	69.0 (55.0, 83.1)	
About once a day	59.1 (44.9, 73.2)	
Several times a day	68.9 (59.7, 78.0)	
Enabling		
Has health insurance		<.001
No	77.6 (69.8, 85.3)	
Yes	64.2 (54.2, 74.3)	
Distance to SSP from residence		<.001
In walking distance	72.3 (62.2, 82.3)	
<30-min drive	60.7 (50.2, 71.2)	
30–60-min drive	72.3 (62.2, 82.3)	
>60-min drive	88.8 (76.2, 101.3)	
No SSP in reasonable distance	89.0 (79.6, 98.4)	
SUD treatment[b,d]		.03
No	65.5 (56.5, 74.5)	

Continued

by law enforcement (PR = 1.14; 95% confidence interval [CI] = 1.04, 1.24), arrested (PR = 1.12; 95% CI = 1.04, 1.21), or incarcerated (PR = 1.08; 95% CI = 1.01, 1.16) but not with community supervision (Table 3).

These relationships did not persist in the fully adjusted models (Table 3). Either the magnitude of relationships weakened, as occurred with arrest (adjusted PR [APR] = 0.95; 95% CI = 0.78, 1.15) and incarceration (APR = 1.01; 95% CI = 0.89, 1.14), or the CI widened to include no effect, as is the case for stops (APR = 1.13; 95% CI = 0.97, 1.32). The nonsignificant relationship between community supervision and unmet need persisted. Rerunning the model without potential mediators (i.e., health insurance, housing status, injection frequency, employment status, HCV infection, drug treatment) did not substantively change associations (Table 3).

Of the 48 relationships assessed between the 4 kinds of criminal–legal encounters and 12 reasons for unmet need, just 7 were statistically significant in fully adjusted models (Table C, available as a supplement to the online version of this article at http://www.ajph.org). Participants who were stopped and searched were more likely to report having an unmet need because they were too high to seek care (APR = 1.51; 95% CI = 1.14, 2.01), were concerned about poor treatment by providers (APR = 1.51; 95% CI = 1.25, 1.82), had experienced poor treatment in the past (APR = 1.49; 95% CI = 1.09, 2.03), or had sought lay care (APR = 1.31; 95% CI = 1.05, 1.63).

Arrests were inversely associated with unmet need that occurred because participants had experienced poor past treatment (APR = 0.62; 95% CI = 0.40, 0.98). People on community supervision

TABLE 2— Continued

Variable	% With Unmet Need for Care (95% CI)	P^a
Yes	71.3 (61.6, 81.0)	
Needs		
HCV diagnosis		.03
No	64.9 (54.6, 75.1)	
Yes	71.7 (63.3, 80.0)	
Prescription opioid misuse[c]		<.01
No	63.1 (54.3, 71.9)	
Yes	71.1 (61.3, 80.8)	
MOUD treatment misuse[c]		.21
No	65.9 (56.3, 75.5)	
Yes	69.5 (60.2, 78.7)	
Illicit opioid use[c]		.01
No	63.0 (53.1, 72.9)	
Yes	69.9 (60.8, 79.0)	
Stimulant use[c]		<.001
No	55.3 (42.5, 68.1)	
Yes	70.5 (62.2, 78.8)	
Injection drug use frequency[c]		<.001
Never	52.5 (37.8, 67.2)	
Weekly or less	72.1 (61.4, 82.9)	
More than weekly	75.7 (60.5, 91.0)	
Daily	73.6 (64.9, 76.9)	
More than once daily	70.0 (63.0, 76.9)	
Study site		<.001
Kentucky	40.1 (35.2, 45.0)	
North Carolina	83.2 (78.6, 87.9)	
Ohio	80.8 (75.1, 86.5)	
West Virginia	83.7 (77.7, 89.7)	

Note. CI = confidence interval; HCV = hepatitis C virus; MOUD = medications for opioid use disorder; SSP = syringe service program; SUD = substance use disorder.
[a]*P* values are derived from the *t* test because of aggregation across multiple imputation sets. The underlying test in each set varies across variables. The Rao–Scott χ^2 statistic adjusted for respondent-driven sampling (RDS) clustering were used for categorical variables, and *z* scores derived from generalized estimating equations models adjusted for RDS clustering were used for the continuous variable (i.e., age).
[b]In past 6 mo.
[c]In past 30 d.
[d]Includes outpatient counseling, inpatient or residential treatment, oral buprenorphine or injections, methadone maintenance treatment, or naltrexone injections.

were more likely to report cost-related unmet need (APR = 1.38; 95% CI = 1.14, 1.67) or childcare barriers (APR = 1.71; 95% CI = 1.01, 2.89). All but 2 of these relationships (arrests and poor past treatment, and community supervision and inability to pay) retained significance when potential mediators were removed (Table C).

DISCUSSION

In our sample of White PWUD in a rural Appalachian sacrifice zone, rates of unmet need for medical care and of criminal–legal encounters were high and testify to the escalation of the War on Drugs in the region and to the multiple barriers that PWUD face when seeking essential care. These phenomena were, however, statistically unrelated in the multivariable model. Multivariable models also found no relationships between these encounters and the component reasons for unmet need in 41 of the 48 relationships tested.

Nonsignificant results persisted across models when we removed potential mediators and contrast with decades of research with PWUD in the predominantly Black impoverished urban neighborhoods where the War on Drugs originated. We dedicate this section to considering these findings, with the goal of generating possible avenues for future research in this emergent arena—emergent because little research has explored the impacts of the War on Drugs in this region and because little research has considered racialized capitalism and White health.

Existing research with residents of predominantly Black urban neighborhoods posits that a psychological distress pathway mediates established relationships between criminal–legal encounters and health and health care utilization. Specifically, residents experience pervasive criminal–legal encounters as crystallizations of contemporary anti-Black structural discrimination that directly link to historical systems of White supremacy.[3,4] The consequent psychological distress undermines health care engagement,[36] which might be especially pronounced because of well-earned distrust of health care systems.[37] This pathway is unlikely to operate among White Appalachian PWUD: a persistent hallmark of Appalachian Whiteness has been freedom

TABLE 3— Associations Between Composite Measure of Unmet Need for Medical Care and Criminal–Legal Encounters: Kentucky, West Virginia, Ohio, North Carolina, 2018–2020

	Overall Composite Measure of Unmet Need for Care		
Criminal–Legal Encounter[a]	Crude PR (95% CI)	Full Model,[b] APR (95% CI)	Possible Mediators Removed,[c] APR (95% CI)
Stop and search	1.14 (1.04, 1.24)	1.13 (0.97, 1.32)	1.12 (0.97, 1.29)
Arrest	1.12 (1.04, 1.21)	0.95 (0.78, 1.15)	0.97 (0.80, 1.18)
Incarceration	1.08 (1.01, 1.16)	1.01 (0.89, 1.14)	1.02 (0.90, 1.15)
Community supervision	1.01 (0.94, 1.10)	0.99 (0.90, 1.09)	0.98 (0.89, 1.08)

Note. APR = adjusted prevalence ratio; CI = confidence interval; HCV = hepatitis C virus; MOUD = medications for opioid use disorder; PR = prevalence ratio; SUD = substance use disorder. We determined associations using Poisson regression.
[a]Within past 6 mo.
[b]Model adjusted for predisposing characteristics (i.e., age, education, gender, houselessness status, employment, selling sex or drugs for money, cell phone, Internet use frequency), enabling characteristics (i.e., health insurance, distance to a syringe service program from residence, SUD treatment), needs (i.e., HCV diagnosis, prescription opioid misuse, MOUD treatment misuse, illegalized opioid use, stimulant use, injection drug use frequency), and study site.
[c]Model excludes health insurance, houselessness status, injection frequency, HCV status, employment status, SUD treatment, and MOUD treatment misuse.

from such saturating and persistent criminal–legal control.[22] PWUD in this sample are thus unlikely to experience these criminal–legal encounters as a form of racial subjugation.

A corollary possibility is that social networks in these 22 counties may be better able to buffer the psychological distress that does arise from criminal–legal encounters. Waves of forced migration have systematically eroded social networks in Black communities; in the past century alone, the 40-plus years of network disruptions catalyzed by mass incarceration are sedimented atop the disruptions of the 1910 to 1970 Great Northward Migration, urban renewal, and gentrification.[38] A defining characteristic of Appalachian Whiteness, by contrast, is the capacity to wield sovereignty over home and community[22]; ongoing qualitative research in this area indicates that PWUD and other residents have lived in the region for generations. This sovereignty has allowed strong, stable local networks to thrive.[39] The relative recency of mass incarceration in the region, coupled with the absence of systematic, generations-long disruptions, may allow White Appalachian networks to provide essential support—emotional and otherwise—that buffers the effects of criminal–legal encounters. Future research should explore this possibility.

Cause-specific analyses also indicate that stops were associated with multiple reasons for unmet need (i.e., participant was too high, received provider mistreatment in the past or feared future mistreatment, sought care from a layperson). Two previous analyses of rural Appalachian PWUD corroborate the power of stops in the region (one analyzed data from the Rural Opioid Initiative North Carolina sample but analyzed a different outcome and the full sample, so we cite it here): they found that these encounters, or concerns about them, were associated with unsterile injecting practices and with impeding syringe service program participation.[40,41]

Freedom from these stops has long been a defining feature of Whiteness in the United States. The American Revolution was catalyzed, in part, by White colonists' rage that British soldiers could stop and search them with impunity, and protections against such unreasonable search and seizure were inscribed in the Constitution's Fourth Amendment.[3,42,43] Both this rage and the Fourth Amendment were, however, limited to White people: enslaved individuals, freemen, freewomen, and their descendants have been routinely stopped and searched by slave patrols and their successors.

The Supreme Court legalized this practice in 1968 when it created "*Terry* stops," a novel form of legal police–civilian encounter that police can instigate when they harbor a "reasonable suspicion" of criminalized activity—a far lower threshold than the "probable cause" standard required for an arrest.[3,42] These stops have subsequently become an essential, pervasive, and racialized War on Drugs strategy.[3,42] The erosion of this protection from these police encounters—protections long a property of Whiteness—may lead to psychological distress among this White sample of PWUD, an experience that in turn might generate the deeper addiction cited as a barrier to health care. Future qualitative research should explore this possibility as well as whether experiences of "unreasonable" stops and searches undermine PWUD's trust in other local systems, including health care providers.

Limitations

Findings should be interpreted in light of several limitations. We could not use probability-based sampling methods, and so samples might not generalize to the underlying PWUD population. Rural Appalachia is home to BILPOC people, who may have strikingly different criminal–legal encounters and unmet need; relationships between the 2 may vary in this population as well. Future research should oversample BILPOC who use drugs to analyze these possibilities.

Criminal–legal constructs were operationalized solely as individual-level phenomena but are deployed in municipalities. Future multilevel research should establish criminal–legal exposures as both place-based and individual-level constructs.

Qualitative methods could also explore these contextual features and investigate essential questions about perceived pathways through which criminal–legal encounters might or might not affect health care utilization. A widely used measure of unmet need for health care exists[44] and was not included in the harmonized survey. Future research with this population should incorporate this measure.

Public Health Implications

Multivariable models found no relationship between indicators of the expanding War on Drugs and our overall measure of health care utilization among White PWUD in 22 rural Appalachian counties, by contrast to decades of research conducted in the impoverished predominantly Black urban neighborhoods where this war originated.

Racialized capitalism and critical Whiteness studies raise the possibility that the War on Drugs is deployed in both areas to reinforce the ongoing codification of race and class but that health and health care effects may diverge because the races and classes it creates differ. Specifically, findings raise the possibility that the psychological distress pathway may be severed in Appalachia, where the War on Drugs is devoid of the weight of racial subjugation and where Whiteness has protected local social networks through sovereignty over home and community. As part of broader engagement in the impacts of racialized capitalism on White health, future research should explore these possibilities and the impacts of the War on Drugs on other drug-related harms in Appalachia. AJPH

ABOUT THE AUTHORS

At the time of writing, Hannah L. F. Cooper, Melvin "Douglas" Livingston, Natalie D. Crawford, Chandra L. Ford, Umed Ibragimov, Tasfia Jahangir, Anna Mullany, and Snigdha Peddireddy were with the Emory University Rollins School of Public Health, Atlanta, GA. Judith Feinberg and Gordon Smith were with the West Virginia University School of Medicine, Morgantown. Vivian Go and William C. Miller were with the University of North Carolina School of Public Health, Chapel Hill. Leslie Salas-Hernandez was with the Center for Policing Equity, Denver, CO. April M. Young was with the University of Kentucky College of Public Health, Lexington. William Zule was with the Research Trial Institute, Research Triangle Park, NC. Ali Sewell was with the Emory University College of Arts and Science, Atlanta.

CORRESPONDENCE

Correspondence should be sent to Hannah L. F. Cooper, 1518 Clifton Rd NE, Room 520, Atlanta, GA 30322 (e-mail: hcoope3@emory.edu). Reprints can be ordered at https://www.ajph.org by clicking the "Reprints" link.

PUBLICATION INFORMATION

Full Citation: Cooper HLF, Livingston MD, Crawford ND, et al. The war on drugs, racialized capitalism, and health care utilization among White people who use drugs in 22 rural Appalachian counties. *Am J Public Health*. 2024;114(10):1086–1096.

Acceptance Date: May 24, 2024.

DOI: https://doi.org/10.2105/AJPH.2024.307744

ORCID iDs:

Hannah L. F. Cooper https://orcid.org/0000-0002-0521-2438

Leslie Salas-Hernandez https://orcid.org/0000-0002-2700-8892

Gordon Smith https://orcid.org/0000-0002-2911-3071

CONTRIBUTORS

H. L. F. Cooper led the conceptualization of the article and the initial writing of the introduction and discussion. M. D. Livingston led the analyses and wrote the initial draft of the results. J. Feinberg, V. Go, W. C. Miller, G. Smith, A. M. Young, and W. Zule led site-specific data collection. S. Peddireddy developed the tables. All authors reviewed and revised the article and approved the submission.

ACKNOWLEDGMENTS

This work was funded by the National Institutes of Health (NIH; grants T32DA050552 to H. L. F. C.; UG3DA044798 to H. L. F. C. and A. M. Y.; UG3DA044825 to J. F. and G. S.; UG3DA044822 to V. G. and W. C. M.; UH3DA044823 to W. Z.).

We are grateful to the participants who took part in the survey and to the staff who led the data collection.

Note. The content of this article is solely the responsibility of the authors and does not necessarily represent the official views of NIH.

CONFLICTS OF INTEREST

The authors have no conflicts of interest to declare.

HUMAN PARTICIPANT PROTECTION

The institutional review board of each participating research site approved the component studies.

REFERENCES

1. Kang-Brown J, Subramanian R. *Out of Sight: The Growth of Jails in Rural America*. New York, NY: Vera Institute of Justice; 2017.
2. Cooper HL, Cloud DH, Freeman PR, et al. Buprenorphine dispensing in an epicenter of the US opioid epidemic: a case study of the rural risk environment in Appalachian Kentucky. *Int J Drug Policy*. 2020;85:102701. https://doi.org/10.1016/j.drugpo.2020.102701
3. Cooper HL, Fullilove MT. *From Enforcers to Guardians: A Public Health Primer on Ending Police Violence*. Baltimore, MD: Johns Hopkins University Press; 2020.

4. Alexander M. *The New Jim Crow: Mass Incarceration in the Age of Colorblindness.* New York, NY: New Press; 2020.
5. Alang S, McAlpine D, McClain M, Hardeman R. Police brutality, medical mistrust and unmet need for medical care. *Prev Med Rep.* 2021; 22:101361. https://doi.org/10.1016/j.pmedr.2021.101361
6. Li-Rodenborn ER, Navarro-Serer B, Pitts S, Anchuri K. Improving healthcare access among the newly decarcerated. *J Sci Policy Gov.* 2020;17(2). Available at: https://www.sciencepolicyjournal.org/article_1038126_jspg170209.html. Accessed July 31, 2024. https://doi.org/10.38126/JSPG170209
7. National Academies of Sciences, Engineering, and Medicine. *The Effects of Incarceration and Reentry on Community Health and Well-Being: Proceedings of a Workshop.* Washington, DC: National Academies Press; 2020. https://doi.org/10.17226/25659
8. Cooper H, Moore L, Gruskin S, Krieger N. The impact of a police drug crackdown on drug injectors' ability to practice harm reduction: a qualitative study. *Soc Sci Med.* 2005;61(3):673–684. https://doi.org/10.1016/j.socscimed.2004.12.030
9. Cooper HL, Des Jarlais DC, Tempalski B, Bossak BH, Ross Z, Friedman SR. Drug-related arrest rates and spatial access to syringe exchange programs in New York City health districts: combined effects on the risk of injection-related infections among injectors. *Health Place.* 2012;18(2):218–228. https://doi.org/10.1016/j.healthplace.2011.09.005
10. Mital S, Wolff J, Carroll JJ. The relationship between incarceration history and overdose in North America: a scoping review of the evidence. *Drug Alcohol Depend.* 2020;213:108088. https://doi.org/10.1016/j.drugalcdep.2020.108088
11. Beletsky L, LaSalle L, Newman M, Pare J, Tam J, Tochka A. Fatal re-entry: legal and programmatic opportunities to curb opioid overdose among individuals newly released from incarceration. *NEULJ.* 2015;7:149.
12. Hernández A, Lan M, MacKinnon NJ, Branscum AJ, Cuadros DF. "Know your epidemic, know your response": epidemiological assessment of the substance use disorder crisis in the United States. *PLoS One.* 2021;16(5):e0251502. https://doi.org/10.1371/journal.pone.0251502
13. Goldberg D, Ross-Driscoll K, Lynch R. County differences in liver mortality in the United States: impact of sociodemographics, disease risk factors, and access to care. *Gastroenterology.* 2021; 160(4):1140–1150.e1. https://doi.org/10.1053/j.gastro.2020.11.016
14. Schalkoff CA, Lancaster KE, Gaynes BN, et al. The opioid and related drug epidemics in rural Appalachia: a systematic review of populations affected, risk factors, and infectious diseases. *Substance Abuse.* 2020;41(1):35–69. https://doi.org/10.1080/08897077.2019.1635555
15. Robinson CJ. Capitalismo racial: el carácter no objetivo del desarrollo capitalista [Racial capitalism: the nonobjective character of capitalist development]. *Tabula Rasa.* 2018;(28):23–56. https://doi.org/10.25058/20112742.n28.2
16. Vasudevan P, Smith S. The domestic geopolitics of racial capitalism. *Environ Plan C: Polit Space.* 2020;38(7–8):1160–1179. https://doi.org/10.1177/2399654420901567
17. Fluri JL, Hickcox A, Frydenlund S, Zackary R. Accessing racial privilege through property: geographies of racial capitalism. *Geoforum.* 2022;132:238–246. https://doi.org/10.1016/j.geoforum.2020.06.013
18. Danewid I. The fire this time: Grenfell, racial capitalism and the urbanisation of empire. *Eur J Int Relat.* 2020;26(1):289–313. https://doi.org/10.1177/1354066119858388
19. Roediger DR. *Working Toward Whiteness: How America's Immigrants Became White: The Strange Journey From Ellis Island to the Suburbs.* New York, NY: Basic Books; 2006.
20. Jacobson MF. *Whiteness of a Different Color.* Cambridge, MA: Harvard University Press; 1999. https://doi.org/10.2307/j.ctvjk2w15
21. Roediger DR. The wages of Whiteness: race and the making of the American working class. In: Aronowitz S, Roberts MJ, eds. *Class: The Anthology.* Hoboken, NJ: Wiley-Blackwell; 2017:41–55.
22. Smith BE. De-gradations of Whiteness: Appalachia and the complexities of race. *J Appalach Stud.* 2004;10(1/2):38–57.
23. Kozlowski M, Perkins HA. Environmental justice in Appalachia Ohio? An expanded consideration of privilege and the role it plays in defending the contaminated status quo in a White, working-class community. *Local Environ.* 2016;21(10):1288–1304. https://doi.org/10.1080/13549839.2015.1111316
24. Stoll S. *Ramp Hollow: The Ordeal of Appalachia.* New York, NY: Hill and Wang; 2017.
25. Andrews TG. *Killing for Coal: America's Deadliest Labor War.* Cambridge, MA: Harvard University Press; 2008. https://doi.org/10.4159/9780674020214
26. Muhammad KG. *The Condemnation of Blackness: Race, Crime, and the Making of Modern Urban America.* 2nd ed. Cambridge, MA: Harvard University Press; 2019. https://doi.org/10.4159/9780674240919
27. Gilmore R, Kumanyika C. Ruth Wilson Gilmore makes the case for abolition. *The Intercept.* June 10, 2020. Available at: https://theintercept.com/2020/06/10/ruth-wilson-gilmore-makes-the-case-for-abolition. Accessed July 31, 2024.
28. Billings DB, Blee KM. *The Road to Poverty: The Making of Wealth and Hardship in Appalachia.* Cambridge, UK: Cambridge Books; 2000.
29. Schept J. *Coal, Cages, Crisis: The Rise of the Prison Economy in Central Appalachia.* New York, NY: New York University Press; 2022.
30. Liu M, Luce C, Orevba M, Sebastian S, Shupe C. *Consumer Finances in Rural Appalachia.* Washington, DC: Consumer Financial Protection Bureau; 2022.
31. Van Winkle WW. *Appealing to the Rust Belt and Appalachian Voter—Trump and the Rhetoric of Nostalgia and Race.* Dayton, OH: University of Dayton; 2020.
32. Gray R. Trump defends White-nationalist protesters: "Some very fine people on both sides." *Atlantic.* August 2017;320(2):15. Available at: https://www.theatlantic.com/politics/archive/2017/08/trump-defends-white-nationalist-protesters-some-very-fine-people-on-both-sides/536940. Accessed July 31, 2024.
33. Appalachian Regional Commission. Creating a culture of health in Appalachia: healthcare systems. 2021. Available at: https://www.arc.gov/wp-content/uploads/2021/02/Health_Disparities_in_Appalachia_Health_Care_Systems_Domain.pdf. Accessed July 31, 2024.
34. Skaggs P, Bell SB, Scutchfield FD, Robinson LE. Providers' stigmas and the effects on patients with opioid use disorder: a scoping review. *J Appalach Health.* 2023;4(3):87. https://doi.org/10.13023/jah.0403.04
35. Gelberg L, Andersen RM, Leake BD. The behavioral model for vulnerable populations: application to medical care use and outcomes for homeless people. *Health Serv Res.* 2000;34(6):1273.
36. Witt WP, Kahn R, Fortuna L, et al. Psychological distress as a barrier to preventive healthcare among US women. *J Prim Prev.* 2009;30(5):531–547. https://doi.org/10.1007/s10935-009-0190-z
37. Hall OT, Jordan A, Teater J, et al. Experiences of racial discrimination in the medical setting and associations with medical mistrust and expectations of care among Black patients seeking addiction treatment. *J Subst Abuse Treat.* 2022; 133:108551. https://doi.org/10.1016/j.jsat.2021.108551
38. Fullilove MT. *Root Shock: How Tearing Up City Neighborhoods Hurts America, And What We Can Do About It.* New York, NY: New Village Press; 2016. https://doi.org/10.2307/j.ctt21pxmmc
39. Roberson PN, Tasman J, Renegar R, Cortez G, Lenger KA. The importance of family relationships for the health of underserved Appalachians: an application and extension of the biobehavioral family model. *Fam Syst Health.* 2023;41(4):514–526. https://doi.org/10.1037/fsh0000826
40. Davis SM, Kristjansson AL, Davidov D, Zullig K, Baus A, Fisher M. Barriers to using new needles encountered by rural Appalachian people who inject drugs: implications for needle exchange. *Harm Reduct J.* 2019;16(1):1–8. https://doi.org/10.1186/s12954-019-0295-5
41. Carpenter DM, Zule WA, Hennessy CM, Evon DM, Hurt CB, Ostrach B. Factors associated with perceived ease of access to syringes in Appalachian North Carolina. *J Rural Health.* 2023;39(1):212–222. https://doi.org/10.1111/jrh.12698
42. Cooper HL. War on drugs policing and police brutality. *Subst Use Misuse.* 2015;50(8–9):1188–1194. https://doi.org/10.3109/10826084.2015.1007669
43. Saleem O. The age of unreason: the impact of reasonableness, increased police force, and colorblindness on Terry "stop and frisk." *Okla. L. Rev.* 1997;50(4):451.
44. National Center for Health Statistics. National Health Interview Survey, 1995: access to care supplement. Hyattsville, MD;1998.

Preinjury and Event-Related Characteristics of Pediatric Firearm Injuries: The American College of Surgeons Firearm Study, United States, March 2021–February 2022

Katherine T. Flynn-O'Brien, MD, MPH, Chethan Sathya, MD, MSc, Meera Kotagal, MD, MPH, Samantha Banks, MS, Lauren L. Agoubi, MD, MA, Deborah A. Kuhls, MD, Avery Nathens, MD, PhD, MPH, Ashley B. Hink, MD, MPH, and Frederick P. Rivara, MD, MPH

Objectives. To assess differences in contextual factors by intent among pediatric firearm injury patients and determine factors associated with data missingness.

Methods. We retrospectively queried the American College of Surgeons Firearm Study database (March 1, 2021–February 28, 2022) for patients aged 18 years or younger. We stratified preinjury, firearm-related, and event-related factors by intent and compared them by using Fisher exact, χ^2, or 1-way analysis of variance testing. Secondary analysis estimated the adjusted odds of missingness by using generalized linear modeling with binominal logit link.

Results. Among 17 395 patients, 2974 (17.1%) were aged 18 years or younger; 1966 (66.1%) were injured by assault, 579 (19.5%) unintentionally, and 76 (2.6%) by self-inflicted means. Most contextual factors differed by intent, including proportion of youths with previous adverse childhood experiences, mental illness, and violent assaults or injury, firearm type and access, perpetrator relationship, and injury location. In adjusted analyses, age, trauma center designation, intent, and admission status were associated with missingness.

Conclusions. Contextual factors related to pediatric firearm injury vary by intent. Specific predictors associated with missingness may inform improved future data collection.

Public Health Implications. Contextual factors related to pediatric firearm injury can be obtained in a systematic manner nationally to inform targeted interventions. (*Am J Public Health*. 2024;114(10):1097–1109. https://doi.org/10.2105/AJPH.2024.307754)

AJPH October 2024, Vol. 114, No. 10

Firearm injury is the leading cause of death in children and adolescents in the United States, overtaking motor vehicle–related deaths in 2019.[1] Pediatric nonfatal firearm injury has been increasing steadily as well.[2] Little is known about the contextual factors associated with these injuries.

Epidemiological data on previous adverse childhood experiences (ACEs) and neighborhood distress, for example, may allow for identification of youth at risk for injury. Data such as firearm access, storage, and ownership may help clarify the context in which injuries occur and may identify modifiable risk factors to guide prevention. Data on intent and the extent to which assault, suicide, and unintentional injuries are associated with specific patient characteristics may also assist with prevention.[3–5]

Comprehensive data pertaining to nonfatal firearm injuries in the

United States are scarce, limiting rigorous study. Existing data systems utilizing hospital billing data lack granularity. The National Violent Death Reporting System captures some victim characteristics, risks, and contextual factors; however, it is limited to fatal events.[6] The National Electronic Injury Surveillance System Firearm Surveillance Study captures data on nonfatal injury including firearm type, criminal incident, and location but does not include contextual data important for youths such as ACEs, details related to firearm access and ownership, or information about hospital care.[7] The American College of Surgeons (ACS) collects data on injury characteristics for fatal and nonfatal injury, but the data are limited to patients who are admitted, die in the emergency department (ED), or are transferred to a trauma center; thus, it does not capture patients who are treated and released.[8] Altogether, existing data systems are limited in their ability to provide important contextual information related to both fatal and nonfatal firearm injuries.

With these challenges in mind, the ACS Committee on Trauma utilized the Trauma Quality Improvement Project (TQIP) infrastructure to pilot a data surveillance strategy to capture more complete data on firearm injuries in all patients presenting to participating hospitals.[9] The objective of the ACS Firearm Study was to describe the patient and injury characteristics and the pre-event, firearm, and event-related factors associated with firearm injuries.[9] The primary aim of the current study was to characterize pediatric patients treated at trauma centers for firearm injuries, explore differences based on injury intent among pediatric patients, and examine characteristics of their care. Our secondary aim was to determine what factors might be related to data missingness for novel variables. We hypothesized there would be differences in patient and contextual factors by injury intent and that predictors of missingness could be identified, potentially providing a process and systems-based approach to improve data collection in the future.

METHODS

TQIP collects data from more than 700 centers in the United States for performance improvement and risk-adjusted benchmarking. All TQIP centers were invited to participate in the ACS Firearm Study, and 165 volunteered to participate, with 128 centers contributing data (17.3% of TQIP centers). Among TQIP trauma centers that only treat pediatric patients, 20 of 51 centers were included (39.2%). TQIP captures high-fidelity data as trained abstractors capture the data from the medical record.

The ACS Firearm study was a cross-sectional study that captured data for firearm-injured patients of any age who arrived alive at a participating center between March 1, 2021, and February 28, 2022. Methods specific to the ACS Firearm study protocol and data acquisition have been described in detail elsewhere.[9] This study focused on patients aged 18 years or younger, and followed Strengthening the Reporting of Observational Studies in Epidemiology (STROBE) guidelines (Appendix A, available as a supplement to the online version of this article at https://ajph.org).

Demographic, injury, and hospital characteristics were captured through the TQIP infrastructure using the National Trauma Data Standard data dictionary.[8] Additional data elements were extracted from the medical record. Novel demographic variables included the primary caregiver and the Distressed Community Index (DCI).[10] Caregivers were defined as individuals the patient lives with and who provide oversight or caregiving responsibilities. The DCI is a tool for measuring economic well-being of US communities[10] and was captured relative to residence zip code. Overall, injury severity was defined by Injury Severity Scale (ISS) score. Severe injury based on anatomic location was defined by abbreviated injury score of 3 or greater.

Preinjury Factors

Preinjury factors included ACEs, history of mental illness, previous traumatic events, previous violent assault or injury, and previous suicide attempt or self-harm. For each type of preinjury factor confirmed by a patient or caregiver, details were then queried on the subtypes, such as type of ACE, mental illness, and traumatic event. Definitions for each main variable and answer options are provided (Appendix A, Table A).

Firearm and Event-Related Factors

We abstracted firearm type, ownership, storage, and access, in addition to relationship between the patient and shooter, and event-related factors included the setting of injury and the context of injury. We collapsed the injury settings into 8 categories most applicable to youth: residence, motor vehicle, school or childcare, street, woods or forest, public space, other, and missing. Definitions for each question are provided (Appendix A, Tables B and C).

Data Analysis

We stratified all variables by injury intent. We made comparisons with the

Fisher exact test or χ^2 test for categorical variables and 1-way analysis of variance (ANOVA) for continuous variables, with a significance level set at 0.05.

To understand the missingness of specific data elements, we chose 7 of the main novel variables with the highest missingness for secondary analysis. These included preinjury factors (ACEs, mental illness, previous assault or injury, previous suicide attempt or self-harm) and firearm-factors (firearm access and type). We calculated mean percent missingness by patient and facility ID. For patient-level missingness, we used the ggplot package in R version 4.2.2 (RStudio PBC, Boston, MA) to create a heat map, demonstrating variability by patient.[11] Facility-level missingness was reflected in a caterpillar plot with error bars reflecting standard deviation.[11] To understand predictors of missingness, we estimated the adjusted odds of missingness by using generalized linear modeling with binominal logit link. This missingness analysis was limited to survivors, hypothesizing that patients who died in the ED or hospital may have less data available.

We determined predictors a priori based on our hypothesis that they would be associated with missingness, and they included age, admission status (admitted vs ED discharge), ISS, DCI, hospital trauma designation (adult only, pediatric only, combined adult and pediatric), and intent of injury. We hypothesized that there would be less data available (higher missingness) for more severely injured patients because of their inability to share information, and for older patients, those from distressed communities, and for victims of assault, all of which may be associated with less information gathering and sharing on behalf of clinician and patient, respectively. We also hypothesized that center type may impact how comprehensively data are captured related to preinjury factors and injury circumstances.

RESULTS

Among the 17 395 patients in the study overall, 2974 (17.1%) were aged 18 years or younger and were included in this analysis. The majority of injured children and adolescents (referred to as "youths") were injured by assault (n = 1966; 66.1%), with 579 (19.5%) injured unintentionally and 76 (2.6%) with self-inflicted injuries. An additional 353 (11.9%) did not have an intent reported in the medical record. Differences by intent were present by age, race, urbanicity, primary method of payment, and DCI quintile (Table 1). Only 32.6% of youth injured by assault reported living with both parents; however, there was 26.9% missingness. In contrast, 55.3% and 48.5% of youths injured by self-inflicted and unintentional means had both parents at home, respectively.

ISS differed by intent, with severe injury (ISS > 25) affecting 28.9% of youths injured by self-inflicted means, compared with 8.7% of assault- and 4.3% of unintentionally injured youths. Location of injury also varied, particularly among severe injuries (Appendix A, Table D). For example, among assault-injured youths, 12.7% had severe chest injury and 12.0% had severe abdominal injury. Among youths with self-inflicted injury, 63.2% had severe head injury. Differences by intent were also identified by transport mode, ED disposition, facility type, intensive care unit length of stay (LOS), hospital LOS, hospital discharge disposition, and mortality (Table 1). Mean intensive care unit LOS was lowest for unintentional and self-inflicted injury, the latter potentially reflecting a bias introduced by those who die early. Youths with self-inflicted injuries had the longest mean total LOS, possibly reflecting injury severity and rehabilitation needs. While a minority of youths injured by assault or unintentional means died from their injury (6.5% and 4.0%, respectively), more than half of all youths with self-inflicted injury died (51.3%). Overall ISS, head abbreviated injury score, and mortality were correlated and associated with self-inflicted injury.

Preinjury Factors

Preinjury factors varied by intent; however, findings were limited by missingness in more than 50% of many variables (Table 2). At least 1 ACE was identified in the medical records of 18.9% of youths with assault injury, 32.9% with self-inflicted injury, and 22.6% with unintentional injury, with the type of ACE varying by intent. History of mental illness and type of mental illness reported also varied: 12.0% of assault-injured youths had a mental illness documented compared with 46.1% of youths with self-inflicted injury. The most common mental illnesses recorded across all intents were major depression and attention-deficit disorder or attention-deficit/hyperactivity disorder. Overall, history of at least 1 previous traumatic event varied from 15% to 22% across intent groups; however, the most notable difference was the proportion of youths with exposure to community violence in the assault-injured group (26.3%) compared with 5.3% and 6.9% in self-inflicted and unintentional injury groups, respectively. Missingness varied by intent for "previous violent assault/injury" and for "prior suicide attempt/self-harm";

AJPH October 2024, Vol. 114, No. 10

TABLE 1— Demographic and Injury Characteristics Among Children Aged 18 Years or Younger Presenting to the Emergency Department With Firearm Injury: United States, March 1, 2021–February 28, 2022

	Overall	Assault[a]	Self-Inflicted	Unintentional	Missing	P[b]
Overall sample size	2974	1966	76	579	353	
Age, y						<.001
Mean (SD)	14.7 (4.17)	15.3 (3.66)	15.6 (2.48)	12.2 (5.09)	15.2 (3.90)	
Median (range)	16 (0.00–18.00)	16 (0.00–18.00)	16 (0.00–18.00)	14 (1.00–18.00)	16 (0.00–18.00)	
Sex, no. (%)						.19
Female	511 (17.2)	348 (17.7)	18 (23.7)	86 (14.9)	59 (16.7)	
Male	2358 (79.3)	1544 (78.5)	58 (76.3)	477 (82.4)	279 (79.0)	
Missing	105 (3.5)	74 (3.8)	0 (0)	16 (2.8)	15 (4.2)	
Race, no. (%)						<.001
Black	1951 (65.6)	1412 (71.8)	14 (18.4)	260 (44.9)	265 (75.1)	
White	701 (23.6)	349 (17.8)	46 (60.5)	254 (43.9)	52 (14.7)	
AI, Asian, PI/Native Hawaiian, multiracial, other	264 (8.9)	164 (8.3)	14 (18.4)	58 (10.0)	28 (7.9)	
Missing	58 (2.0)	41 (2.1)	2 (2.6)	7 (1.2)	8 (2.3)	
Ethnicity, no. (%)						.07
Hispanic/Latino	481 (16.2)	333 (16.9)	16 (21.1)	89 (15.4)	43 (12.2)	
Not Hispanic/Latino	2399 (80.7)	1564 (79.6)	57 (75.0)	478 (82.6)	300 (85.0)	
Missing	94 (3.2)	69 (3.5)	3 (3.9)	12 (2.1)	10 (2.8)	
Urban/rural, no. (%)						<.001
Rural	352 (11.8)	143 (7.3)	21 (27.6)	163 (28.2)	25 (7.1)	
Urban	2591 (87.1)	1796 (91.4)	54 (71.1)	415 (71.7)	326 (92.4)	
Missing	31 (1.0)	27 (1.4)	1 (1.3)	1 (0.2)	2 (0.6)	
Primary method of payment, no. (%)						<.001
Medicaid/Medicare/other government	2043 (68.7)	1379 (70.1)	38 (50.0)	401 (69.3)	225 (63.7)	
Private/commercial insurance	523 (17.6)	325 (16.5)	27 (35.5)	111 (19.2)	60 (17.0)	
Self-pay/not billed/other	312 (10.5)	200 (10.2)	8 (10.5)	52 (9.0)	52 (14.7)	
Missing	96 (3.2)	62 (3.2)	3 (3.9)	15 (2.6)	16 (4.5)	
DCI quintiles, no. (%)						<.001
1, prosperous	209 (7.0)	131 (6.7)	13 (17.1)	52 (9.0)	13 (3.7)	
2, comfortable	281 (9.4)	163 (8.3)	12 (15.8)	74 (12.8)	32 (9.1)	
3, midtier	416 (14.0)	275 (14.0)	12 (15.8)	81 (14.0)	48 (13.6)	
4, at-risk	730 (24.5)	481 (24.5)	17 (22.4)	134 (23.1)	98 (27.8)	
5, distressed	1282 (43.1)	875 (44.5)	21 (27.6)	230 (39.7)	156 (44.2)	
Missing	56 (1.9)	41 (2.1)	1 (1.3)	8 (1.4)	6 (1.7)	
Patient caregiver,[c] no. (%)						NA
Parents	1063 (35.7)	641 (32.6)	42 (55.3)	281 (48.5)	99 (28.0)	
Single mother	771 (25.9)	522 (26.6)	16 (21.1)	147 (25.4)	86 (24.4)	
Single father	69 (2.3)	44 (2.2)	3 (3.9)	17 (2.9)	5 (1.4)	
Grandparents/other family member/adult friend	283 (9.5)	188 (9.6)	6 (7.9)	69 (11.9)	20 (5.7)	
Other[d]	138 (4.6)	98 (5.0)	1 (1.3)	12 (2.1)	27 (7.6)	
Missing	745 (25.1)	528 (26.9)	12 (15.8)	80 (13.8)	125 (35.4)	

Continued

TABLE 1— Continued

	Overall	Assault[a]	Self-Inflicted	Unintentional	Missing	P[b]
ISS score, no. (%)						<.001
0–15	2218 (74.6)	1486 (75.6)	28 (36.8)	461 (79.6)	243 (68.8)	
16–25	345 (11.6)	222 (11.3)	26 (34.2)	53 (9.2)	44 (12.5)	
>25	256 (8.6)	171 (8.7)	22 (28.9)	25 (4.3)	38 (10.8)	
Missing	155 (5.2)	87 (4.4)	0 (0)	40 (6.9)	28 (7.9)	
Transport mode,[e] no. (%)						<.001
Ground ambulance	2040 (68.6)	1393 (70.9)	51 (67.1)	359 (62.0)	237 (67.1)	
Private/public vehicle/walk-in	572 (19.2)	371 (18.9)	1 (1.3)	127 (21.9)	73 (20.7)	
Police	72 (2.4)	63 (3.2)	0 (0)	4 (0.7)	5 (1.4)	
Air	272 (9.1)	129 (6.6)	24 (31.6)	86 (14.9)	33 (9.3)	
Missing	18 (0.6)	10 (0.5)	0 (0)	3 (0.5)	5 (1.4)	
ED discharge disposition, no. (%)						<.001
Home	947 (31.8)	641 (32.6)	0 (0)	183 (31.6)	123 (34.8)	
Floor/observation unit	689 (23.2)	466 (23.7)	3 (3.9)	158 (27.3)	62 (17.6)	
ICU/SDU	393 (13.2)	247 (12.6)	37 (48.7)	60 (10.4)	49 (13.9)	
OR	689 (23.2)	462 (23.5)	19 (25.0)	134 (23.1)	74 (21.0)	
Other	99 (3.3)	61 (3.1)	3 (3.9)	21 (3.6)	14 (4.0)	
Died in ED	118 (4.0)	71 (3.6)	12 (15.8)	10 (1.7)	25 (7.1)	
Missing	39 (1.3)	18 (0.9)	2 (2.6)	13 (2.2)	6 (1.7)	
Length of ICU stay, d[f]						.92
Sample size, no.	717	464	49	124	80	
Mean (SD)	6.41 (8.65)	6.51 (9.62)	6.06 (7.14)	5.99 (5.93)	6.69 (7.03)	
Median (range)	3 (1.00–94.00)	3 (1.00–94.00)	3 (1.00–37.00)	3 (1.00–33.00)	4 (1.00–28.00)	
Missing, no. (%)	11 (1.5)	7 (1.5)	1 (2.0)	1 (0.08)	2 (2.5)	
Length of stay among admitted, d						<.001
Sample size, no.	1808	1192	61	365	190	
Mean (SD)	5.77 (8.79)	5.93 (9.04)	9.62 (15.6)	4.82 (6.49)	5.60 (8.19)	
Median (range)	3.00 (1.00–123.00)	3.00 (1.00–123.00)	3.50 (1.00–88.00)	2.00 (1.00–54.00)	2.00 (1.00–58.00)	
Missing	34 (1.9)	22 (1.8)	4 (6.6)	5 (1.4)	3 (1.6)	
Hospital discharge disposition among admitted, no. (%)						<.001
Sample size	1808	1192	61	365	190	
Home	1470 (81.3)	990 (83.1)	14 (23.0)	320 (87.7)	146 (76.8)	
Transferred to acute care	18 (1.0)	9 (0.8)	3 (4.9)	4 (1.1)	2 (1.1)	
SNF or other long-term care	140 (7.7)	84 (7.0)	16 (26.2)	19 (5.2)	21 (11.1)	
Died	110 (6.1)	56 (4.7)	27 (44.3)	13 (3.6)	14 (7.4)	
Other	57 (3.2)	46 (3.9)	0 (0)	6 (1.6)	5 (2.6)	
Missing	13 (0.7)	7 (0.6)	1 (1.6)	3 (0.8)	2 (1.1)	
Mortality, no. (%)						<.001
Deceased	228 (7.7)	127 (6.5)	39 (51.3)	23 (4.0)	39 (11.0)	
Survived	2746 (92.3)	1839 (93.5)	37 (48.7)	556 (96.0)	314 (89.0)	
Facility designation by state, ACS criteria, or both, no. (%)						<.001
Adult only	1382 (46.5)	972 (49.4)	31 (40.8)	172 (29.7)	207 (58.6)	
Both adult and pediatric	718 (24.1)	487 (24.8)	25 (32.9)	142 (24.5)	64 (18.1)	

Continued

TABLE 1— Continued

	Overall	Assault[a]	Self-Inflicted	Unintentional	Missing	P^b
Pediatric only	873 (29.4)	506 (25.7)	20 (26.3)	265 (45.8)	82 (23.2)	
Missing	1 (0.0)	1 (0.1)	0 (0)	0 (0)	0 (0)	

Note. ACS = American College of Surgeons; AI = American Indian; DCI = Distressed Community Index; ED = emergency department; ICU/SDU = intensive care unit/step down unit; ISS = Injury Severity Scale; NA = not applicable; OR = operating room; PI = Pacific Islander; SNF = skilled nursing facility.

[a]Assault includes those who had an "injury intent" of "law enforcement" (n = 6).

[b]Comparisons were made using the Fisher exact test or χ^2 test for categorical variables, and 1-way analysis of variance for continuous variables, with a significance level set at .05.

[c]Categories are not mutually exclusive.

[d]Includes foster parents, lives in a facility, independent/emancipated.

[e]Mutually exclusive categories. Primary mode of transport, meaning mode of transport that delivered patient to the hospital. It is possible that multiple modes were used, but only the last mode is reported here.

[f]Among patients who were admitted to the ICU from the ED or who had a nonmissing length of ICU stay variable. Those missing are patients who were discharged from the ED to the ICU but have a missing length of ICU stay variable.

however, "previous violent assault/injury," particularly by firearms, was most prevalent among assault-injured youths, and "prior suicide attempt/self-harm" was most prevalent among youths with self-inflicted injury.

Firearm and Event-Related Factors

Data related to the firearm and event-related factors were often missing; however, among nonmissing data, a handgun was the most common firearm reported across all intents (Table 3). The shooter was most often a stranger among assault-injured youths, and almost evenly split between self and friend or family for unintentional injury. Overall, firearm assaults generally occurred on the street (36.3%), at home (25.9%), or in a motor vehicle (12.5%). Most self-inflicted injuries and unintentional injuries occurred at home (76.3% and 73.1%, respectively). Results stratified by age and intent are provided (Appendix A, Tables Ea–c).

Missing Data Analysis

The patient-level missingness heat map for ACEs, mental illness, history of previous assault or injury, history of previous traumatic event, previous suicide or self-harm attempt, firearm access, and firearm type demonstrated a lack of patterned findings and "hot spots," suggesting missingness was pervasive (Appendix A, Figure A). Facility-level missingness (Appendix A, Figure B) demonstrated that some centers did better than others at capturing data elements. It was rare to have complete data, and only 7 centers had greater than 80% data capture.

In adjusted analyses, age, trauma center designation, injury intent, and admission status were associated with missingness for select variables, while injury severity and DCI were not (Table 4; Appendix A, Figure C). In particular, the adjusted odds that any key variable was missing (compared with not missing) for adolescents aged 15 to 18 years as compared with children aged 10 years and younger varied from 1.47 (95% confidence interval [CI] = 1.09, 1.99) for firearm type to 4.75 (95% CI = 3.36, 46.85) for previous suicide attempt or self-harm. In addition, the adjusted odds that firearm type was missing (compared with not missing) at pediatric-only centers compared with adult centers was 1.83 (95% CI = 1.45, 2.30). However, for all other variables, the adjusted odds that data were missing was significantly less than 1, suggesting pediatric centers captured other variables of interest better than adult centers. Compared with youths with assault injuries, there was less missingness for youths with self-inflicted injuries across 5 of the 7 variables, and for youths with unintentional injuries for 2 of the 7 variables. Missing intent was strongly associated with missingness in all 7 variables of interest. Not being admitted was associated with missingness (adjusted odds of mean missingness ranged from 1.32; 95% CI = 1.09, 1.62 to 1.89; 95% CI = 1.57, 2.29).

DISCUSSION

This study was the first attempt, to our knowledge, at nationwide systematic collection of contextual factors related to pediatric firearm injury, including pre-event, firearm, and event-related factors. Concordant with our hypothesis, there were notable differences in many of these variables depending on the intent of the injury. Unfortunately, missingness was high, limiting the inference from some data elements.

TABLE 2— Preinjury Factors Among Children Aged 18 Years or Younger Presenting to the Emergency Department With Firearm Injury: United States, March 1, 2021–February 28, 2022

	Overall, No. (%) (n = 2974)	Assault[a], No. (%) (n = 1966)	Self-Inflicted, No. (%) (n = 76)	Unintentional, No. (%) (n = 579)	Missing, No. (%) (n = 353)	P[b]
Adverse childhood experience						.02
No	759 (25.5)	484 (24.6)	16 (21.1)	204 (35.2)	55 (15.6)	
Yes	557 (18.7)	372 (18.9)	25 (32.9)	131 (22.6)	29 (8.2)	
Missing	1658 (55.7)	1110 (56.5)	35 (46.1)	244 (42.1)	269 (76.2)	
Adverse childhood experiences[c]						NA
Emotional abuse	31 (2.4)	19 (2.2)	4 (9.8)	5 (1.5)	3 (3.6)	
Physical abuse	38 (2.9)	28 (3.3)	3 (7.3)	4 (1.2)	3 (3.6)	
Intimate partner violence exposure	32 (2.4)	24 (2.8)	1 (2.4)	5 (1.5)	2 (2.4)	
Household substance misuse	59 (4.5)	35 (4.1)	2 (4.9)	18 (5.4)	4 (4.8)	
Household mental illness	50 (3.8)	36 (4.2)	2 (4.9)	10 (3.0)	2 (2.4)	
Parental divorce	409 (31.1)	269 (31.4)	21 (51.2)	98 (29.3)	21 (25.0)	
Incarcerated household member	88 (6.7)	52 (6.1)	0 (0)	30 (9.0)	6 (7.1)	
Emotional neglect	31 (2.4)	14 (1.6)	3 (7.3)	12 (3.6)	2 (2.4)	
Physical neglect	29 (2.2)	14 (1.6)	1 (2.4)	12 (3.6)	2 (2.4)	
Mental illness present						<.001
No	1962 (66.0)	1314 (66.8)	25 (32.9)	437 (75.5)	186 (52.7)	
Yes	370 (12.4)	236 (12.0)	35 (46.1)	67 (11.6)	32 (9.1)	
Missing	642 (21.6)	416 (21.2)	16 (21.1)	75 (13.0)	135 (38.2)	
Mental illness[c]						NA
Major depression	90 (3.9)	45 (2.9)	21 (35.0)	16 (3.2)	8 (3.7)	
Anxiety	71 (3.0)	41 (2.6)	9 (15.0)	14 (2.8)	7 (3.2)	
Bipolar disorder	37 (1.6)	25 (1.6)	2 (3.3)	7 (1.4)	3 (1.4)	
Posttraumatic stress disorder	22 (0.9)	14 (0.9)	1 (1.7)	4 (0.8)	3 (1.4)	
Schizophrenia	9 (0.4)	7 (0.5)	2 (3.3)	0 (0)	0 (0)	
ADD/ADHD	199 (8.5)	132 (8.5)	9 (15.0)	38 (7.5)	20 (9.2)	
Other[d]	66 (2.8)	43 (2.8)	6 (10.0)	12 (2.4)	22 (10.1)	
Traumatic events						<.001
No	904 (30.4)	574 (29.2)	24 (31.6)	247 (42.7)	59 (16.7)	
Yes[e]	564 (19.0)	428 (21.8)	14 (18.4)	87 (15.0)	35 (9.9)	
1 traumatic event	448 (79.4)	341 (79.7)	11 (78.6)	68 (78.2)	28 (80.0)	
≥ 2 traumatic events	111 (19.7)	83 (19.4)	3 (21.4)	19 (21.8)	6 (17.1)	
Missing	1506 (50.6)	964 (49.0)	38 (50.0)	245 (42.3)	259 (73.4)	
Traumatic events[c]						NA
Major illness/injury	54 (3.7)	43 (4.3)	2 (5.3)	6 (1.8)	3 (3.2)	
Child protective services	130 (8.9)	80 (8.0)	4 (10.5)	34 (10.2)	12 (12.8)	
Community violence	301 (20.5)	264 (26.3)	2 (5.3)	23 (6.9)	12 (12.8)	
Homelessness	51 (3.5)	38 (3.8)	0 (0)	12 (3.6)	1 (1.1)	
Food insecurity	21 (1.4)	13 (1.3)	0 (0)	8 (2.4)	0 (0)	
Other traumatic event	153 (10.4)	99 (9.9)	12 (31.6)	30 (9.0)	12 (12.8)	
Previous violent assaults/injuries						<.001
No	1197 (40.2)	761 (38.7)	36 (47.4)	337 (58.2)	63 (17.8)	
Yes	188 (6.3)	153 (7.8)	4 (5.3)	14 (2.4)	17 (4.8)	
Missing	1589 (53.4)	1052 (53.5)	36 (47.4)	228 (39.4)	273 (77.3)	

Continued

TABLE 2— Continued

	Overall, No. (%) (n = 2974)	Assault[a], No. (%) (n = 1966)	Self-Inflicted, No. (%) (n = 76)	Unintentional, No. (%) (n = 579)	Missing, No. (%) (n = 353)	P[b]
Previous violent assault/injury events[c]						NA
Gunshot wound	103 (7.4)	87 (9.5)	1 (2.5)	5 (1.4)	10 (12.5)	
Knife stabbing	10 (0.7)	7 (0.8)	0 (0)	1 (0.3)	2 (2.5)	
Sexual assault	6 (0.4)	3 (0.3)	0 (0)	2 (0.6)	1 (1.3)	
Blunt mechanism	69 (5.0)	56 (6.1)	3 (7.5)	6 (1.7)	4 (5.0)	
Strangulation or suffocation	1 (0.1)	1 (0.1)	0 (0)	0 (0)	0 (0)	
Prior suicide attempt/self-harm						< .001
No	1454 (48.9)	959 (48.8)	25 (32.9)	387 (66.8)	83 (23.5)	
Yes	99 (3.3)	55 (2.8)	22 (28.9)	15 (2.6)	7 (2.0)	
Missing	1421 (47.8)	952 (48.4)	29 (38.2)	177 (30.6)	263 (74.5)	
Prior suicide attempt/self-harm events[c]						NA
Suicide attempt	40 (2.6)	20 (2.0)	13 (27.7)	5 (1.2)	2 (2.2)	
Suicidal ideation	61 (3.9)	39 (3.8)	10 (21.3)	8 (2.0)	4 (4.4)	
Suicide threat	14 (0.9)	7 (0.7)	2 (4.3)	3 (0.7)	2 (2.2)	
Self-harm	23 (1.5)	10 (1.0)	8 (17.0)	4 (1.0)	1 (1.1)	

Note. ADD = attention-deficit disorder; ADHD = attention-deficit/hyperactivity disorder; NA = not applicable. All subvariables (specific types of events or illnesses) are not mutually exclusive, and percentages are calculated out of those who answered either "yes" or "no" to the parent variable (i.e., nonmissing data).
[a]Assault includes those who had an "injury intent" of "law enforcement" (n = 6).
[b]Comparisons were made using the Fisher exact test or χ^2 test for categorical variables, and 1-way analysis of variance for continuous variables, with a significance level set at .05.
[c]Among nonmissing (no/yes) data from parent variable.
[d]Other mental illness included obsessive–compulsive disorder, eating disorders, personality disorders, and other.
[e]Five patients answered "yes" to having a traumatic event but then had no further subvariable information (4 in assault, 1 with missing injury intent); hence, the totals in 1 and ≥ 2 traumatic event rows do not add to the number of people who said "yes" to a traumatic event.

Overall, this 12-month study included data on almost 3000 firearm-injured youth. This compares to a yearly average of 4016 pediatric firearm-related injuries reported to the National Trauma Data Bank (NTDB) between 2013 and 2017, despite only capturing 17% of the total NTDB TQIP centers.[12] Our sample size was shy of the yearly average of 4753 pediatric firearm injuries captured between 2003 and 2012 by the Healthcare Cost and Utilization Project (HCUP) Kids database, an all-payer database that samples up to 80% of pediatric discharges from more than 4000 US hospitals.[13] In a study of the HCUP Nationwide Emergency Department Sample, which provides all ages weighted national estimates of hospital-based ED visits, a yearly average of 7351 patients aged younger than 18 years was described (2009–2016).[14] These estimates are all greater than the yearly average of 470 pediatric firearm injuries in the single payer MarketScan database (2010–2016)[15] and the yearly average of 627 in the Pediatric Health Information Systems data (2017–2020), which is limited to 44 US children's hospitals.[16] Altogether, these findings suggest the NTDB TQIP platform performs well to capture pediatric firearm injury (4016 NTDB vs 4753 HCUP during comparable years) and yet captures higher-fidelity data with trained abstractors and more detailed data on hospital care processes and outcomes. In addition, it is critical to note that the Nationwide Emergency Department Sample estimates more than 50% of patients (up to 21 years) are discharged from the ED, and 32% were discharged home from the ED in our study.[14] This highlights the importance of including ED discharges in any surveillance data focused on firearm injuries.

When focused on intent, firearm injury by assault was most common, affecting 66% of the population. Less than 3% of youths were injured by self-harm or suicide, likely because of the high lethality of these injuries, most of which result in death in the field. This is

TABLE 3— Firearm and Event-Related Factors Among Children Aged 18 Years or Younger Presenting to the Emergency Department With Firearm Injury: United States, March 1, 2021–February 28, 2022

	Overall, No. (%) (n = 2974)	Assault,[a] No. (%) (n = 1966)	Self-Inflicted, No. (%) (n = 76)	Unintentional, No. (%) (n = 579)	Missing, No. (%) (n = 353)	P[b]
Firearm type						< .001
BB gun	190 (6.4)	28 (1.4)	2 (2.6)	145 (25.0)	15 (4.2)	
Handgun	1154 (38.8)	736 (37.4)	59 (77.6)	301 (52.0)	58 (16.4)	
Rifle	45 (1.5)	19 (1.0)	2 (2.6)	24 (4.1)	0 (0)	
Shotgun	35 (1.2)	13 (0.7)	2 (2.6)	19 (3.3)	1 (0.3)	
Missing	1550 (52.1)	1170 (59.5)	11 (14.5)	90 (15.5)	279 (79.0)	
Relationship to shooter						< .001[c]
Friend/family/partner	416 (14.0)	148 (7.5)	0 (0)	259 (44.7)	9 (2.5)	
Self	355 (11.9)	3 (0.2)	76 (100)	273 (47.2)	3 (0.8)	
Stranger	1052 (35.4)	1019 (51.8)	0 (0)	12 (2.1)	21 (5.9)	
Law enforcement	7 (0.2)	7 (0.4)	0 (0)	0 (0)	0 (0)	
Relationship not disclosed	106 (3.6)	98 (5.0)	0 (0)	5 (0.9)	3 (0.8)	
Missing	1038 (34.9)	691 (35.1)	0 (0)	30 (5.2)	317 (89.8)	
Firearm access						< .001
No	644 (21.7)	514 (26.1)	3 (3.9)	89 (15.4)	38 (10.8)	
Yes	433 (14.6)	71 (3.6)	40 (52.6)	319 (55.1)	3 (0.8)	
Missing	1897 (63.8)	1381 (70.2)	33 (43.4)	171 (29.5)	312 (88.4)	
Firearm owner access (among those with access)						NA
Self	99 (22.9)	19 (26.8)	5 (12.5)	74 (23.2)	1 (33.3)	
Cohabitant	216 (49.9)	35 (49.3)	25 (62.5)	154 (48.3)	2 (66.7)	
Close residence/neighboring house	102 (23.6)	13 (18.3)	3 (7.5)	86 (27.0)	0 (0)	
Owner of firearm						.001
Stranger	25 (0.8)	1 (0.1)	1 (1.3)	13 (2.2)	10 (2.8)	
Patient (self)	93 (3.1)	0 (0)	8 (10.5)	84 (14.5)	1 (0.3)	
Intimate partner/other family member	248 (8.3)	0 (0.0)	29 (38.2)	216 (37.3)	3 (0.8)	
Acquaintance, friend, or colleague	117 (3.9)	0 (0)	1 (1.3)	113 (19.5)	3 (0.8)	
Missing	2491 (83.8)	1965 (99.9)	37 (48.7)	153 (26.4)	336 (95.2)	
Method of firearm storage						.06[d]
Locked in gun safe, lockbox, or gun lock	22 (0.7)	0 (0)	5 (6.6)	17 (2.9)	0 (0)	
Locked in a stored unit (e.g., drawer, glove box) that is not specifically meant for firearm storage	5 (0.2)	0 (0)	1 (1.3)	4 (0.7)	0 (0)	
Unlocked	315 (10.6)	0 (0)	30 (39.5)	282 (48.7)	3 (0.8)	
Missing	2632 (88.5)	1966 (100)	40 (52.6)	276 (47.7)	350 (99.2)	
Injury setting						< .001
Residence	1071 (36.0)	510 (25.9)	58 (76.3)	423 (73.1)	80 (22.7)	
School/childcare	13 (0.4)	11 (0.6)	0 (0)	1 (0.2)	1 (0.3)	
Motor vehicle	307 (10.3)	246 (12.5)	5 (6.6)	35 (6.0)	21 (5.9)	
Street	816 (27.4)	714 (36.3)	5 (6.6)	23 (4.0)	74 (21.0)	
Woods/forest	33 (1.1)	6 (0.3)	2 (2.6)	24 (4.1)	1 (0.3)	
Public space	268 (9.0)	228 (11.6)	2 (2.6)	17 (2.9)	21 (5.9)	

Continued

TABLE 3— Continued

	Overall, No. (%) (n = 2974)	Assault,[a] No. (%) (n = 1966)	Self-Inflicted, No. (%) (n = 76)	Unintentional, No. (%) (n = 579)	Missing, No. (%) (n = 353)	P^b
Other	20 (0.7)	11 (0.6)	0 (0)	9 (1.6)	0 (0)	
Missing	446 (15.0)	240 (12.2)	4 (5.3)	47 (8.1)	155 (43.9)	

Note. NA = not applicable.
[a]Assault includes those who had an "injury intent" of "law enforcement" (n = 6).
[b]Comparisons were made using the Fisher exact test or χ^2 test for categorical variables, and 1-way analysis of variance for continuous variables, with a significance level set at .05.
[c]*P* value calculated comparing assault, unintentional, and missing intents only.
[d]*P* value calculated comparing self-inflicted and unintentional intents only.

similar to other NTDB analyses in patients aged 0 to 18 years, which have estimates of 71% injured by assault,[12] but notably lower than estimates from other national samples. For example, a recent analysis of the Nationwide Emergency Department Sample estimated 38% of all firearm injuries were from assault, despite the inclusion of patients up to age 21.[14] The differences are likely related to the fidelity of coding by trained registrars as compared with administrative and billing data.

Youths with firearm injuries from assault were predominantly urban, Black,

TABLE 4— Adjusted Odds Ratios of Missingness Among Select Preinjury and Firearm-Related Factors Among Children Aged 18 Years or Younger Presenting to the Emergency Department With Firearm Injury: United States, March 1, 2021–February 28, 2022

	Outcomes, AOR (95% CI)						
Predictors	Adverse Childhood Experiences	Mental Illness	Traumatic Event	Prior Assault/ Injury	Firearm Access	Prior Suicide Attempt/Self Harm	Firearm Type
Age, y (ref: 0–10)							
11–14	1.24 (0.89, 1.73)	1.10 (0.68, 1.80)	1.25 (0.89, 1.76)	2.26 (1.59, 3.23)	1.84 (1.31, 2.58)	3.27 (2.21, 4.92)	1.37 (0.97, 1.94)
15–18	1.97 (1.48, 2.63)	1.52 (1.02, 2.32)	1.88 (1.41, 2.52)	3.78 (2.79, 5.18)	2.61 (1.95, 3.49)	4.75 (3.36, 6.85)	1.47 (1.09, 1.99)
ISS (ref: 0–15)							
16–25	0.92 (0.69, 1.22)	0.81 (0.55, 1.17)	1.06 (0.80, 1.41)	1.01 (0.76, 1.34)	1.02 (0.75, 1.38)	0.84 (0.62, 1.12)	1.25 (0.94, 1.68)
> 25	1.03 (0.71, 1.49)	0.75 (0.45, 1.22)	0.76 (0.52, 1.10)	0.80 (0.55, 1.16)	0.82 (0.56, 1.22)	0.94 (0.64, 1.37)	0.96 (0.66, 1.40)
DCI (ref: low)							
Medium	1.03 (0.71, 1.49)	0.75 (0.45, 1.22)	0.76 (0.52, 1.10)	0.80 (0.55, 1.16)	0.82 (0.56, 1.22)	0.94 (0.64, 1.37)	0.96 (0.66, 1.40)
High	0.99 (0.77, 1.28)	1.08 (0.78, 1.50)	1.00 (0.78, 1.29)	0.98 (0.76, 1.27)	0.96 (0.73, 1.26)	1.24 (0.96, 1.61)	1.26 (0.97, 1.64)
Designation (ref: adult)							
Pediatric and adult	0.63 (0.51, 0.78)	0.49 (0.37, 0.65)	0.79 (0.65, 0.97)	1.45 (1.17, 1.80)	1.20 (0.95, 1.52)	1.20 (0.97, 1.48)	1.41 (1.13, 1.75)
Pediatric	0.26 (0.21, 0.32)	0.44 (0.33, 0.59)	0.26 (0.21, 0.33)	0.43 (0.35, 0.54)	0.48 (0.39, 0.60)	0.36 (0.28, 0.45)	1.83 (1.45, 2.30)
Injury intent (ref: assault)							
Self-Inflicted	0.40 (0.18, 0.84)	0.57 (0.14, 1.64)	0.66 (0.31, 1.34)	0.29 (0.13, 0.62)	0.16 (0.07, 0.34)	0.35 (0.15, 0.77)	0.12 (0.05, 0.28)
Unintentional	0.86 (0.69, 1.08)	0.84 (0.61, 1.14)	1.21 (0.97, 1.52)	0.92 (0.74, 1.16)	0.24 (0.19, 0.30)	0.76 (0.60, 0.97)	0.12 (0.09, 0.15)
Missing	2.84 (2.09, 3.90)	2.15 (1.61, 2.86)	3.20 (2.39, 4.32)	3.58 (2.64, 4.91)	3.58 (2.47, 5.34)	3.95 (2.92, 5.40)	2.60 (1.93, 3.55)
Admission status (ref: admitted)							
Not admitted	1.89 (1.57, 2.29)	1.33 (1.06, 1.66)	1.32 (1.09, 1.58)	1.32 (1.09, 1.59)	1.33 (1.09, 1.62)	1.46 (1.21, 1.76)	1.13 (0.93, 1.36)

Note. AOR = adjusted odds ratio; CI = confidence interval; DCI = Distressed Community Index; ISS = Injury Severity Scale. Results among surviving patients. Each outcome of interest is represented by a column, with AORs and 95% CIs reported for each predictor of interest. The odds ratio for each predictor is adjusted for all other predictors in the table.

and male. This is concordant with multiple national and regional data sources.[3,5,17,18] In addition, DCI quintiles varied by intent, with a greater proportion of assault-injured youths living in at-risk or distressed communities. Trinidad et al. found similar results when exploring socioeconomic deprivation and its relationship to pediatric firearm injury.[18] The authors found that neighborhood deprivation was associated with assault and that youths from the neighborhoods in the highest quintile of deprivation accounted for 57% of all firearm-related injuries and 70% of all firearm-related injuries from assault.[18] This compares to 43% and 45% in our population, respectively. Importantly, while DCI and neighborhood deprivation are both measures of socioeconomic status and neighborhood context, they differ in their component variables, which may explain differences in estimates.[19–21]

Unique to this study was the systematic capture of preinjury risk factors. Among youths with nonmissing data, 42% report at least 1 ACE, 16% a prior mental illness, 38% at least 1 traumatic event (distinct from the defined ACEs), 14% a previous violent assault, and 6% a previous suicide attempt. When comparing to precedent literature, there are similarities and differences. For example, in a study of youths aged 3 to 17 years, Ehrlich et al. looked at Medicaid claims and reported that 20% of the firearm-injured population had a claim related to a mental health diagnosis before their injury.[22] Oddo et al. analyzed Medicaid and commercial claims in youths aged 0 to 17 years injured by firearms and, in the 12-month preinjury period, reported 39% had a mental health diagnosis.[23]

Our estimates differ, however, when comparing to the general youth population. For example, among ACE subtypes, in the 2016 National Survey of Children's Health (NSCH), 21.9% respondents reported parental divorce compared with 31.1% in our study.[24] About 7% of children in the NSCH reported a parent or guardian served time in jail, which is similar to the 6.7% of youths in our study who reported an incarcerated household member. Finally, NSCH estimates for intimate partner violence exposure, household substance misuse, and mental illness were 5.0%, 8.1%, and 7.1%, respectively, compared with 2.4%, 4.5%, and 3.8% in our study for similar variables. Only 3.9% of youths had documented major depression in our study (at any point before their injury); an estimated 15.7% of youths aged 12 to 17 years nationally had at least 1 major depressive episode in 2019.[25] Many of these differences in estimates are likely related to differences in study design, including survey versus chart review, sampling frame, and data capture methods.

Our study was also novel in its attempt to systematically capture contextual factors related to the firearm injury event, including firearm type, relationship to shooter, firearm access, firearm storage, and injury setting, among others. While the National Violent Death Reporting System does collect some of these data elements, there are high rates of missingness in those data as well.[26] Choi et al. extracted the circumstances of shooting, relationship of shooter, and type of firearm from the charts at a level I pediatric trauma center in the Midwest; however, the type of firearm was not reported in the results, and how missingness for each data element was addressed was not described.[27] Interestingly, in the study by Choi et al., patients aged 12 years or younger were often injured by someone who was known to them (44%) and from an accidental shooting (62%), while older patients, aged 13 to 17 years, were usually injured by an "unknown assailant" (59%) and as an assault (62%).[27] Presumably, unknown assailant indicates a stranger and not missing data from the authors' chart review. Overall, however, the findings by Choi et al. corroborate our findings in which "family/friend/partner" as perpetrator accounted for 45% of unintentional firearm injuries, while assault-related injuries were reported to be caused by a stranger in 52% of cases.

Perhaps most critical to our findings was the exploration into missing data. Missingness imposes significant challenges to data interpretability and generalizability and hampers the ability of researchers to make meaningful and valid conclusions. Despite its importance in data inference, missingness is rarely reported as evidenced by recent studies in pediatric firearm injury from the NTDB,[12] institutional data,[27,28] and other national samples.[14] Others report and appropriately acknowledge missingness as a limitation, though with low rates and little exploration into the type of, and reason for, missingness.[29]

As hypothesized, certain patient, injury, and hospital characteristics played a role in missingness. For example, assault was associated with more missing data than self-inflicted and unintentional injuries, as was older age, even when we controlled for intent. This may reflect a discomfort by providers and staff to ask questions or by patients to share information when asked, perhaps because of a concern that information may be used against them or reflect an overall lack of trust of the health care system. Missing intent was strongly associated with missingness in all variables of interest, which may reflect overall hospital and trauma program resources. In addition, lack of admission, even while controlling for injury severity, was associated with higher missingness. In addition, pediatric-only centers had more missingness for firearm type but had less missingness for all other variables. This may reflect more limited resources or may reflect comfort level with specific questions by the care team.

Limitations

This study had a number of limitations. First, and most importantly, the extent of missingness significantly limits the inference possible within the data—hence, the dedicated missingness analysis. The study captured only what was recorded in the electronic medical record, so it is very likely, particularly for the novel data elements, that the missingness or unknown reflects not being asked about specific circumstances or a lack of clear documentation. This may be attributable to lack of comfort or time, biases and assumptions, and more. Second, this study captured only those patients who presented to a participating center, limiting its generalizability. That being said, it is the largest study on pediatric firearm injury that captures pre-existing risk factors and contextual factors related to the incident, for both fatal and nonfatal injury. Third, this study did not capture patients who died at the scene, which likely biases the results toward intents that are less fatal (i.e., assault and unintentional injury).

Public Health Implications

Our study highlights notable findings related to pediatric firearm injury. Preinjury factors such as ACEs and previous mental health diagnoses, traumatic events, assaults, suicide attempts, and self-harm events are common but not ubiquitous, and, while there is variability by intent in terms of patient demographics, the data indicate that no child is immune to firearm injury. The data also suggest that health care systems nationally must focus on improved documentation and data collection, specifically for elements related to the injury context, including firearm and event-related factors. Overall, the variability and high rates of missingness suggest both systems and process measures must be targeted for improved data collection. Clinicians and other care team members should understand that such information is key to providing and improving the care provided to children and adolescents sustaining firearm injuries. AJPH

ABOUT THE AUTHORS

Katherine T. Flynn-O'Brien is with the Department of Surgery, Medical College of Wisconsin, Milwaukee. Chethan Sathya is with the Division of Pediatric Surgery, Cohen Children's Medical Center, New Hyde Park, NY. Meera Kotagal is with the Division of Pediatric General and Thoracic Surgery, Cincinnati Children's Hospital Medical Center, Cincinnati, OH. Samantha Banks is with the Firearm Injury and Policy Research Program, University of Washington, Seattle. Lauren L. Agoubi is with the Department of Surgery, University of Washington, Seattle. Deborah A. Kuhls is with the Department of Surgery, Kirk Kerkorian School of Medicine, Las Vegas, NV. Avery Nathens is with Sunnybrook Health Sciences Center, Toronto, Ontario, Canada. Ashley B. Hink is with the Department of Surgery, Medical University of South Carolina, Charleston. Frederick P. Rivara is with the Departments of Pediatrics and Epidemiology, University of Washington, Seattle.

CORRESPONDENCE

Correspondence should be sent to Katherine Flynn-O'Brien, MD, MPH, Medical College of Wisconsin and Children's Wisconsin, 999 N 92nd St, Milwaukee, WI 53226 (e-mail: kflynnobrien@mcw.edu). Reprints can be ordered at https://www.ajph.org by clicking the "Reprints" link.

PUBLICATION INFORMATION

Full Citation: Flynn-O'Brien KT, Sathya C, Kotagal M, et al. Preinjury and event-related characteristics of pediatric firearm injuries: The American College of Surgeons Firearm Study, United States, March 2021–February 2022. *Am J Public Health.* 2024;114(10):1097–1109.

Acceptance Date: June 6, 2024.

DOI: https://doi.org/10.2105/AJPH.2024.307754

ORCID iDs:

Katherine T. Flynn-O'Brien https://orcid.org/0000-0001-5450-7278

Chethan Sathya https://orcid.org/0000-0003-4846-7673

Samantha Banks https://orcid.org/0009-0007-2677-6594

Lauren L. Agoubi https://orcid.org/0000-0003-0727-4365

CONTRIBUTORS

K. T. Flynn-O'Brien, C. Sathya, M. Kotagal, S. Banks, and L. L. Agoubi contributed to the data analysis, data interpretation, and writing and critical revision of the article. F. P. Rivara contributed to the study design, data analysis, data interpretation, and writing and critical revision of the article. D. A. Kuhls, A. Nathens, and A. B. Hink contributed to the study design, data interpretation, and writing and critical revision of the article. All authors approve of the final version to be published.

ACKNOWLEDGMENTS

This study was funded by the National Collaborative on Gun Violence Research by a grant to the American College of Surgeons.

We would like to acknowledge all participating institutions and their leaders who contributed data for this study as represented in Appendix B (available as a supplement to the online version of this article at https://ajph.org).

CONFLICTS OF INTEREST

The authors have no conflicts of interest to report.

HUMAN PARTICIPANT PROTECTION

The study was approved by Advarra Center for Institutional Review Board Intelligence.

REFERENCES

1. Goldstick JE, Cunningham RM, Carter PM. Current causes of death in children and adolescents in the United States. *N Engl J Med.* 2022;386(20):1955–1956. https://doi.org/10.1056/NEJMc2201761
2. Centers for Disease Control and Prevention, National Center for Injury Prevention and Control. Web-based Injury Statistics Query and Reporting System (WISQARS). 2023; Available at: https://www.cdc.gov/injury/wisqars. Accessed April 1, 2023.
3. Fowler KA, Dahlberg LL, Haileyesus T, Gutierrez C, Bacon S. Childhood firearm injuries in the United States. *Pediatrics.* 2017;140(1):e20163486. https://doi.org/10.1542/peds.2016-3486

4. Hendry PL, Suen A, Kalynych CJ, Lott M, Paul J, Smotherman C. A 6-year retrospective review of pediatric firearm injuries: do patients < 14 years of age differ from those 15–18 years of age? *J Trauma Acute Care Surg*. 2014;77(3, suppl 1):S41–S45. https://doi.org/10.1097/TA.0000000000000384
5. Hughes BD, Cummins CB, Shan Y, Mehta HB, Radhakrishnan RS, Bowen-Jallow KA. Pediatric firearm injuries: racial disparities and predictors of healthcare outcomes. *J Pediatr Surg*. 2020; 55(8):1596–1603. https://doi.org/10.1016/j.jpedsurg.2020.02.021
6. Centers for Disease Control and Prevention. National Violent Death Reporting System. 2023. Available at: https://www.cdc.gov/violenceprevention/datasources/nvdrs/index.html. Accessed May 16, 2023.
7. US Department of Health and Human Services, Centers for Disease Control and Prevention, National Center for Injury Prevention Control. Firearm Injury Surveillance Study, 1993–2021. Ann Arbor, MI: Inter-university Consortium for Political and Social Research; 2023.
8. *National Trauma Data Standard Data Dictionary: 2020 Admissions*. Chicago, IL: American College of Surgeons Committee on Trauma; 2020.
9. Rivara FP, Hink AB, Kuhls DA, et al. Firearm injuries treated at trauma centers in the United States. *J Trauma Acute Care Surg*. 202496(6): 955–964. doi:10.1097/TA.0000000000004172.
10. Economic Innovation Group. Distressed communities. Introduction to the Distressed Community Index. 2023. Available at: https://eig.org/distressed-communities. Accessed May 31, 2023.
11. Wickham H. *ggplot2: Elegant Graphics for Data Analysis*. 2nd ed. New York, NY: Springer-Verlag; 2016.
12. Cheng T, Burjonrappa S. Pediatric firearm injury trends in the United States: a National Trauma Data Bank (NTDB) analysis. *J Pediatr Surg*. 2022; 57(2):278–283. https://doi.org/10.1016/j.jpedsurg.2021.10.040
13. Taylor JS, Madhavan S, Han RW, Chandler JM, Tenakoon L, Chao S. Financial burden of pediatric firearm-related injury admissions in the United States. *PLoS One*. 2021;16(6):e0252821. https://doi.org/10.1371/journal.pone.0252821
14. Patel SJ, Badolato GM, Parikh K, Iqbal SF, Goyal MK. Sociodemographic factors and outcomes by intent of firearm injury. *Pediatrics*. 2021;147(4): e2020011957. https://doi.org/10.1542/peds.2020-011957
15. Pulcini CD, Goyal MK, Hall M, et al. Mental health utilization and expenditures for children pre–post firearm injury. *Am J Prev Med*. 2021;61(1):133–135. https://doi.org/10.1016/j.amepre.2021.01.024
16. Gastineau KAB, Williams DJ, Hall M, et al. Pediatric firearm-related hospital encounters during the SARS-CoV-2 pandemic. *Pediatrics*. 2021; 148(2):e2021050223. https://doi.org/10.1542/peds.2021-050223
17. Goldstick JE, Carter PM, Cunningham RM. Current epidemiological trends in firearm mortality in the United States. *JAMA Psychiatry*. 2021;78(3): 241–242. https://doi.org/10.1001/jamapsychiatry.2020.2986
18. Trinidad S, Vancil A, Brokamp C, et al. Relationships between socioeconomic deprivation and pediatric firearm-related injury at the neighborhood level. *J Trauma Acute Care Surg*. 2022;93(3): 283–290. https://doi.org/10.1097/TA.0000000000003679
19. Trinidad S, Brokamp C, Mor Huertas A, et al. Use of area-based socioeconomic deprivation indices: a scoping review and qualitative analysis. *Health Aff (Millwood)*. 2022;41(12):1804–1811. https://doi.org/10.1377/hlthaff.2022.00482
20. Trinidad S, Kotagal M. Social determinants of health as drivers of inequities in pediatric injury. *Semin Pediatr Surg*. 2022;31(5):151221. https://doi.org/10.1016/j.sempedsurg.2022.151221
21. Dalve K, Gause E, Mills B, Floyd AS, Rivara FP, Rowhani-Rahbar A. Neighborhood disadvantage and firearm injury: does shooting location matter? *Inj Epidemiol*. 2021;8(1):10. https://doi.org/10.1186/s40621-021-00304-2
22. Ehrlich PF, Pulcini CD, De Souza HG, et al. Mental healthcare following firearm and motor vehicle related injuries: differences impacting our treatment strategies. *Ann Surg*. 2022;276(3):463–471. https://doi.org/10.1097/SLA.0000000000005557
23. Oddo ER, Maldonado L, Hink AB, Simpson AN, Andrews AL. Increase in mental health diagnoses among youth with nonfatal firearm injuries. *Acad Pediatr*. 2021;21(7):1203–1208. https://doi.org/10.1016/j.acap.2021.06.003
24. Crouch E, Probst JC, Radcliff E, Bennett KJ, McKinney SH. Prevalence of adverse childhood experiences (ACEs) among US children. *Child Abuse Negl*. 2019;92:209–218. https://doi.org/10.1016/j.chiabu.2019.04.010
25. Behavioral Health Barometer: United States, Volume 6: Indicators as measured through the 2019 National Survey on Drug Use and Health and the National Survey of Substance Abuse Treatment Services. Rockville, MD: Substance Abuse and Mental Health Services Administration; 2020.
26. Hink AB, Bonne S, Levy M, et al. Firearm injury research and epidemiology: a review of the data, their limitations, and how trauma centers can improve firearm injury research. *J Trauma Acute Care Surg*. 2019;87(3):678–689. https://doi.org/10.1097/TA.0000000000002330
27. Choi PM, Dekonenko C, Aguayo P, Juang D. Pediatric firearm injuries: a Midwest experience. *J Pediatr Surg*. 2020;55(10):2140–2143. https://doi.org/10.1016/j.jpedsurg.2020.06.027
28. Carter PM, Walton MA, Roehler DR, et al. Firearm violence among high-risk emergency department youth after an assault injury. *Pediatrics*. 2015; 135(5):805–815. https://doi.org/10.1542/peds.2014-3572
29. Vasan A, Mitchell HK, Fein JA, Buckler DG, Wiebe DJ, South EC. Association of neighborhood gun violence with mental health–related pediatric emergency department utilization. *JAMA Pediatr*. 2021;175(12):1244–1251. https://doi.org/10.1001/jamapediatrics.2021.3512

Structural Stigma and Disparities in Long-Term Health Conditions Among Australians in Same-Sex Relationships: 2021 Australian Census

Karinna Saxby, PhD, Yuting Zhang, PhD, and Zoe Aitken, PhD

Objectives. To explore the extent to which structural stigma (sociocultural and institutional constraining factors) is associated with sexual orientation disparities in long-term health conditions.

Methods. We measured structural stigma using the regional percentage of votes against same-sex marriage from Australia's 2017 Marriage Equality Survey and mapped this to the 2021 Census survey of 10 093 399 and 136 988 individuals in different-sex and same-sex relationships, respectively. Controlling for individual and area-level confounders, we used logistic regression analyses to examine the association between quartiles of structural stigma and sexual orientation disparities in long-term health conditions (e.g., any, mental health, asthma, cardiovascular).

Results. In the lowest stigma quartile, individuals in same-sex relationships had 56% higher odds of reporting any long-term health condition (odds ratio [OR] = 1.56; 95% confidence interval [CI] = 1.53, 1.59) and this increased to 63% in the highest stigma quartile (OR = 1.63; 95% CI = 1.58, 1.68). Effects were particularly pronounced for cardiovascular, respiratory, and mental health conditions as well as for men, younger populations, and those living in socioeconomically deprived regions.

Conclusions. Living in stigmatizing environments may have deleterious health effects for sexual minorities in Australia. Policy action and enhanced protections for sexual minorities are urgently required. (*Am J Public Health*. 2024;114(10):1110–1122. https://doi.org/10.2105/AJPH.2024.307759)

AJPH October 2024, Vol. 114, No. 10

Sexual orientation has unequivocally emerged as a risk factor for poorer health outcomes. Compared with their heterosexual counterparts, sexual minorities are at higher risk of mental health disorders[1]; acute respiratory and inflammatory illnesses, such as asthma and arthritis[2,3]; and circulatory conditions, such as heart disease and hypertension.[4] There is also evidence suggesting that these health disparities may translate into premature mortality among sexual minorities.[5]

Structural stigma, which encompasses institutional and societal-level conditions that disadvantage or constrain sexual minorities, is postulated to be a critical factor contributing to these health disparities by inducing heightened social stress, risky health behaviors, and reduced health care seeking.[6] Previous research has demonstrated that structural stigma is associated with poorer mental health,[7,8] higher rates of cigarette smoking and drug use,[9–11] and reduced use of primary and preventive health care among sexual minorities.[12–14]

The impact of structural stigma on long-term health conditions has been less explored. The paucity of research in this space is due, in part, to the lack of population-level data containing information on both sexual identity and health outcomes.[15] Plausibly, stigma could predict poorer health among sexual minorities for some conditions more than others. This could, in turn, provide some evidence on the mechanisms leading to sexual orientation health disparities. For instance, consistent with a large body of previous work, experiences of discrimination and psychological distress are likely to predict a greater prevalence of mental health disorders among sexual minorities.[16] Furthermore, there is some evidence that exposure to stigma and associated stressors can detrimentally impact circulatory conditions among sexual minorities via elevated heart rates and higher blood pressure.[17] Moreover, given stigma has been associated with smoking and heavy alcohol consumption[9–11]—known risk factors for cardiovascular and respiratory diseases—we may expect to see that stigma predicts disparities in heart and lung conditions. More broadly, structural stigma could impact health via reduced access to health care. This could occur via stigma-induced reductions in self-care or reduced availability of inclusive health care.[6,12,18] Reduced access to primary and preventive health care could, in turn, lead to poorer health trajectories and potentially preventable long-term chronic health conditions. Altogether, the extent to which structural stigma is associated with long-term health conditions, and which condition types, remains an important empirical question.

Addressing this important gap in the literature, this study exploits recent innovations in Australian data linkage infrastructure to investigate the extent to which structural stigma is associated with disparities in long-term health conditions among Australians in same-sex relationships. We additionally contribute to the evidence base by exploring whether stigma effects vary by type of chronic condition and key sociodemographic characteristics including sex, age, and socioeconomic deprivation.

METHODS

The data sourced for this analysis come from the Person Level Integrated Data Asset (PLIDA; https://www.abs.gov.au/about/data-services/data-integration/integrated-data/person-level-integrated-data-asset-plida). PLIDA is an individual-level linked data set that combines information from population Census and various administrative records including health care, income and taxation, government payments, location, employment, and mortality.[12,19] The majority of individuals' demographic information is sourced from the Census, and this is a key source of linkage to other data sets included within PLIDA. This study sourced data from the 2021 Australian Census. Completing the Census is mandatory in Australia, and, in 2021, approximately 96% of dwellings completed the Census.[20] Critically, for our study, the 2021 Census contains information on individuals' relationship status, their health outcomes, and their residential location.

Measures

Sexual orientation classification. Information on sexual orientation, gender diversity, or innate variations of sex characteristics is currently not available in PLIDA. Individuals in same-sex and heterosexual relationships were therefore identified based on responses to the Census question on household relationships. Individuals in "de facto marriage, same-sex couple" or "registered marriage, same-sex couple" were classified as being in a same-sex relationship while individuals in different-sex relationships were identified from being either "in de facto marriage, opposite-sex couple" or "in a registered marriage, opposite-sex couple." The baseline sample comprised all individuals linked to the PLIDA spine and aged 18 years and older and in either a same-sex or different-sex relationship at the time of the 2021 Census. Full details of the sample construction are provided in Figure A (available as a supplement to the online version of this article at https://ajph.org). Our final sample of cohabiting adults in relationships (n = 10 230 387) comprises 10 093 399 (98.7%) and 136 988 (1.3%) individuals in different-sex and same-sex relationships, respectively. A comparison of the sample to the Census sample is provided in Table A (available as a supplement to the online version of this article at https://ajph.org).

Long-term health conditions. The Australian 2021 Census included a question on long-term health conditions: "Have you been told by a doctor or nurse that you have any of these long-term health conditions" with the following details: "include health conditions that have lasted or are expected to last for six months or more; include health conditions that may recur from time to time, or are controlled by medication; or are in remission."[21] The following response options were provided: arthritis, asthma, cancer (including remission), dementia, diabetes (excluding gestational diabetes), heart disease (including heart attack or angina), kidney disease, lung condition (including chronic obstructive pulmonary disorder or emphysema), mental health condition (including depression or anxiety), stroke, any other long-term health condition, or no long-term health condition. The selected health conditions were chosen based on outcomes of stakeholder consultation and were explicitly included based upon "relevance to inform services, policy, and research."[21]

Structural stigma. In 2017, the Australian government conducted a national survey on the legalization of same-sex marriage (the Australian Marriage Law Postal Survey [AMLPS]). The AMLPS asked the question "Should the law be changed to allow same-sex couples to marry?" allowing only a "yes" or "no" response. All Australian citizens aged 18 years and older and on the electoral roll were eligible to vote, and, although voting was not mandatory, 79.5% of eligible Australians participated. The results showed that the majority of voting Australians (61.6%) thought the law should be changed to allow same-sex couples to marry.[22] This led to eventual policy change in December 2017.

There was, however, significant regional variation in the responses to the AMLPS. Quartiles of votes against marriage equality are presented in Figure 1. For example, the highest and lowest regional percentage of votes against legalizing same-sex marriage out of the eligible voting population (55.5% and 13.1% respectively, compared with 38.4% overall) were both found in metropolitan regions within Australia's most populous state, New South Wales.

Following previous research,[7,12,13] we defined structural stigma as the regional proportion of votes against legalizing same-sex marriage. Specifically, we calculated the percentage of votes against legalizing same-sex marriage (total number of votes against legalizing same-sex marriage out of the total eligible voting population) for each of the 150 electoral divisions across Australia. These are then categorized into quartiles based on the national distribution as "low stigma" (representing [13.1%–26.3%] votes against same-sex marriage), "low–moderate stigma" [representing (26.3%–30.1%] votes against same-sex marriage], "moderate–high stigma" [representing (30.1%–34.3%] votes against same-sex marriage], and "high stigma" [representing (34.3%–55.5%] votes against same-sex marriage].

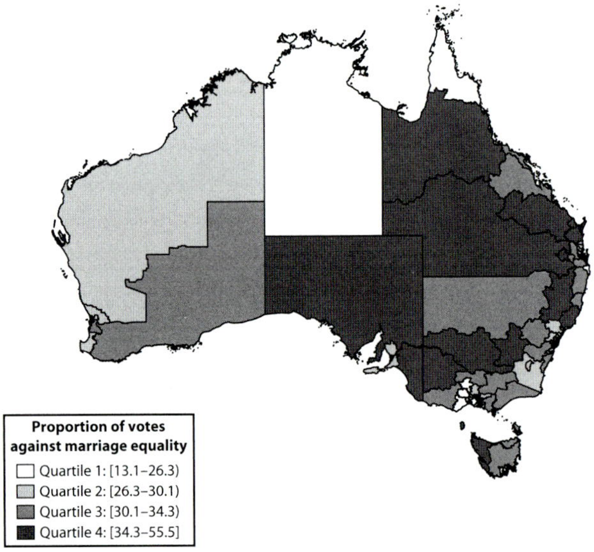

FIGURE 1— Percentage of Votes Against Legalizing Same-Sex Marriage by Electoral Districts: Australian Marriage Law Postal Survey, 2017

Note. Figure shows proportion of votes against legalizing same-sex marriage out of total eligible voting population. Categories are presented in quartiles. In these categories, square brackets (e.g., "[a–b]") indicate that the range includes the endpoint values, while a round bracket indicates exclusion of that endpoint value (e.g., "(a–b]" includes b but not a).

Statistical Analysis

For all individuals in our sample, we first assigned their regional level of stigma (quartiles of votes against same-sex marriage) based on their electorate of residence at the time of the Census. To test whether sexual orientation disparities in health outcomes vary across different levels of structural stigma, we conducted a series of logistic regression models of the following form (one for any long-term health condition and each type of long-term health condition excluding dementia, which had only 256 individuals in same-sex relationships reporting dementia):

$$\ln\left(\frac{p_{y_{ir}}}{1-p_{y_{ir}}}\right) = \alpha_0 + \sum_{k=1}^{4} \beta_k (SSR_i \times \mathbf{S_{kr}}) + \theta_l \gamma_r + \zeta_m \mathbf{X}_i \quad (1)$$

where $p_{y_{ir}}$ represents the probability that individual i living in electorate r reports the outcome of interest, SSR_i is a binary indicator equal to 1 if the individual is in a same-sex relationship, and $\mathbf{S}_r$ is a categorical variable representing the quartile of structural stigma in electorate r. We include an interaction term in the model between the exposure variable (in same-sex relationship) and the stigma quartile variable to examine how sexual orientation disparities in outcomes differ across levels of structural stigma.

To control for potential regional-level confounders of the relationship between structural stigma and health, we controlled for region fixed effects at the electoral level (γ_r). This captures differences in regional-level factors that could impact health such as access and supply of health care, air pollution, socioeconomic status, and crime. As the measure of structural stigma is a fixed measure (i.e., based off responses to the AMLPS in 2017), the region fixed effects also capture the influence of structural stigma on outcomes among those in different-sex relationships.

In $\boldsymbol{X}_i$, we controlled for a vector of individual-level characteristics that could impact health and have been applied in similar analyses[7,8,12]—namely, age, sex (male, female), educational attainment (less than high school, high school, professional, or university or above), country of birth, and equivalized household income.

The main coefficients of interest are captured in β_k and represent the odds of an individual in a same-sex relationship reporting outcome *y* compared with an individual in a different-sex relationship across different levels of structural stigma. We used the Wald test to assess whether disparities in quartiles 2 to 4 were statistically different from quartile 1 (i.e., the lowest level of stigma). We applied the Romano–Wolf multiple-hypothesis correction to account for familywise error.[23]

We then explored whether associations between stigma and sexual orientation disparities in long-term health conditions varied by key demographic subgroups. This was achieved by running subgroup analyses that have been used in similar studies in the Australian context.[7,12] Specifically, we separately estimated whether there was variation by age group (< 40 years, 40–64 years, ≥ 65 years), sex (male, female), rurality (metropolitan, rural), area-level deprivation (bottom five deciles of socioeconomic disadvantage: "low"; top five deciles of socioeconomic disadvantage: "high"), and education (less than university, university level). Similar to our baseline analysis, for each subgroup, we used the Wald test to assess whether disparities in quartiles 2 to 4 were statistically different from quartile 1 and applied the Romano–Wolf multiple-hypothesis correction.[23]

For all models, we handled missing data for covariates by using the missing-indicator method. We conducted all analyses with Stata version 17 (StataCorp LP, College Station, TX).

RESULTS

The descriptive characteristics of the study sample are presented in Table 1.

Descriptive Characteristics

Compared with individuals in different-sex relationships, on average, individuals in same-sex relationships were younger (mean 43 vs 51 years), had higher levels of educational attainment, had higher household incomes, and were less likely to be married (29% vs 81%).

A slightly higher proportion of individuals in same-sex relationships reported 1 or more long-term health condition at the time of the Census (41% vs 38%). Among all long-term health conditions, the largest observed difference was the proportion of individuals who reported mental health conditions; 17% of individuals in same-sex relationships reported a mental health condition compared with 8% of individuals in different-sex relationships. Asthma was also slightly higher among sexual minorities (12% vs 9%).

Compared with individuals in different-sex relationships, individuals in same-sex relationships were more likely to live in metropolitan areas, areas with a lower proportion of votes against Marriage Equality (mean 27% vs 31% no votes), and areas with less area-level deprivation. On average, individuals in same-sex relationships were less likely to have missing data on individual-level characteristics than those in different-sex relationships (e.g., 6% missing educational attainment for those in same-sex relationships compared with 12% for those in different-sex relationships). Missing information for long-term health conditions was similar across both groups (3%).

Compared with other adults in the Census, the study sample had higher levels of educational attainment, had higher household incomes, and were more likely to live in areas with less area-level deprivation (Table A).

Regression Analyses

The results of the regression analyses for reporting a long-term health condition are presented in Table 2. The results for each type of long-term health condition are presented in Table B (available as a supplement to the online version of this article at https://ajph.org). These show, for each quartile of structural stigma (votes against marriage equality), the relative odds of an individual in a same-sex relationship reporting a health condition, compared with those in different-sex relationships. Across all different levels of stigma, individuals in same-sex relationships had higher odds of reporting any long-term health condition compared with those in different-sex relationships. Greater levels of stigma were associated with widening sexual orientation disparities

TABLE 1— Descriptive Characteristics of Individuals in Same-Sex and Different-Sex Relationships: 2021 Australian Census

	In Different-Sex Relationship (n = 10 093 399), Mean (SD) or Proportion (No.)	In Same-Sex Relationship (n = 136 988), Mean (SD) or Proportion (No.)
Individual characteristics		
Age, y	50.60 (15.8)	43.29 (13.9)
Female	0.50 (5 085 594)	0.50 (67 853)
In registered marriage	0.81 (8 193 348)	0.29 (39 405)
Educational attainment		
Less than high school	0.13 (1 270 708)	0.07 (9 547)
Year 12	0.12 (1 206 786)	0.13 (18 091)
Professional	0.31 (3 124 297)	0.27 (37 553)
University or above	0.33 (3 330 358)	0.47 (63 941)
Missing	0.12 (1 161 250)	0.06 (7 856)
Equivalized household income	73 994 (43 646)	98 367 (48 258)
Country of birth		
Australia	0.63 (6 316 203)	0.69 (94 212)
New Zealand	0.03 (266 764)	0.04 (4 905)
Melanesia, Micronesia, Polynesia	0.01 (85 687)	0.00 (628)
United Kingdom	0.06 (645 288)	0.07 (9 157)
Ireland	0.00 (45 546)	0.01 (813)
Western Europe	0.01 (126 856)	0.01 (1 809)
Northern Europe	0.00 (17 524)	0.00 (239)
Southern Europe	0.01 (131 059)	0.01 (1 013)
Southeastern Europe	0.02 (176 278)	0.00 (660)
Eastern Europe	0.01 (69 222)	0.00 (618)
North Africa	0.00 (36 506)	0.00 (148)
Middle East	0.02 (198 470)	0.01 (902)
Mainland Southeast Asia	0.02 (213 434)	0.02 (2 658)
Maritime Southeast Asia	0.03 (309 594)	0.04 (5 532)
Chinese Asia	0.03 (349 088)	0.03 (4 246)
Japan and the Koreas	0.01 (74 271)	0.00 (661)
Southern Asia	0.05 (553 723)	0.01 (1 444)
Central Asia	0.00 (32 235)	0.00 (131)
North America	0.01 (75 175)	0.02 (2 353)
South America	0.01 (68 571)	0.01 (1 644)
Central America	0.00 (10 235)	0.00 (221)
Caribbean	0.00 (2975)	0.00 (59)
Central and West Africa	0.00 (14 830)	0.00 (91)
Southern and East Africa	0.02 (181 497)	0.02 (2 088)
Missing	0.01 (92 368)	0.01 (756)
Health conditions		
One or more long-term health condition(s)	0.38 (3 813 846)	0.41 (56 683)
Arthritis	0.11 (1 102 042)	0.08 (10 550)
Asthma	0.09 (864 968)	0.12 (16 736)
Cancer (including remission)	0.04 (414 839)	0.03 (4 002)
Diabetes (excluding gestational diabetes)	0.06 (650 811)	0.04 (5 248)

Continued

TABLE 1— Continued

	In Different-Sex Relationship (n = 10 093 399), Mean (SD) or Proportion (No.)	In Same-Sex Relationship (n = 136 988), Mean (SD) or Proportion (No.)
Heart disease (including heart attack or angina)	0.05 (521 236)	0.03 (3 904)
Kidney disease	0.01 (106 457)	0.01 (954)
Lung condition (including COPD and emphysema)	0.02 (189 129)	0.01 (1 732)
Mental health condition (including depression or anxiety)	0.08 (840 007)	0.17 (23 291)
Other long-term health condition(s)	0.09 (915 195)	0.12 (16 007)
Stroke	0.01 (106 783)	0.01 (826)
Missing	0.03 (315 340)	0.03 (3 551)
	Regional characteristics	
Regional percentage of "no" votes	30.7 (7.0)	27.2 (8.0)
Quartile of "no" votes out of eligible population		
Q1 (lowest)	0.23 (2 321 176)	0.42 (57 255)
Q2	0.28 (2 777 579)	0.25 (34 562)
Q3	0.24 (2 380 725)	0.17 (23 346)
Q4 (highest)	0.26 (2 613 919)	0.16 (21 825)
Low socioeconomic deprivation	0.45 (4 578 171)	0.39 (53 504)
Missing socioeconomic deprivation score	0.11 (1 083 090)	0.12 (15 907)
Rurality		
Metropolitan	0.73 (7 335 233)	0.79 (108 589)
Rural	0.27 (2 758 166)	0.21 (28 399)

Note. COPD = chronic obstructive pulmonary disease. Characteristics based on values reported at the time of the 2021 Census. All differences in characteristics between individuals in different-sex and same-sex relationships were statistically significant at the 1% level ($P < .001$), with the exception of those born in Western Europe ($P = .04$), Northern Europe ($P = .94$), and the Caribbean ($P < .01$). Low socioeconomic deprivation represents top five quintiles of socioeconomic disadvantage based on the Index of Relative Socio-economic Disadvantage (IRSD) score. IRSD is a general socioeconomic index that summarizes a range of information about the economic and social conditions of people and households within an area.
Source. Data are from the Person Level Integrated Data Asset[19] and 2017 Australian Marriage Law Postal Survey.[22]

in outcomes. For example, in the lowest-stigma regions (quartile 1 votes against marriage equality [Q1]) individuals in same-sex relationships had 56% higher odds of reporting any long-term health condition than those in different-sex relationships (odds ratio [OR] = 1.56; 95% confidence interval [CI] = 1.53, 1.59), and this increased to 63% increased odds in the highest-stigma regions (quartile 4 votes against marriage equality [Q4]; OR = 1.63; 95% CI = 1.58, 1.68). The differences in sexual orientation disparities between the lowest- and highest-stigma regions were also statistically significant ($P = .02$).

There was evidence of sexual orientation disparities in the odds of long-term health conditions for most long-term health conditions, though the magnitude of these effects varied across different health conditions (Table B). Absolute disparities were largest for mental health conditions (1.74; 95% CI = 1.70, 1.78 in Q1), asthma (1.24; 95% CI = 1.21, 1.27 in Q1), and other long-term health conditions (1.39; 95% CI = 1.36, 1.43 in Q1).

The differences in sexual orientation disparities between low-stigma (Q1) and high-stigma (Q4) regions were largest for heart disease (1.13; 95% CI = 1.05, 1.21), lung conditions (1.12; 95% CI = 1.04, 1.22), stroke (1.12; 95% CI = 1.03, 1.22), cancer (1.10; 95% CI = 1.03, 1.18), mental health conditions (1.09; 95% CI = 1.05, 1.14), and asthma (1.07; 95% CI = 1.02, 1.12) but did not vary as substantially for kidney disease (1.10; 95% CI = 1.00, 1.19), arthritis (1.04; 95% CI = 0.99, 1.10), diabetes (1.06; 95% CI = 1.00, 1.13), or other long-term health conditions (0.96; 95% CI = 0.92, 1.01).

Heterogeneity analyses results for any long-term health condition and

TABLE 2— Differences in Reporting Long-Term Health Condition for Individuals in a Same-Sex Relationship Compared With Those in a Different-Sex Relationship by Quartiles of Structural Stigma (Votes Against Marriage Equality): 2021 Australian Census

Subgroup	Structural Stigma Quartile	Relationship	No. With Long-Term Health Condition (% Subgroup)	OR (95% CI)	Test for Equivalence to Quartile 1, OR (95% CI)
Quartile 1					. . .
In different-sex relationship	1	0	840 924 (36)	1 (Ref)	
In same-sex relationship	1	1	22 461 (39)	1.56 (1.53, 1.59)	
Quartile 2					1.02 (0.99, 1.05)
In different-sex relationship	2	0	1 073 503 (39)	1 (Ref)	
In same-sex relationship	2	1	14 819 (43)	1.56 (1.56, 1.63)	
Quartile 3					1.04 (1.01, 1.08)
In different-sex relationship	3	0	948 327 (40)	1 (Ref)	
In same-sex relationship	3	1	10 499 (45)	1.63 (1.59, 1.68)	
Quartile 4					1.04 (1.01, 1.08)
In different-sex relationship	4	0	951 092 (36)	1 (Ref)	
In same-sex relationship	4	1	21 825 (41)	1.63 (1.58, 1.68)	

Note. CI = confidence interval; OR = odds ratio. Subgroups are based on structural stigma quartile (categorical; 1 = first quartile; 2 = second quartile; 3 = third quartile; 4 = fourth quartile) and relationship type (0 = different-sex relationship; 1 = same-sex relationship). Quartile 1 represents [13.12%–26.27%] votes against same-sex marriage; quartile 2 represents (26.27%–30.13%] votes against same-sex marriage; quartile 3 represents (30.13%–34.27%] votes against same-sex marriage; and quartile 4 represents (34.27%–55.47%] votes against same-sex marriage. Each interaction term indicates the odds of an individual in a same-sex relationship reporting a given health condition relative to an individual in a different-sex relationship living in the same electorate (i.e., β_k in equation 1). All models control for region fixed effects at the electorate level, sex, age, educational attainment, country of birth, and equivalized household income. OR results are from logistic regression analyses. Tests for equivalence tested whether ORs between those in same-sex versus different-sex relationships in quartile 2, quartile 3, and quartile 4, respectively, were equivalent to the ORs between those in same-sex versus different-sex relationships in quartile 1. The results for each type of long-term health condition are presented in Table B (available as a supplement to the online version of this article at https://ajph.org), along with *P* values for the test for equivalence to quartile 1.
Source. Data are from the Person Level Integrated Data Asset[19] and 2017 Australian Marriage Law Postal Survey.[22]

each different type of health condition are presented in Table 3 and Table C (available as a supplement to the online version of this article at https://ajph.org), respectively. These results show sexual orientation disparities in low-stigma (Q1) and high-stigma (Q4) regions by sex, age group, education, socioeconomic deprivation, and rurality. Absolute sexual orientation disparities in reporting any long-term health condition were more pronounced for individuals with lower educational attainment (OR = 1.66; 95% CI = 1.61, 1.71 in Q1), women (OR = 1.59; 95% CI = 1.55, 1.63 in Q1), younger populations (OR = 1.62; 95% CI = 1.58, 1.66 for individuals younger than 40 years in Q1), and those living in more metropolitan regions (OR = 1.57; 95% CI = 1.58, 1.66 in Q1). Further disaggregation by condition type shows that sexual orientation disparities in asthma, arthritis, heart, and lung conditions were larger for women than men (Table C). Overall disparities in mental health conditions were largest for younger populations and were slightly larger for men than women.

The differences in sexual orientation disparities in reporting any long-term health condition between low-stigma (Q1) and high-stigma (Q4) regions were larger for men (OR = 1.06; 95% CI = 1.01, 1.11) and younger populations (OR = 1.14; 95% CI = 1.08, 1.20). These patterns were similar across most condition types but were additionally larger for those living in metropolitan areas and areas with greater socioeconomic deprivation (Table C).

DISCUSSION

Prejudice and discrimination toward sexual minorities remain commonplace. While sexual orientation health disparities have been documented,

TABLE 3— Differences in Reporting Long-Term Health Condition for Individuals in a Same-Sex Relationship Compared With Those in a Different-Sex Relationship: 2021 Australian Census

Subgroup	Structural Stigma Quartile	Relationship	No. With Long-Term Health Condition (% Subgroup)	OR (95% CI)	Test for Equivalence to Quartile 1, OR (95% CI)
Sex: male					
Quartile 1					. . .
In different-sex relationship	1	0	411 140 (36)	1 (Ref)	
In same-sex relationship	1	1	12 201 (36)	1.56 (1.52, 1.59)	
Quartile 4					1.06 (1.01, 1.11)
In different-sex relationship	4	0	477 214 (37)	1 (Ref)	
In same-sex relationship	4	1	3 955 (39)	1.65 (1.58, 1.72)	
Sex: female					
Quartile 1					. . .
In different-sex relationship	1	0	429 784 (37)	1 (Ref)	
In same-sex relationship	1	1	10 260 (44)	1.59 (1.55, 1.63)	
Quartile 4					1.00 (0.95, 1.05)
In different-sex relationship	4	0	473 878 (36)	1 (Ref)	
In same-sex relationship	4	1	4 949 (43)	1.59 (1.53, 1.65)	
Age group: < 40 y					
Quartile 1					. . .
In different-sex relationship	1	0	186 240 (25)	1 (Ref)	
In same-sex relationship	1	1	9 507 (35)	1.62 (1.58, 1.66)	
Quartile 4					1.14 (1.08, 1.20)
In different-sex relationship	4	0	153 057 (20)	1 (Ref)	
In same-sex relationship	4	1	3 643 (35)	1.84 (1.77, 1.92)	
Age group: 40–64 y					
Quartile 1					. . .
In different-sex relationship	1	0	365 735 (33)	1 (Ref)	
In same-sex relationship	1	1	10 353 (40)	1.50 (1.46, 1.54)	
Quartile 4					0.99 (0.94, 1.04)
In different-sex relationship	4	0	434 816 (34)	1 (Ref)	
In same-sex relationship	4	1	3 909 (42)	1.49 (1.43, 1.55)	
Age group: ≥ 65 y					
Quartile 1					. . .
In different-sex relationship	1	0	288 949 (61)	1 (Ref)	
In same-sex relationship	1	1	2 601 (62)	1.19 (1.11, 1.23)	
Quartile 4					1.08 (0.96, 1.21)
In different-sex relationship	4	0	363 219 (63)	1 (Ref)	
In same-sex relationship	4	1	1 352 (66)	1.27 (1.16, 1.40)	
Education: less than university					
Quartile 1					. . .
In different-sex relationship	1	0	407 350 (39)	1 (Ref)	
In same-sex relationship	1	1	9 055 (38)	1.66 (1.61, 1.71)	
Quartile 4					1.01 (0.96, 1.06)
In different-sex relationship	4	0	546 837 (38)	1 (Ref)	
In same-sex relationship	4	1	4 963 (43)	1.67 (1.61, 1.74)	

Continued

TABLE 3— Continued

Subgroup	Structural Stigma Quartile	Relationship	No. With Long-Term Health Condition (% Subgroup)	OR (95% CI)	Test for Equivalence to Quartile 1, OR (95% CI)
Education: university or above					
Quartile 1					. . .
In different-sex relationship	1	0	338 849 (32)	1 (Ref)	
In same-sex relationship	1	1	12 502 (38)	1.51 (1.47, 1.54)	
Quartile 4					1.06 (1.00, 1.12)
In different-sex relationship	4	0	222 993 (28)	1 (Ref)	
In same-sex relationship	4	1	3 102 (37)	1.59 (1.52, 1.67)	
High area-level deprivation					
Quartile 1					. . .
In different-sex relationship	1	0	214 671 (40)	1 (Ref)	
In same-sex relationship	1	1	5 097 (41)	1.50 (1.44, 1.56)	
Quartile 4					1.08 (1.03, 1.14)
In different-sex relationship	4	0	621 160 (38)	1 (Ref)	
In same-sex relationship	4	1	5 645 (43)	1.63 (1.57, 1.69)	
Low area-level deprivation					
Quartile 1					. . .
In different-sex relationship	1	0	446 829 (36)	1 (Ref)	
In same-sex relationship	1	1	13 032 (39)	1.55 (1.52, 1.59)	
Quartile 4					1.08 (1.02, 1.14)
In different-sex relationship	4	0	258 943 (33)	1 (Ref)	
In same-sex relationship	4	1	2 773 (38)	1.67 (1.59, 1.76)	
Rurality: metropolitan					
Quartile 1					. . .
In different-sex relationship	1	0	676 268 (36)	1 (Ref)	
In same-sex relationship	1	1	19 554 (39)	1.57 (1.54, 1.60)	
Quartile 4					1.04 (1.00, 1.07)
In different-sex relationship	4	0	578 851 (33)	1 (Ref)	
In same-sex relationship	4	1	5 641 (38)	1.62 (1.57, 1.67)	
Rurality: rural					
Quartile 1					. . .
In different-sex relationship	1	0	164 656 (39)	1 (Ref)	
In same-sex relationship	1	1	2 907 (44)	1.48 (1.35, 1.63)	
Quartile 4					1.12 (0.99, 1.26)
In different-sex relationship	4	0	372 241 (44)	1 (Ref)	
In same-sex relationship	4	1	3 263 (48)	1.66 (1.52, 1.79)	

Note. CI = confidence interval; OR = odds ratio. Subgroups are based on structural stigma quartile (categorical; 1 = first quartile; 2 = second quartile; 3 = third quartile; 4 = fourth quartile) and relationship type (0 = different-sex relationship; 1 = same-sex relationship). Quartile 1 represents [13.12%–26.27%] votes against same-sex marriage and quartile 4 represents (34.27%–55.47%] votes against same-sex marriage. Each interaction term indicates the odds of an individual in a same-sex relationship reporting a given health condition relative to an individual in a different-sex relationship living in the same electorate (i.e., β_k in equation 1). All models controlled for region fixed effects at the electorate level, sex, age, educational attainment, country of birth, and equivalized household income. Models were run separately by sex, age, education, area-level deprivation, and rurality. Heterogeneity analyses illustrating OR results are from subgroup logistic regression analyses. Tests for equivalence tested whether ORs between those in same-sex versus different-sex relationships in quartile 4 were equivalent to the ORs between those in same-sex versus different-sex relationships in quartile 1.
Source. Data are from the Person Level Integrated Data Asset[19] and 2017 Australian Marriage Law Postal Survey.[22]

little is known about the extent to which stigma may influence these disparities. This study addresses this gap in the literature by exploring the extent to which structural stigma, as measured by votes against legalizing same-sex marriage, was associated with sexual orientation disparities in long-term health conditions.

We found that higher levels of structural stigma were associated with higher disparities in the odds of long-term health conditions among Australians in same-sex relationships, relative to those in different-sex relationships. Structural stigma was most strongly associated with disparities in circulatory conditions (heart disease, stroke), lung conditions, and mental health conditions.

Our findings support a growing body of research documenting the negative health effects of stigma among sexual minorities[7,8,24] and theories that sexual minorities in more stigmatized regions are at heightened risk of social stressors.[6,25] The association between structural stigma and sexual orientation disparities in lung and circulatory conditions aligns with previous research documenting associations between stigma and risk-taking behavior predictive of these conditions among sexual minorities, including higher levels of smoking, alcohol use, and substance use.[10,11] The results also echo findings outlining how stress pathways can influence health, including allostatic load and stress-related biomarkers, which are relevant for circulatory and inflammatory conditions.[17,26,27] The results also align with another study, which used PLIDA data to show that, compared with those in different-sex relationships, individuals in same-sex relationships were less likely to access primary health care in areas with greater stigma.[12] This would support the hypothesis that delays in preventive health care could lead to deterioration of health and, in turn, the development of long-term health conditions. That stigma and sexual orientation disparities in health conditions were generally more pronounced in regions with higher socioeconomic deprivation suggests that supply-based constraints are indeed important. Altogether, these results could indicate that sexual minorities living in more stigmatized regions may experience higher levels of stress, be more likely to engage in risky health behaviors to cope with these stressors, and be less willing, or able, to access health care.

Our heterogeneity results suggest that structural stigma and sexual orientation disparities in long-term health conditions were generally more pronounced for younger populations, men, and those living in metropolitan and more socioeconomically disadvantaged regions, whereas absolute disparities in asthma and lung conditions were larger for women. This aligns with previous research that has documented a higher prevalence of asthma among lesbian or bisexual women relative to gay or bisexual men.[3,28] Other studies suggest that lesbian and bisexual women are more likely to engage in heavy drinking and smoking relative to gay and bisexual men.[28]

This also aligns with previous research that found that sexual orientation disparities in self-rated health were larger among adolescents and young adults[3] and that positive associations between discrimination and suicidal behavior were largest for younger sexual minority males (younger than 30 years).[29] It is possible that younger people may have less experience in coping with these stressors that may be more common in this stage of the life course such as identity concealment, or parental or peer rejection.[3] Previous studies have also found that, compared with sexual minority females, sexual minority males are more likely to experience victimization and discrimination on the basis of their sexual orientation.[30]

Limitations

The results of this study should be interpreted within the context of several important limitations. First, our sample only identifies individuals in same-sex relationships that were residing in the same household at the time of the 2021 Census. As individuals in relationships tend to share common health traits, this may lead to nonindependence of observations. Compared with others in the Census, this sample has higher incomes and higher levels of education and is more likely to exclude younger people and singles or partnered individuals not living together, for whom the effects of stigma may be greater. Moreover, as the 2021 Census did not capture information on sexual orientation, gender diversity, or innate variations of sex characteristics, there is undoubtedly some misrepresentation of relationship structures. For example, an individual identifying as a transgender man partnered with a cisgender woman might have completed the Census as being in a "opposite sex relationship."

Second, this analysis is based on individuals' exposure to a proxy for structural stigma, as measured in 2017, mapped to health measures reported in 2021 (i.e., 4 years after marriage equality). We therefore cannot fully account for selective migration[12] and other societal-level conditions, including potential changes after marriage equality. It is also likely that differential exposure to stigma and discrimination across the life course could affect sexual minorities' health. Future research should therefore endeavor to develop alternate and "contemporary" measures of structural stigma as well as consider the health effects of individuals' lifetime "exposure" to these conditions.

Third, as our analyses compare people in different-sex and same-sex relationships, there may be residual confounding from poorly measured or unmeasured characteristics, such as education and homophily within relationship dyads.

Despite these limitations, this research provides important empirical evidence on the discrimination–health relationship among sexual minorities. To our knowledge, this study is also the first to document sexual orientation disparities in long-term health conditions in Australia, a setting with universal health care and marriage equality. Our study also boasts important strengths relative to other studies that have investigated sexual orientation health disparities. With our sample comprising more than 130 000 individuals in same-sex relationships, this analysis provides the large sample needed to investigate rare outcomes for sexual minorities. This has also enabled us to provide robust estimates for important subgroups that, to our knowledge, have not been investigated before.

Public Health Implications

Compared with other Organization for Economic Co-operation and Development countries, Australia is generally more progressive for sexual minority rights.[31] More recently, Australia has seen considerable progress in counteracting discriminatory policies, including the strengthening of antidiscrimination protections (e.g., the 2013 Sex Discrimination Amendment), the widespread abolition of conversion therapy, and, notably, the legalization of same-sex marriage. However, despite this progress, here we have documented stark health disparities by sexual orientation and a strong gradient in these health outcomes by stigma. That these disparities remain, even 4 years after marriage equality, highlights the urgent need for action and greater protections for sexual minorities in Australia. Our results suggest that younger populations and those living in more socioeconomically disadvantaged regions are at particular risk of adverse health outcomes and should be prioritized in policy efforts.

When considering these results in the context of similar research on stigma and health care use among sexual minorities,[12,13,18] it is plausible that sexual minorities living in more stigmatizing environments may be less able to access affirming, safe, and inclusive care. Enhancing equitable access to health care, especially mental health services, is therefore crucial. However, addressing the underlying causes of these disparities is equally, if not more, important. As previous research has shown that laws can shape attitudes,[32] it is clear that structural and policy changes will continue to play an important role. Beyond these structural changes, more research is needed to understand what interventions can shape attitudes toward sexual minorities.

Our results also suggest that more knowledge is needed regarding the mechanisms underlying these broader disparities. Future research should aim to assess whether sexual orientation health disparities are changing in response to policy variation, consider the influence of past exposure to social stressors and stigma on health, and investigate other outcomes including mortality and utilization of acute health care services. More research on the pathways through which stigma impacts sexual minority health is also necessary. Finally, expanding this research to consider health outcomes among broader populations of sexuality, gender, and bodily diverse people is crucial. Improving population-level data collections of Australians will be critical for this work. In particular, proposals to include questions on sex, gender, variations of sex characteristics, and sexual orientation in Australia's 2026 Census[33] should be strongly encouraged. Nevertheless, policymakers and community organizations should draw on this and other research to advocate sexual minority health. AJPH

ABOUT THE AUTHORS

Karinna Saxby and Yuting Zhang are with the Melbourne Institute: Applied Economic and Social Research, the University of Melbourne, Melbourne, Australia. Zoe Aitken is with the Melbourne School of Population and Global Health, the University of Melbourne.

CORRESPONDENCE

Correspondence should be sent to Karinna Saxby, PhD, Level 5, Faculty of Business and Economics Building, 111 Barry St, Carlton, The University of Melbourne, Victoria 3010 Australia (e-mail: karinna.saxby@unimelb.edu.au). Reprints can be ordered at https://www.ajph.org by clicking the "Reprints" link.

PUBLICATION INFORMATION

Full Citation: Saxby K, Zhang Y, Aitken Z. Structural stigma and disparities in long-term health conditions among Australians in same-sex relationships: 2021 Australian Census. *Am J Public Health*. 2024;114(10):1110–1122.

Acceptance Date: June 6, 2024.

DOI: https://doi.org/10.2105/AJPH.2024.307759

ORCID iD:
Karinna Saxby https://orcid.org/0000-0003-0100-8437

CONTRIBUTORS

K. Saxby conceptualized the study, conducted the data analysis and community engagement, and led the writing. Z. Aitken and Y. Zhang were involved in the initial conceptualization of the study and reviewed all analytical outputs. All of the authors contributed original ideas and edited drafts of the article.

ACKNOWLEDGMENTS

Y. Zhang is the recipient of an Australian Research Council Australian Future Fellowship award funded by the Australian Government (project ID FT200100630). Zoe Aitken is the recipient of an Australian Research Council Early Career Industry Fellowship (IE230100561).

Findings are based on the use of Person Level Integrated Data Asset data. We would like to thank Talei Parker, Ben Harrington, Rashmin Chitale, Zac Steyn, Humaira Khan, and the rest of the ABS DataLab team for their tireless vetting and assistance. We would like to thank Michelle Escobar Carias, Curtis Chan, Phillip Keen, Dennis Petrie, Luke Munford, Jan Kabatek, Nathan Kettlewell, and David Johnston for their feedback, which greatly improved the article. For useful discussions and comments, we thank participants at seminars at the Kirby Institute Seminar Series, the Economics of LGBTQ+ Individuals Virtual Seminar Series, the 2024 Australian Gender Economics Workshop, the 2023 PLIDA Analytical Working Group Meeting, and the 2024 LGBTIQ+ Health in Difference Conference. We acknowledge the study chief investigators and partners and, in particular, Ian Down from LGBTIQ+ Health Australia for his ongoing guidance and support.

Note. Throughout this study, we collectively use the terminology "sexual minorities." We acknowledge that the framing of questions in the 2021 Census did not adequately capture the experiences of lesbian, gay, bisexual, trans/transgender, intersex, queer, and other sexuality, gender, and bodily diverse people and communities. We understand that the results presented in this article, along with the underlying concepts and theories discussed, may cause sadness or distress. If you need to talk to someone, there are local and national support services available in Australia. Anonymous and free LGBTIQ+ peer support is available through QLife (https://qlife.org.au or phone 1800 184 527) and a list of services and supports is available at LGBTIQ+ Health Australia's Web site (https://www.lgbtiqhealth.org.au/services_and_supports).

CONFLICTS OF INTEREST

The authors have no conflicts of interest.

HUMAN PARTICIPANT PROTECTION

No protocol approval was required for this study because no human participants were involved.

REFERENCES

1. Gilman SE, Cochran SD, Mays VM, Hughes M, Ostrow D, Kessler RC. Risk of psychiatric disorders among individuals reporting same-sex sexual partners in the National Comorbidity Survey. *Am J Public Health*. 2001;91(6):933–939. https://doi.org/10.2105/AJPH.91.6.933
2. Fredriksen-Goldsen KI, Kim H-J, Shui C, Bryan AE. Chronic health conditions and key health indicators among lesbian, gay, and bisexual older US adults, 2013–2014. *Am J Public Health*. 2017; 107(8):1332–1338. https://doi.org/10.2105/AJPH.2017.303922
3. Bränström R, Hatzenbuehler ML, Pachankis JE. Sexual orientation disparities in physical health: age and gender effects in a population-based study. *Soc Psychiatry Psychiatr Epidemiol*. 2016; 51(2):289–301. https://doi.org/10.1007/s00127-015-1116-0
4. Hatzenbuehler ML, McLaughlin K, Slopen N. Sexual orientation disparities in cardiovascular biomarkers among young adults. *Am J Prev Med*. 2013;44(6):612–621. https://doi.org/10.1016/j.amepre.2013.01.027
5. Cochran SD, Björkenstam C, Mays VM. Sexual orientation and all-cause mortality among US adults aged 18 to 59 years, 2001–2011. *Am J Public Health*. 2016;106(5):918–920. https://doi.org/10.2105/AJPH.2016.303052
6. Hatzenbuehler ML. Structural stigma: research evidence and implications for psychological science. *Am Psychol*. 2016;71(8):742–751. https://doi.org/10.1037/amp0000068
7. Perales F, Todd A. Structural stigma and the health and wellbeing of Australian LGB populations: exploiting geographic variation in the results of the 2017 same-sex marriage plebiscite. *Soc Sci Med*. 2018;208:190–199. https://doi.org/10.1016/j.socscimed.2018.05.015
8. Hatzenbuehler ML, McLaughlin K, Keyes KM, Hasin D. The impact of institutional discrimination on psychiatric disorders in lesbian, gay, and bisexual populations: a prospective study. *Am J Public Health*. 2010;100(3):452–459. https://doi.org/10.2105/AJPH.2009.168815
9. Hatzenbuehler ML, Jun H, Corliss H, Austin S. Structural stigma and cigarette smoking in a prospective cohort study of sexual minority and heterosexual youth. *Ann Behav Med*. 2014;47(1): 48–56. https://doi.org/10.1007/s12160-013-9548-9
10. Bryan AEB, Kim H-J, Fredriksen-Goldsen KI. Factors associated with high-risk alcohol consumption among LGB older adults: the roles of gender, social support, perceived stress, discrimination, and stigma. *Gerontologist*. 2017; 57(suppl 1):S95–S104. https://doi.org/10.1093/geront/gnw100
11. Hatzenbuehler ML, Jun H, Corliss H, Austin S. Structural stigma and sexual orientation disparities in adolescent drug use. *Addict Behav*. 2015; 46:14–18. https://doi.org/10.1016/j.addbeh.2015.02.017
12. Saxby K, de New SC, Petrie D. Structural stigma and sexual orientation disparities in healthcare use: evidence from Australian Census-linked-administrative data. *Soc Sci Med*. 2020;255: 113027. https://doi.org/10.1016/j.socscimed.2020.113027
13. Saxby K, Chan C, Bavinton BR. Structural stigma and sexual health disparities among gay, bisexual, and other men who have sex with men in Australia. *J Acquir Immune Defic Syndr*. 2022; 89(3):241–250. doi:10.1097/QAI.0000000000002851
14. Oldenburg CE, Perez-Brumer A, Hatzenbuehler M, et al. State-level structural sexual stigma and HIV prevention in a national online sample of HIV-uninfected MSM in the United States. *AIDS*. 2015;29(7):837–845. https://doi.org/10.1097/QAD.0000000000000622
15. Saxby K. Australia's LGBTIQ research data landscape. *Aust Econ Rev*. 2022;55(2):290–308. https://doi.org/10.1111/1467-8462.12462
16. Meyer IH. Minority stress and mental health in gay men. *J Health Soc Behav*. 1995;36(1):38–56. https://doi.org/10.2307/2137286
17. Juster R-P, Doyle DM, Hatzenbuehler ML, Everett BG, DuBois LZ, McGrath JJ. Sexual orientation, disclosure, and cardiovascular stress reactivity. *Stress*. 2019;22(3):321–331. https://doi.org/10.1080/10253890.2019.1579793
18. Saxby K, Stephens M. Medicare and priority populations: structural and place-based considerations for Aboriginal and Torres Strait Islander peoples and LGBTQ+ Australians. *Aust Econ Rev*. 2024;57(2):149–159. https://doi.org/10.1111/1467-8462.12561
19. Australian Bureau of Statistics. Person Level Integrated Data Asset (PLIDA). 2022. https://www.abs.gov.au/about/data-services/data-integration/integrated-data/person-level-integrated-data-asset-plida. Accessed January 1, 2024.
20. Australian Bureau of Statistics. Participation in the 2021 Census. Canberra, Australia: Australian Government; 2021.
21. Australian Bureau of Statistics. Whether has one or more long-term health condition(s) (HLTHP). Canberra, Australia: Australian Government; 2021.
22. Australian Bureau of Statistics. 1800.0 - Australian Marriage Law Postal Survey, 2017. Available at: https://www.abs.gov.au/ausstats/abs@.nsf/mf/1800.0. Accessed January 12, 2019.
23. Clarke D, Romano JP, Wolf M. The Romano–Wolf multiple-hypothesis correction in Stata. *Stata J*.

2020;20(4):812–843. https://doi.org/10.1177/1536867X20976314

24. Hatzenbuehler ML. The social environment and suicide attempts in lesbian, gay, and bisexual youth. *Pediatrics*. 2011;127(5):896–903. https://doi.org/10.1542/peds.2010-3020
25. Meyer I, Frost D. Minority stress and the health of sexual minorities. In: Patterson CJ, D'Augelli AR, eds. *Handbook of Psychology and Sexual Orientation*. New York, NY: Oxford University Press; 2013:252–266.
26. Wahrendorf M, Chandola T, Goldberg M, Zins M, Hoven H, Siegrist J. Adverse employment histories and allostatic load: associations over the working life. *J Epidemiol Community Health*. 2022;76(4):374–381. https://doi.org/10.1136/jech-2021-217607
27. Hatzenbuehler ML, McLaughlin K. Structural stigma and hypothalamic–pituitary–adrenocortical axis reactivity in lesbian, gay, and bisexual young adults. *Ann Behav Med*. 2013;47(1):39–47. https://doi.org/10.1007/s12160-013-9556-9
28. Dilley JA, Simmons KW, Boysun MJ, Pizacani BA, Stark MJ. Demonstrating the importance and feasibility of including sexual orientation in public health surveys: health disparities in the Pacific Northwest. *Am J Public Health*. 2010;100(3):460–467. https://doi.org/10.2105/AJPH.2007.130336
29. Fish JN, Rice CE, Lanza ST, Russell ST. Is young adulthood a critical period for suicidal behavior among sexual minorities? Results from a US national sample. *Prev Sci*. 2019;20(3):353–365. https://doi.org/10.1007/s11121-018-0878-5
30. Herek GM. Hate crimes and stigma-related experiences among sexual minority adults in the United States: prevalence estimates from a national probability sample. *J Interpers Violence*. 2009;24(1):54–74. https://doi.org/10.1177/0886260508316477
31. Valfort M. *LGBTI in OECD Countries: A Review*. OECD Social, Employment and Migration Working Papers. Vol 198. Paris, France: OECD Publishing; 2017.
32. Aksoy CG, Carpenter CS, De Haas R, Tran KD. Do laws shape attitudes? Evidence from same-sex relationship recognition policies in Europe. *Eur Econ Rev*. 2020;124:103399. https://doi.org/10.1016/j.euroecorev.2020.103399
33. Australian Bureau of Statistics. 2026 Census topic review: phase one directions. Canberra, Australia: Australian Government; 2023.

Community Engagement: The Missing Link in Public Health Leadership

Yanyi Wu, PhD, and Chenghua Lin, PhD

ABOUT THE AUTHORS

Yanyi Wu and Chenghua Lin are with the School of Public Affairs and the Institute of China's Science, Technology, and Policy, Zhejiang University, Hangzhou, Zhejiang, China.

Helm-Murtagh and Erwin provide a timely and insightful examination of the leadership capabilities required to navigate the challenges exposed by the COVID-19 pandemic and astutely identify the importance of such key skills as effective communication, strategic thinking, and the ability to forge partnerships.[1] However, the authors fall short in emphasizing the core position of community engagement in public health leadership, thus missing an important opportunity to underscore the necessity of actively involving and empowering communities in the decision-making processes that shape their health and well-being.

The impact of the COVID-19 pandemic on marginalized communities was disproportionate, with Black, Hispanic, and Indigenous populations experiencing higher rates of COVID-19 cases, hospitalizations, and deaths than their White counterparts.[2] These disparities are rooted in long-standing structural inequities, including limited access to medical resources, housing shortages, and economic fragility.[3] In this context, public health leaders urgently need to elevate community engagement to a strategic priority and recognize it as a key lever to alleviate health inequalities. For example, the Detroit Community–Academic City Research Center has demonstrated the powerful effectiveness of community-based participatory research in overcoming health inequalities. By engaging community members as equal partners in research and intervention design, it has successfully implemented culturally tailored interventions that have improved health outcomes and built community capacity.[4]

What's more, community engagement is the cornerstone of building trust and ensuring the sustainability of public health interventions. During the COVID-19 pandemic, community health workers were a bridge between public health agencies and marginalized communities. The experience of Chicago, Illinois, shows that community health workers were instrumental in providing culturally and linguistically appropriate education, implementing contact tracing, and connecting families to social services.[5] With community members' deep trust, community health workers successfully mitigated the impact of the epidemic on vulnerable groups, highlighting the importance of equipping public health leaders with the skills to effectively engage and partner with communities. However, the authors failed to adequately explore how public health leadership training can be reimagined to prioritize community engagement as a core competency. Facing the future, how can we ensure that leaders are prepared to build authentic, reciprocal relationships with the communities they serve? AJPH

CORRESPONDENCE

Correspondence should be sent to Yanyi Wu, Zhejiang University, No. 866 Yuhangtang Rd, Xihu District, Hangzhou 310058, China (yanyi.wu@hotmail.com). Reprints can be ordered at https://www.ajph.org by clicking the "Reprints" link.

PUBLICATION INFORMATION

Full Citation: Wu Y, Lin C. Community engagement: the missing link in public health leadership. *Am J Public Health*. 2024;114(10):1123–1124.

Acceptance Date: July 8, 2024.

DOI: https://doi.org/10.2105/AJPH.2024.307796

ORCID iD:

Yanyi Wu https://orcid.org/0009-0002-2948-0493

CONTRIBUTORS

Y. Wu conceptualized the letter. Both authors developed, edited, and reviewed the letter.

ACKNOWLEDGMENTS

We would like to extend our heartfelt gratitude to Hongfang Zhou, Weijia Zhang, Weikang Lu, and Xinyu Lu for their invaluable comments and suggestions.

CONFLICTS OF INTEREST

The authors have no competing interests to declare.

REFERENCES

1. Helm-Murtagh SC, Erwin PC. Building a new generation of public health leaders forged in a public health crisis. *Am J Public Health*. 2024;114(6):626–632. https://doi.org/10.2105/AJPH.2024.307633
2. Centers for Disease Control and Prevention. Trends in racial and ethnic disparities in COVID-19 Hospitalizations, by region—United States, March–December 2020. *MMWR Morb Mortal Wkly Rep*. 2021;70(15):560–565. https://doi.org/10.15585/mmwr.mm7015e2
3. Okonkwo NE, Aguwa UT, Jang M, et al. COVID-19 and the US response: accelerating health inequities. *BMJ Evid Based Med*. 2020;26(4):176–179. https://doi.org/10.1136/bmjebm-2020-111426
4. Israel BA, Coombe CM, Cheezum RR, et al. Community-based participatory research: a capacity-building approach for policy advocacy aimed at eliminating health disparities. *Am J Public Health*. 2010;100(11):2094–2102. https://doi.org/10.2105/AJPH.2009.170506
5. Peretz PJ, Islam N, Matiz LA. Community health workers and COVID-19—addressing social determinants of health in times of crisis and beyond. *N Engl J Med*. 2020;383(19):e108. https://doi.org/10.1056/NEJMp2022641

Helm-Murtagh and Erwin Respond

Susan C. Helm-Murtagh, DrPH, MM, and Paul C. Erwin, MD, DrPH

ABOUT THE AUTHORS

Susan C. Helm-Murtagh is with the Gillings School of Global Public Health, University of North Carolina at Chapel Hill. Paul C. Erwin is with the School of Public Health, University of Alabama at Birmingham.

We appreciate Wu and Lin's clarification and amplification of the public health leadership themes we identified as crucial in our recent article "Building a New Generation of Public Health Leaders Forged in a Public Health Crisis."[1] Wu and Lin correctly highlight the importance of community engagement in public health leadership, pointing out that active community involvement and empowerment in the actions and decisions designed to improve their health and well-being is critical to the success of such efforts, particularly in marginalized communities.

We could not agree more, and we suggest that our viewpoints are tightly aligned. As we note in the discussion of one of our seven leadership themes, "Forge, Facilitate, and Promote Partnerships," creating community partnerships is critical to public health practice, especially during a public health crisis. Furthermore, this requires both systems thinking and the discipline to resist the urge to "go it alone." We reference several case studies in our leadership textbook, *Leadership in Practice: Essentials for Public Health and Healthcare Leaders*, in which community partnerships were key in COVID-19 mitigation efforts and in getting CARES (Coronavirus Aid, Relief, and Economic Security Act) aid to highly vulnerable communities of color.[2]

We thank Wu and Lin for providing additional examples of the power of community engagement in the success and sustainability of public health interventions and for providing us with this opportunity to reinforce its criticality as a leadership theme for the next generation of public health leaders. AJPH

CORRESPONDENCE

Correspondence should be sent to Susan Helm-Murtagh, DrPH, MM, Department of Health Policy & Management, Gillings School of Global Public Health, UNC–Chapel Hill, 1101-H McGavran-Greenberg, CB #7411, Chapel Hill, NC 27599-7411 (e-mail: susan.helm-murtagh@unc.edu). Reprints can be ordered at https://www.ajph.org by clicking the "Reprints" link.

PUBLICATION INFORMATION

Full Citation: Helm-Murtagh SC, Erwin PC. Helm-Murtagh and Erwin respond. *Am J Public Health*. 2024;114(10):1124

Acceptance Date: July 8, 2024.

DOI: https://doi.org/10.2105/AJPH.2024.307798

ORCID iD:

Susan C. Helm-Murtagh https://orcid.org/0000-0002-6193-948X

CONTRIBUTORS

The authors contributed equally to this letter.

CONFLICTS OF INTEREST

The authors have no potential or actual conflicts of interest to report.

REFERENCES

1. Helm-Murtagh SC, Erwin PC. Building a new generation of public health leaders forged in a public health crisis. *Am J Public Health*. 2024;114(6):626–632. https://doi.org/10.2105/AJPH.2024.307633
2. Helm-Murtagh SC, Erwin PC. *Leadership in Practice: Essentials for Public Health and Healthcare Leaders*. New York, NY: Springer; 2022.

Strategies to Improve COVID-19 Vaccination in a Pregnant, Marginalized Population: Correspondence

Hinpetch Daungsupawong, PhD, and Viroj Wiwanitkit, MD

ABOUT THE AUTHORS

Hinpetch Daungsupawong is a private academic consultant, Phonhong, Vientiane, Laos. Viroj Wiwanitkit is with the Department of Research Analytics, Saveetha Dental College and Hospitals, Saveetha Institute of Medical and Technical Sciences, Chennai, India.

"Strategies to Improve COVID-19 Vaccination in a Pregnant, Marginalized Population: Quality Improvement Project" by Bakhai et al.[1] is an interesting article. The quality improvement (QI) initiative the authors describe used lean six sigma techniques to increase pregnant women's COVID-19 immunization rates at a western New York State federally certified health center. Knowledge gaps, inadequate health literacy, and multiple preferred languages were among the obstacles that the QI project team discovered. Motivational interviewing sessions, multilingual resource creation, and education for patients and community health workers were among the interventions. Within six months, there was a significant increase in immunization rates: from 30.0% to 48.0% according to data analysis.

The difficulties in delivering interventions across varied populations with different language preferences and literacy levels may be a weakness of the methodologies used in this QI project. The effectiveness and reach of using community health workers as the main channel for informational campaigns and vaccination campaigns may be constrained. Furthermore, the intricacy of factors affecting vaccination rates may not be adequately captured by data analysis techniques, such as statistical process control charts and weekly run charts.

To better understand the unique needs and preferences of the community regarding receiving health information and immunizations, future directions for this project should consider conducting additional community engagement. Expanding the scope of stakeholders to include local leaders and community organizations may help to increase overall immunization rates and the effectiveness of such programs. Furthermore, investigating cutting-edge communication techniques, such as social media campaigns and digital outreach, could help raise the knowledge of and adherence to immunizations of women in marginalized communities.

Sustaining the gains made by this QI initiative will require ongoing assessment and monitoring of vaccination rates in addition to input from patients and community health workers. Building on the effectiveness of the interventions put in place, the QI team should think about stepping up efforts to address more health care inequities in the community and improve the general health outcomes of the people the health center serves. To improve vaccination rates and general health equity, collaboration with public health organizations and other health care professionals may be helpful in developing a more thorough and long-lasting strategy. AJPH

CORRESPONDENCE

Correspondence should be sent to Dr. Hinpetch Daungsupawong, Private Academic Consultant, Lak 52 Phonhong, Vientiane 10000 Laos.

PUBLICATION INFORMATION

Full Citation: Daungsupawong H, Wiwanitkit V. Strategies to improve COVID-19 vaccination in a pregnant, marginalized population: correspondence. *Am J Public Health*. 2024;114(10): 1125–1126.

Acceptance Date: July 15, 2024.

DOI: https://doi.org/10.2105/AJPH.2024.307807

CONTRIBUTORS

H. Daungsupawong analyzed the literature and wrote the letter. V. Wiwanitkit supervised the letter writing. Both authors conceptualized and approved the letter.

CONFLICTS OF INTEREST

The authors declare no conflict of interest.

REFERENCES

1. Bakhai S, Jordan J, Stoll JA. Strategies to improve COVID-19 vaccination in a pregnant, marginalized population: quality improvement project. *Am J Public Health*. 2024;114(suppl 4):S322–S329. https://doi.org/10.2105/AJPH.2024.307665

Bakhai et al. Respond

Smita Bakhai, MD, MPH, Jacquelyn Jordan, MD, MPH, and Jennifer A. Stoll, PhD

ABOUT THE AUTHORS

Smita Bakhai and Jacquelyn Jordan are with the Department of Internal Medicine, Jacobs School of Medicine and Biomedical Sciences, State University of New York at Buffalo. Jennifer A. Stoll is with the Department of Family Medicine, Jacobs School of Medicine and Biomedical Sciences.

The cornerstone of this quality improvement (QI) project, "Strategies to Improve COVID-19 Vaccination in a Pregnant, Marginalized Population," was its individualized, patient-centered approach tailored to multilingual, diverse, and marginalized populations. Central to patient-centered care are the three foundational elements used in this QI project: respect for each patient's values and preferences, providing comprehensive information and education, and offering emotional support to alleviate fear and anxiety.[1] Additionally, the integration of trusted, multilingual women community health workers plays a pivotal role in addressing patients' attitudes and beliefs toward vaccination, which is fundamental to changing health behaviors.[2]

The QI study highlights the crucial role of community health workers in enhancing vaccination rates and improving health outcomes locally, which can be expanded globally, emphasizing their importance in achieving immunization access and equity in underserved communities worldwide. Policymakers should advocate that community health workers be integrated into national health systems as formal health workers, improve data collection for better health system planning, and strengthen supply chain planning and management.[3]

Although we appreciate the comments of Daungsupawong and Wiwanitkit on the limits of the selected statistical process, the statistical process control charts and run charts are the analytic tools recommended for QI projects.[4] Future directions could include a control group from a similar patient population to overcome this limitation. We commend the merits of public health campaigns to increase health equity. However, we believe these initiatives might inadvertently exclude our target population because of significant language barriers and disparities in digital access.

Factors such as low patient digital literacy and limited broadband access, collectively called the "digital divide," may affect the viability of health care solutions involving digital technologies and tools.[5] An equitable digital health care approach acknowledges that different populations may need a tailored approach to ensure equity. Despite the potential benefits of digital health care technologies and public health campaigns in addressing health care disparities, we must be mindful of substantial disparities stemming from digital access, language barriers, and socioeconomic status.

Furthermore, we agree with Daungsupawong and Wiwanitkit's recommendations for continued engagement with stakeholders to identify the unique needs and preferences of the community and develop targeted digital campaigns that will resonate with the intended audience. We acknowledge the limitations of a QI project in a primary care setting in relation to sustainable public health initiatives to improve health equity. To address these limitations we intend to broaden the stakeholders' base to include local leaders and community organizations. AJPH

CORRESPONDENCE

Correspondence should be sent to Smita Bakhai, MD, MPH, FACP, Clinical Professor, Department of Internal Medicine University at Buffalo, The State University of New York UB Department of Medicine, Erie County Medical Center, David K. Miller Bldg, 2nd floor, Rm C205, 462 Grider St, Buffalo, NY 14215 (sybakhai@buffalo.edu). Reprints can be ordered at https://www.ajph.org by clicking the "Reprints" link.

PUBLICATION INFORMATION

Full Citation: Bakhai S, Jordan J, Stoll JA. Bakhai et al. respond. *Am J Public Health*. 2024;114(10): 1126–1127.

Acceptance Date: July 15, 2024.

DOI: https://doi.org/10.2105/AJPH.2024.307812
ORCID iD:
Smita Bakhai https://orcid.org/0000-0002-9212-4478

CONTRIBUTORS

S. Bakhai contributed to the design, implementation, analysis, writing, and completion of this response and was responsible for the overall content as guarantor. J. Jordan contributed to implementation. J.A. Stoll contributed to analysis and writing.

ACKNOWLEDGMENTS

This work was funded by the Health Resources and Services Administration (HRSA; Primary Care and Enhancement Community Prevention and Maternal Health award T34HP42144-0200). This publication was supported by the HRSA of the US Department of Health and Human Services (HHS) as part of an award totaling $2,840,574 with zero percentage financed with nongovernmental sources.

We would like to thank the directors and staff at Jericho Road Community Health Center for their support. We would also like to thank the HRSA project manager and staff for their guidance.

Note. The contents of this response are those of the authors and do not necessarily represent the official views of, nor an endorsement by, HRSA, HHS, or the US government.

CONFLICTS OF INTEREST

The authors have no conflicts of interest to disclose.

REFERENCES

1. Davis K, Schoenbaum SC, Audet AM. A 2020 vision of patient-centered primary care. *J Gen Intern Med.* 2005;20(10):953–957. https://doi.org/10.1111/j.1525-1497.2005.0178.x
2. Koesnoe S, Siddiq TH, Pelupessy DC, et al. Using integrative behavior model to predict COVID-19 vaccination intention among health care workers in Indonesia: a nationwide survey. *Vaccines (Basel).* 2022;10(5):719. https://doi.org/10.3390/vaccines10050719
3. Gibson E, Zameer M, Alban R, Kouwanou LM. Community health workers as vaccinators: a rapid review of the global landscape, 2000–2021. *Glob Health Sci Pract.* 2023;11(1):e2200307. https://doi.org/10.9745/GHSP-D-22-00307
4. Brady PW, Tchou MJ, Ambroggio L, Schondelmeyer AC, Shaughnessy EE. Quality improvement feature series article 2: displaying and analyzing quality improvement data. *J Pediatric Infect Dis Soc.* 2018;7(2):100–103. https://doi.org/10.1093/jpids/pix077
5. Agency for Healthcare Research and Quality Digital Healthcare Equity Framework. *A Practical Guide for Implementation.* Rockville, MD; 2024. AHRQ publication no. 24-0020-2-EF.

APHA 2024

ANNUAL MEETING & EXPO

Minneapolis | Oct. 27-30

Rebuilding Trust in Public Health and Science

CAN'T TRAVEL?

We're hosting a digital version of APHA2024 from Oct. 26-30. This will include on-demand content and recordings. Recordings will be available through the end of the year.

CAN'T-MISS SESSIONS

CHAMPION CONVERSATION
Democracy and Health: How Did We Get Here? Where Are We Going?
Sunday, Oct. 27 | 2:30–4 p.m.

LIVE TAPING OF THE AMERICA DISSECTED PODCAST
Trauma, Trust and Why We Still Haven't Processed the Pandemic With Professor Eric Klinenberg
Sunday, Oct. 27 | 4:30–6 p.m.
Host: Abdul El-Sayed

CHAMPION CONVERSATION
AJPH Session: Ensuring Inclusivity for the Quality of Scientific Publication
Monday, Oct. 28 | 2:30–4 p.m.

CHAMPION CONVERSATION
Empathy in Action: Transforming Public Health Messaging in a Polarized Era
Tuesday, Oct. 29 | 8:30–10 a.m.

CHAMPION CONVERSATION
Ending Unequal Treatment: Achieving Optimal Health For All
Tuesday, Oct. 29 | 10:30 a.m.–12 p.m.

CLOSING SESSION
Partnering to Make Health a Top Priority for Our Nation
Wednesday, Oct. 30 | 2:30–4 p.m.

Explore the full schedule, presenters and sessions at

APHA.org/Program

OPENING GENERAL SESSION
Sunday, Oct. 27 | 11 a.m. CT

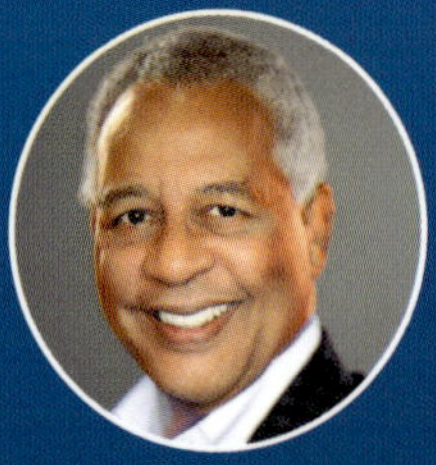

Reed V. Tuckson, MD, FACP
Managing Director,
Tuckson Health Connections, LLC
Co-Convener,
Coalition For Trust in Health & Science
Co-Founder, Black Coalition Against COVID

MONDAY GENERAL SESSION
The Invisible Shield: Clips & Conversation
Monday, Oct. 28 | 4:30-6 p.m.

Presentation of CDC Foundation's 2024 Fries Awards for Health

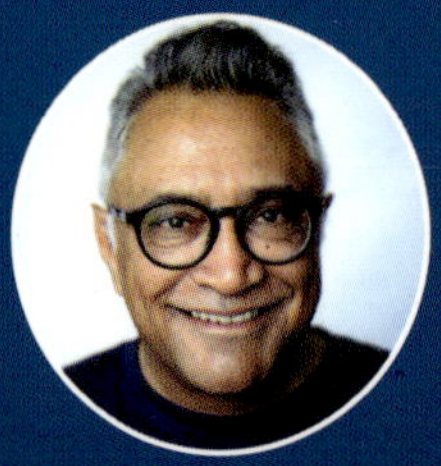

Zackie Achmat
Achmat, a renowned activist, will be honored with the James & Sarah Fries Prize for Improving Health for his work to increase access to lifesaving therapies for people with HIV/AIDS in South Africa and other countries.

REGISTER NOW AT
APHA.org/AnnualMeeting